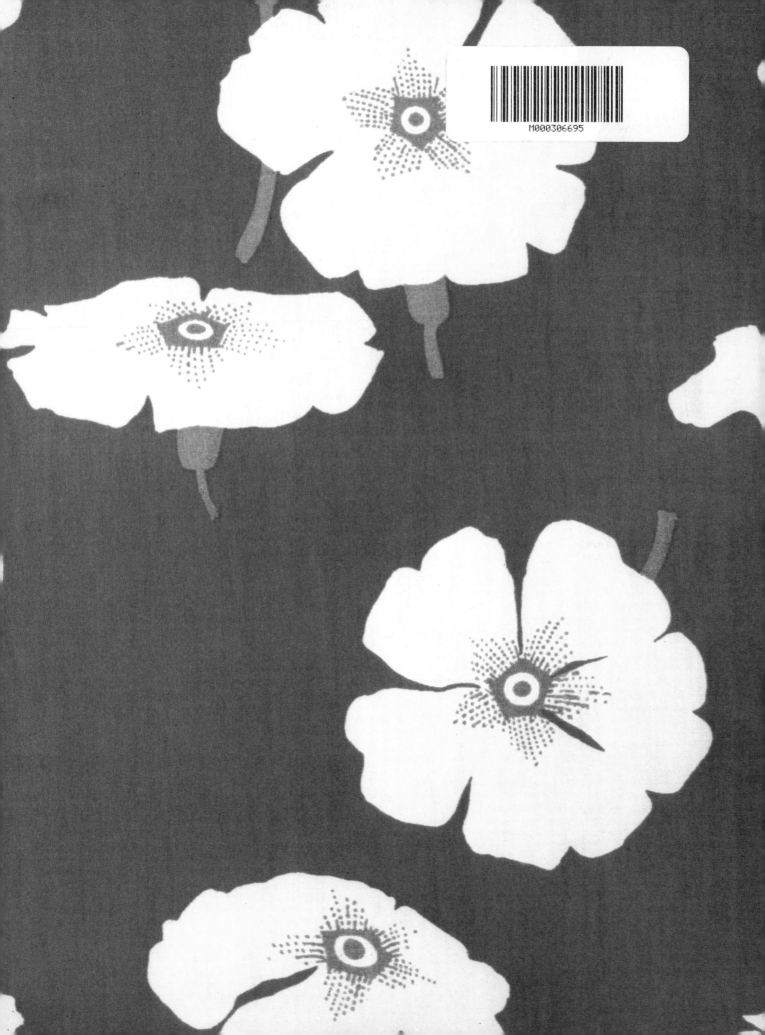

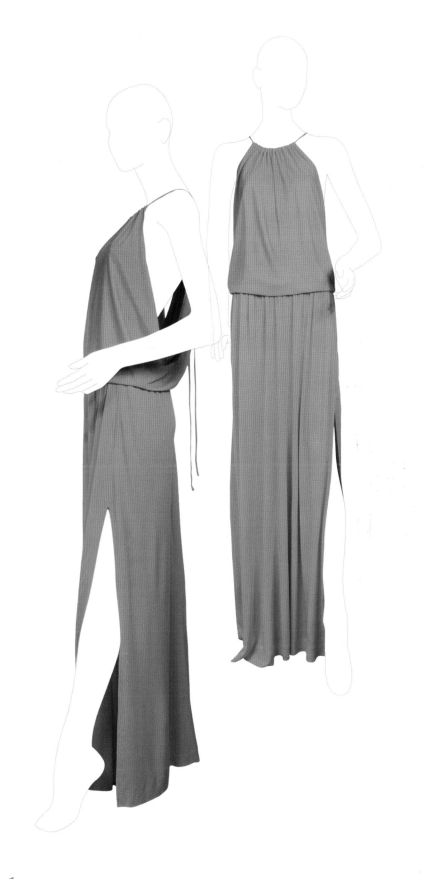

Vintage Fashion

THIS IS A CARLTON BOOK

First published in 2006.
This updated edition published in 2013 by
Carlton Books Limited,
20 Mortimer Street, London W1T 3JW

Text, design and special photography
copyright © 2006, 2013 Carlton Books Limited.

ISBN 978 1 84796 064 1

Printed and bound in China

Senior Executive Editor: Lisa Dyer
Senior Art Editor: Emma Wicks
Designer: Adam Wright
Copy Editors: Nicky Gyopari, Diana Craig and Libby Willis
Picture Researchers: Paul Langan and Jenny Meredith
Production: Janette Burgin
Special Photography: Emma Wicks

CARLTON
BOOKS

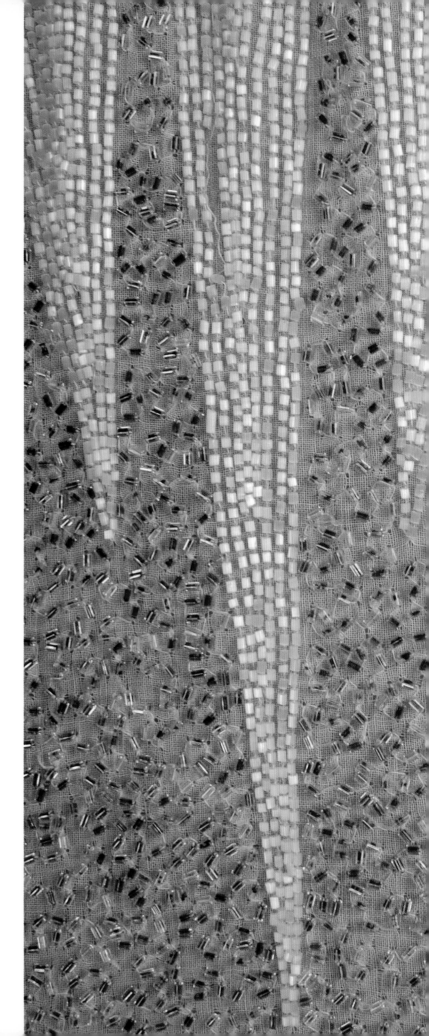

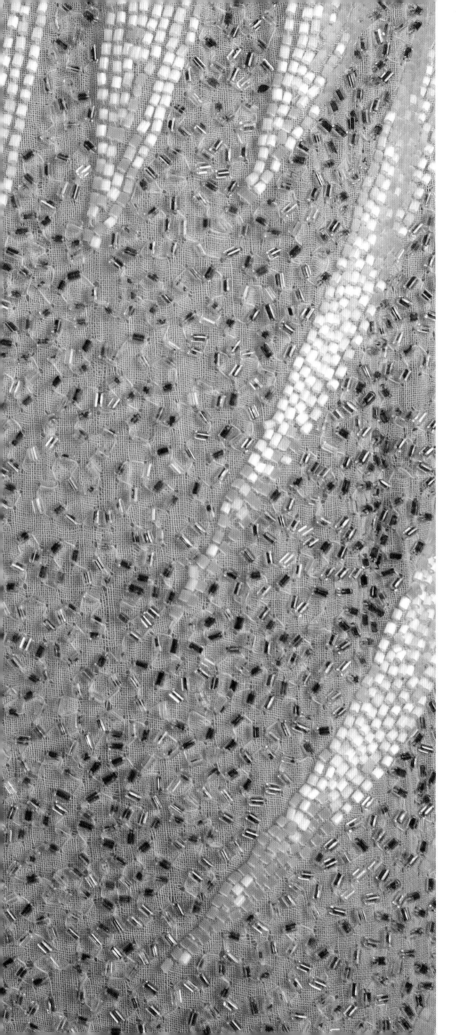

Vintage Fashion

Collecting and wearing designer classics

FOREWORD BY
ZANDRA RHODES

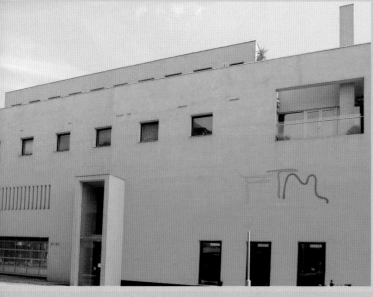
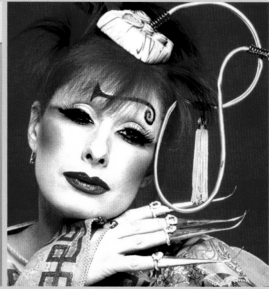

Foreword

Vintage – what wonders this word now conjures up when linked with fashion! A magical harvest of wearable art! A wine from a past season that must be dipped into, sampled and tasted; old yes, but the garment is a survivor of the twentieth century and as such has become a classic of importance.

The world is just realizing that fashion (meaning the clothes and the fabrics they are made from) has been lifted from the status of what we just wear to being an art form. It is the most recent of the acknowledged art forms. Towards the second half of the twentieth century the designers have been acknowledged and are no longer unknowns in the background behind the manufacturer's label. Even more recently textile designers and their contribution to the final garment have started to be acknowledged.

I founded the Fashion and Textile Museum in Bermondsey, London, to ensure that British designers would be remembered and because textile designersmust be memorialized for their contribution. Seeing so many of these vintage examples creates an awareness and hope that these will now be preserved for posterity, perhaps magically framed and carefully displayed.

The vintage clothes pictured in this book must have had adventures and they have survived ill treatment and the toll of years. They have passed through the time warp of being considered outmoded and, God forgive, old-fashioned, and have come through with flying colours into the twenty-first century. These vintage clothes represent what is best, and show the distinctive characteristics of each designer. Exactly as vintage wine, they represent what is outstanding and special about their particular period. Here within this book so many of the key looks of the fast-moving twentieth century have been painstakingly hunted down and researched, with photographs from the relevant decade, or the actual clothes themselves have been photographed, captured in print like gorgeous pressed flowers, indicating just what richness these garments and their designers have given the world.

Suddenly here is a book laying vintage out clearly and chronologically. The genius of Dior and his New Look; the flowering of the Swinging '60s in London side by side with the Parisian movement of Courrèges; the surrealistic approach started by Schiaparelli but continued later in the century by designers such as Moschino; vandalism or unusual treatment to fabrics or even raw edges have entered the design vocabulary while incredible pleating techniques tentatively started by Fortuny have been pioneered and taken to new heights by Issey Miyaki and his school. This book clearly shows periods without print, where sculptural, unsolvable, incredible shapes have been made with fabric twisting around the body, sometimes figure-hugging sometimes not (how did the designer ever come up with that?). So, too, can be seen the early Chanel, who used woven cloth and contained her garment edges with woven braid borders or ribbons, a look of such strength and simplicity that its seeds have endured and grown into a whole empire worldwide.

Zandra Rhodes

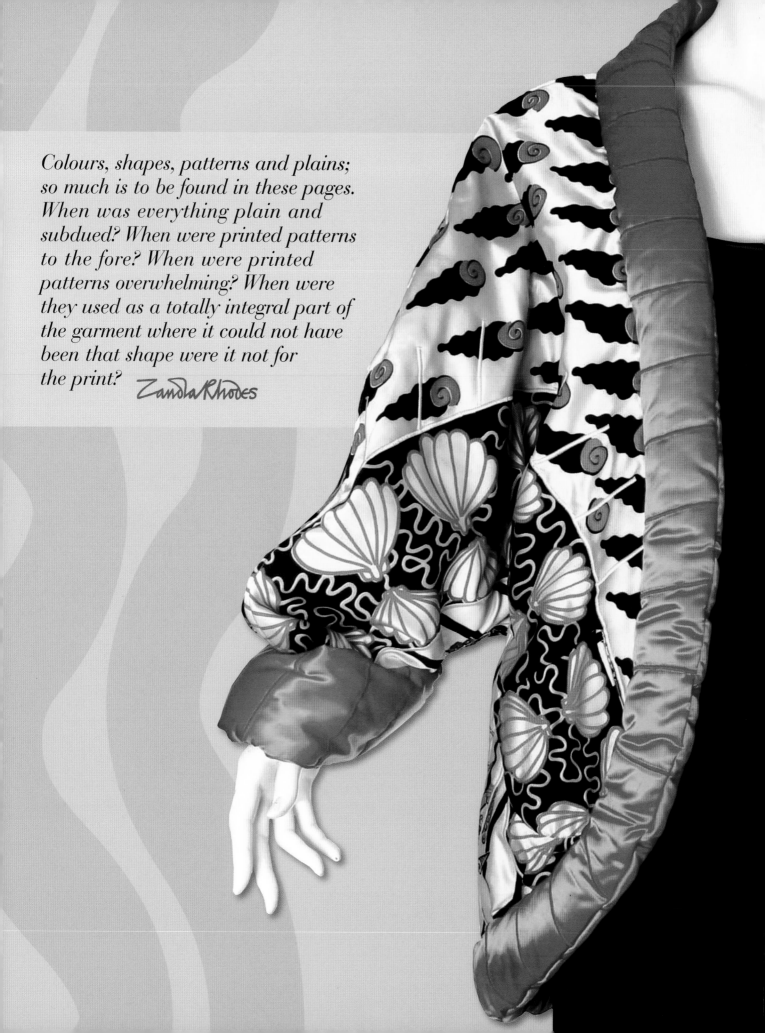

*Colours, shapes, patterns and plains;
so much is to be found in these pages.
When was everything plain and
subdued? When were printed patterns
to the fore? When were printed
patterns overwhelming? When were
they used as a totally integral part of
the garment where it could not have
been that shape were it not for
the print?* Zandra Rhodes

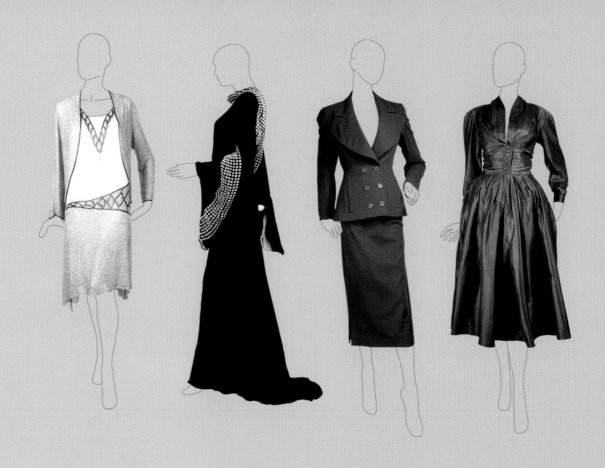

'20s '30s '40s '50s

Introduction

A historical record, a cherished possession, a personal belonging that may be described as a 'second skin': favourite items of clothing have the power to transform the body and spirit of women the world over and always have. The interest in vintage clothing ties deeply into this almost physical response to fashion. Vintage pieces capture not only a historical moment in time, but in themselves can be works of absolute and unique beauty. The techniques and handworking of previous decades, before mass production, can be seen on early pieces up until the end of the Second World War in 1945. After this, factories had learned to mass-produce clothes and a vast number of off-the-rack styles became available to the public. Gone were the days when a handful of couturiers set the pace for style and local seamstresses copied patterns

from Paris or fashion magazines. In becoming reliant upon the manufacturers that produced the clothes, individuality was lost to some extent. However vintage pieces reclaim this by transcending the limitations of what's stylish or available today – a 1930s bias-cut Vionnet gown or a 1950s Christian Dior dress can be stand-out stunning any time. Why choose from the ready-to-wear options produced for you, when the whole history of fashion is available?

Several trends set in earlier decades have developed into classics: the shift dress, the twin set, the tailored suit, the bias-cut gown, the little black dress and many more have not drastically changed since their inception. Even today couture designers plunder the back catalogues in order to study, copy and learn from the masters of years before, often mimicking details, such as pin tucks or seam-finishing,

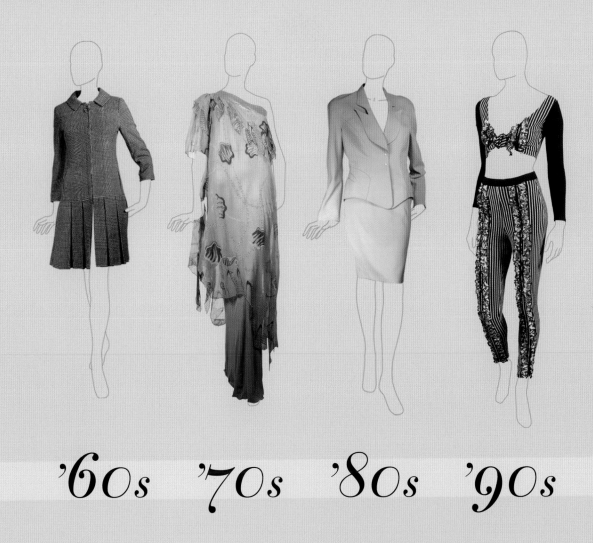

'60s '70s '80s '90s

as well as prints, pattern-cuts or surface decoration, such as beading, lacework or ribbonwork, in their own designs.

In this book vintage pieces are charted through a framework of fashion history over ninety years of the last century, celebrating the most significant designers, developments and movements of each decade, which have contributed to fashion as we know it. Starting from the time when Parisian haute couture houses led the way at the onset of the twentieth century, four writers chronicle the arrival of the flapper, the 'make do and mend' fashions of the war years, Christian Dior's New Look, the 'Swinging '60s', punk and antifashion movements, new romanticism and the power-suited 1980s, the 1990s grunge – all in examples of collectible vintage samples from the time. Giving an overview of

changing trends, the book invests the reader with the knowledge necessary to identify pieces as belonging to specific time periods, to distinguish between various fashion movements, and to understand how and why certain fashions were worn at the time.

In many ways today's fashions evolve from the needs and desires of women rather than the social diktats, conventions and mores that once set the tone of the day. Although fashion has been liberated from the constraints of society and tradition, at this particular vantage point in the twenty-first century we can look back, learn and reinvent, taking what we like from fashions that have gone before, wearing clothing in different ways than originally intended, or simply collecting favourite pieces for the sheer unadulterated pleasure of owning something incomparably beautiful, rare and elusive.

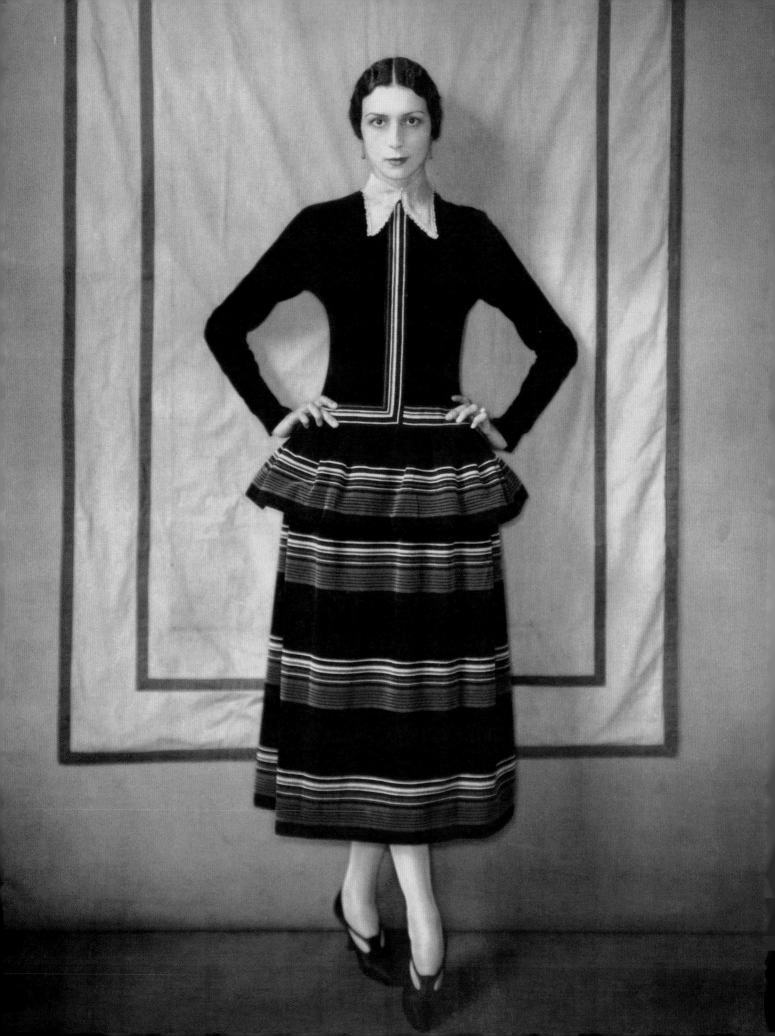

1900-29

At the turn of the century, the Edwardian sun shone for a privileged few. Fashion was dictated from the top and the decorative female in her frills and flounces seemed to waft through society while caged in an ironclad corset. As modernism gathered pace, both the corset and the suffocating Victorian values of the time were torn apart, and in 1909 a new linear silhouette came into fashion. Societal norms were challenged, and an explosion of originality and progressive ideas in art, film, psychology and the role of women were established.

Ethnic elements — oriental themes, ancient Greece and Japanese prints — all influenced fashion, shown in exotic-styled motifs, the natural form and the curvilinear designs of the avant-garde. Added to this, following the tragedy of the First World War and post-1918 fashion, women went wild. Hemlines went up, waistlines went down and flappers boogied to the Charleston, the Bunny Hop and the new hot sound of jazz. Fringes, beads and tassels ornamented short dresses worn above the knee and the accent was on youth and 'misbehaving'.

By the 1920s the media age was beginning. People acquired their sartorial ideas not from their 'betters' but from listening to the radio, copying stars in the cinema and reading about the fashions in *Vogue* and *Vanity Fair*. The growing popularity of sports such as tennis and cycling prompted a new and simpler look. Jean Patou, Madeleine Vionnet and Coco Chanel were among the designers who created the first modern style for women still seen today.

The Belle Epoque

The _belle époque_ – a time of untrammelled gaiety and luxury – covered the period from 1890 to 1914 and was characterized by the Edwardian style, much influenced by King Edward VII, who was on the throne from 1900-10. Against the backdrop of high society and indulgence, Edwardian fashions were status symbols, as well as having an erotic element due to the restrictive silhouette. The constricting dress and the exuberance of frills and flounces were testimony to the leisured life of the wearer. The Edwardian silhouette, with its tiny waist, could not have been created without the corset. Straight-fronted, it pushed the pelvis back and the bosom forward, achieving the fashionable S-shape balanced by a protruding hipline that was svelte and padded. Prominent but low, the bust seemed to overhang and was then festooned with various frills, laces and ribbons. The skirt fitted very tightly over the hips so there was no room for pockets (small bags came into fashion) and then fanned out toward the ground.

Corsets were made of whalebone and encased the wearer in ironclad dignity. They were then covered in satin, brocade, silk and coutil (a close-woven canvas). Trimmed with lace and small roses, they could be bought in black for evening or the pretty Edwardian palettes of pale blue, pinks and mauves. Suspenders were attached to the corset or worn on a separate belt and even these were covered in ribbons and gilt clasps.

By the 1900s the froufrou sound of rustling lace petticoats was enough to stir the minds of ardent men. Patterned machine laces, in particular Valencienne and black Chantilly, were most popular of all and eagerly bought by those who could not afford the real thing. Among the 'chemical' or 'burnt' laces, guipures (lace having an embossed pattern) were very popular.

Net dresses were fashionable (machine-made bobbin net was easy to make) and often worn with a silk underdress. Embroidered on this plain net canvas were chenille floral motifs: roses, lilies and other flowers appeared on necklines, sleeves and bodices. Bunches of lace (jabots) attached to the front of bodices, and gilt braid and seams bound with silk satin, rounded off this pretty look. Intricate lacework with floral patterns, pin tucks and insertions created contrasting texture on

PAGE 10 Black peplum-bodiced velvet dress, trimmed with bands of velvet, with a white batiste turnover collar, by Paul Poiret, 1924. A fine example of modernism in fashion, it is worn by model Dinarzade (Petra Clive).

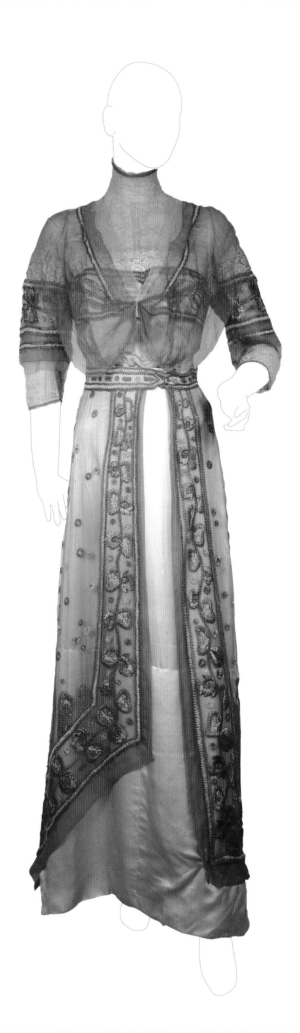

lawn fabric. All fulfilled the Edwardians' love of fussy detail and were dominant characteristics of the period.

The all-important blouse

Figuring largely in Edwardian ladies' sartorial repertoire, the blouse varied from the severely tailored masculine style with detachable starched collars and cuffs replete with tie to highly elaborate confections. Close-fitting, front-buttoned, with lace-edged yoke and leg-of-mutton sleeves, the blouse was often worn for the new female pursuit of cycling, as immortalized by the 'Gibson Girl'.

Romantic-style, hand-embroidered lace blouses were back-buttoned and usually white. They had finely tucked bodices and tucked sleeves. Often edged with white embroidery or machine-made lace, they were made from flimsy muslin, Japanese silk and zephyr and conveyed a fragile femininity. Three-quarter-length sleeves were in the fashionable Magyr style – tight-fitting with undersleeves that matched the neckline, puffed at the shoulders and laced at the cuff.

The Edwardian neck was often tightly enclosed in a high collarette of boned chiffon and lace, giving the wearer a regal bearing. Catalogues featured both the V-neck and the round neck, worn with little modesty squares in the neckline. Over the blouse a woman may have worn a bolero *visite*, generally of chiffon and lace.

Frocks and teagowns

Store catalogues of the era featured afternoon frocks made out of muslin with white cotton foundation bodices fastened with hooks at the front and frilled with machine-made Valencienne lace. Embroidered motifs, flowers or piping were also popular. Tucked gathers at the neckline gave a square, ruched-yoke effect and draped banks of silk at the waist.

SIGNATURE EDWARDIAN ELEMENTS:

* Long trailing skirts that fitted tightly over the hips, flowed to the knees, then fanned out
* High necks enclosed in stiff lace
* Wide puffed sleeves with close-fitting undersleeves
* Fully boned bodices to the neckline
* Ruffles, frills and spangles as all-over decoration on dresses
* Pin tucks as detailing, and used in blouses and dresses
* Low-cut necklines and bare backs for eveningwear
* Machine net used as a fabric in its own right, from which whole dresses were made

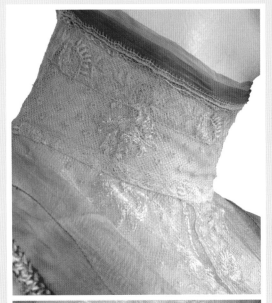

LEFT With layers of lace for structure, a high, slimline collar forced the neck to be held erect, contributing to the long, curved torso line and a well-bred manner. Edwardian collars were shaped to reach as high as possible at the back of the jaw, behind the ear, and this uneven shaping is characteristic of the era, persisting throughout the first decade of the century until the First World War.

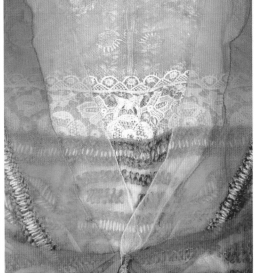

LEFT The deep V construct of the lace bodice accentuates the low bustline. The delicate rose colour of the dress is also a period detail, as the palette was generally subdued and shades had names such as 'ashes of rose'.

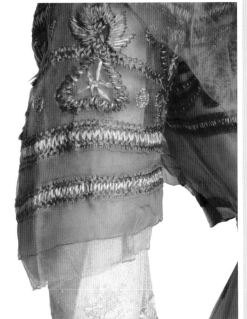

LEFT Three-quarter-length Magyr lace sleeves are overlaid by the ornately embroidered bodice sleeves.

OPPOSITE Edwardian vintage lace dress, by G E Spitzer, Vienna, circa 1905. Worn with a straight-fronted corset that moulded the torso into an S-bend, the dress created a silhouette of a full bottom, narrow waist and low single bustline. The straighter skirt replaced the full Victorian skirt.

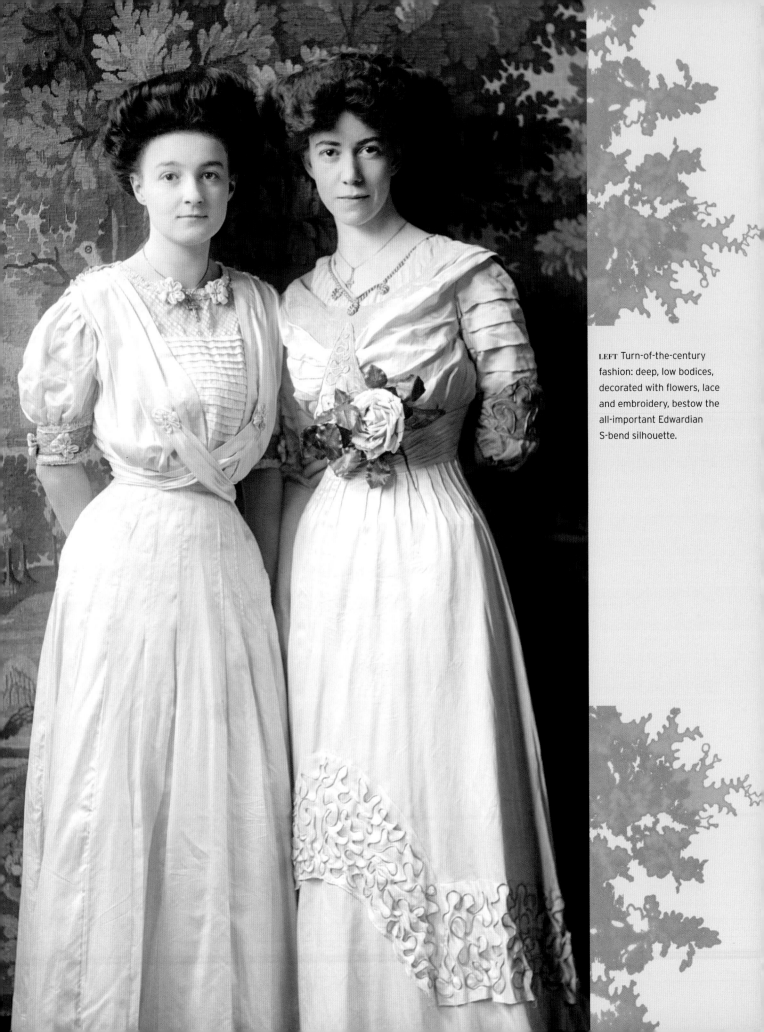

The deification of all that is feminine was embodied in the Edwardian evening dress. Floating dresses of sheer net, a froth of chiffons and soft faille, with bands of pleated silk draped over the shoulder and crossed at the waist, came in sweet pea and sugar almond delicacies of tone. A rounded décolleté was scooped low off the shoulders and filled in with a modesty frill of white chiffon. This would be festooned with ruffles, tulles, ruches, lace and glass beads forming sprays of leaves, flowers and ribbons.

By this time teagowns were usually very elaborate confections of silk or wool and lavish lace trimmings. Worn to entertain visitors for tea, they featured the modest high neck. Often draped or pleated they had deep gathered flounces and lace-edged frills.

The tailormade costume

Appealing to the independent woman, tailored suits became a sort of uniform for the enlightened. Made of tweed, serge or linen, the skirts were high-waisted, shorter than before, and trimmed with braid and buttons. Worn with the starched blouse (see page 13), the suit was completed by a smart tailored jacket, often made in silk, serge or wool and lined with plain fabric or appliqué. Often worn with a waistcoat, this severe jacket style sometimes featured leather cuffs and collars.

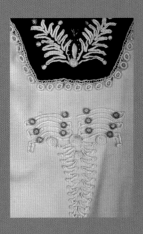

ABOVE AND LEFT An Edwardian ladies jacket, circa 1905, is ornately decorated with military-style frogging and embroidered epaulettes. The back view, above, is richly detailed with a black yoke that recalls a military uniform.

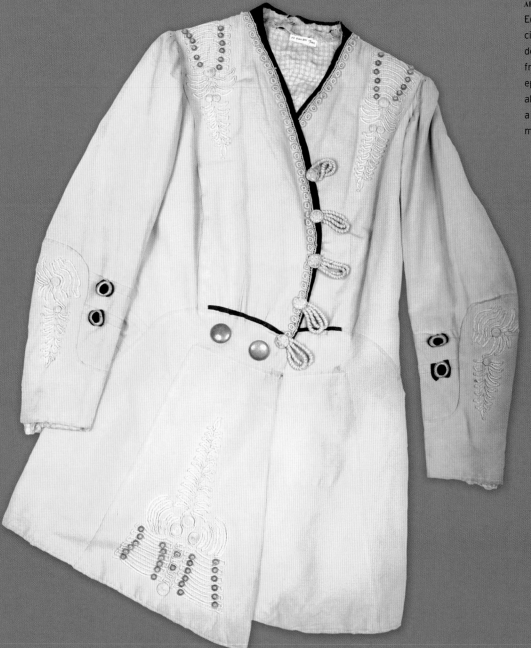

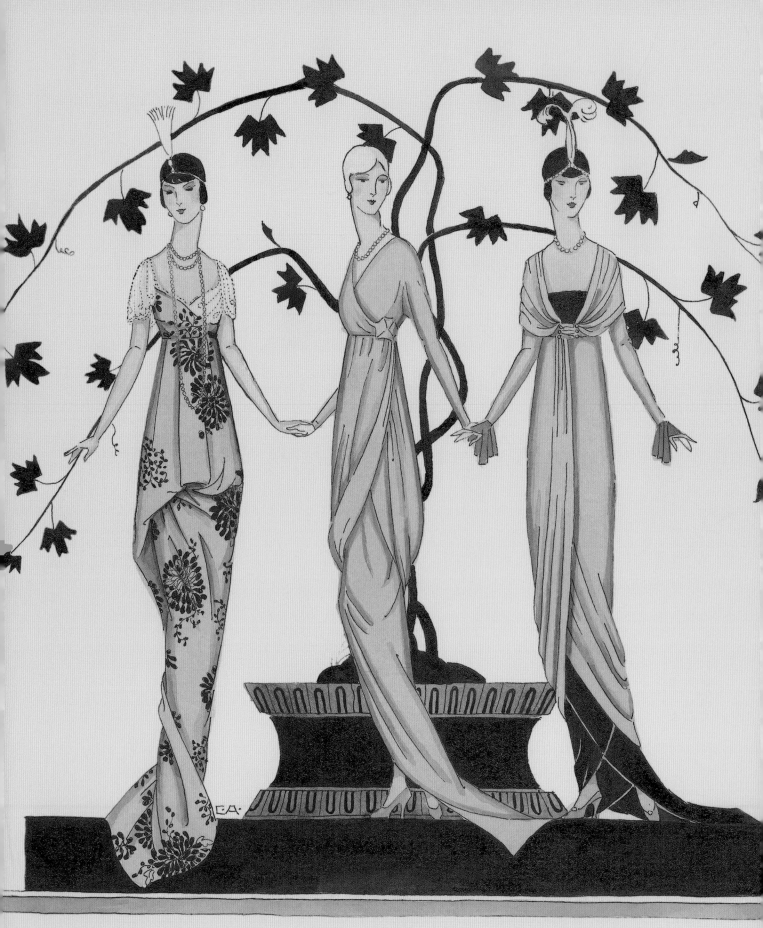

1912   1913   1913

The First Couture Houses

By the turn of the century, 'gay Paree' was the epicentre of fashion and became a regular stop for the leisured classes and 'royals' visiting the new couture houses of Doucet, Paquin, Callot Soeurs, Poiret, Lucile and Redfern. Charles Worth had elevated the status of the dressmaker to that of an artist. In his new luxurious showrooms in 7 rue de Paix, Paris – the first couture house to open – his creations were snapped up.

Charles Worth's lavish evening and reception gowns were almost as important as the events to which they were worn. His ingenuity in combining different fabrics and his creation of the backswept bustle skirt allowed a unique fall of fabric, while his singular cut and sense of ornament are his hallmarks. His work with large-scale, vivid floral motifs was woven to follow the figure once cut into a dress.

By 1908 Paul Poiret had revolutionized the silhouette and over-ornamented crinolines gave way to a high-waisted empire-line dress. A 'natural' style inspired by the Art Deco and Les Fauves movements, with their bold colours and surface decoration, came in. Poiret's Hellenic dresses were designed in the manner of classical Greek drapery to reveal the natural contours of the body and, hanging from the shoulders, would drape around the female form. Materials with fluid qualities such as muslin, light silk, satin and tulle were used to create the draped effect. Poiret's gowns were simple and either in plain colours or with geometric designs. His revolutionary *jupe culotte* (harem skirt) and kimonos were just as outré.

Colour and artistry, beautiful draped dresses, evening wraps, opulent furs and extravagant outerwear are all hallmarks of the house of Paquin, founded by Jeanne Beckers, who became known as Jeanne Paquin, and Isidore Jacobs. In materials such as muslin and voile, Paquin created exciting visual effects with light and texture. Beads and sequins, shirring and ruching, spotted net ribbon trim and padded appliqué were used to create a heightened visual quality, and she loved to combine unconventional materials, such as fur on a light pastel gown or chiffon and serge.

Other designers were clothing the new rich clients. Callot Soeurs favoured individuality and had a superb understanding of old velvet and lace, which they used for elaborate day dresses, and heavy satin for evening. Jacque Doucet meanwhile was known for his excellent workmanship and quality, and the British house of Redfern developed tailored yachting suits, riding habits, dresses, shawls and mantles for the great and the good.

OPPOSITE Illustration of dresses by Jacques Doucet, Lucile (Lucy Kennedy, later Lady Duff Gordon) and Charles Worth, dated 1912, 1913 and 1913 respectively.

LEFT, BELOW AND BELOW LEFT Black 1920s Paquin dress with pink embroidery. Paquin's signature colour was pink but she was also known for her dramatic use of black. Deep slits on the bodice and the back sleeves, a handkerchief hem, and vertical ruching at the waist mark some of the unique details on this rare piece.

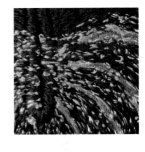

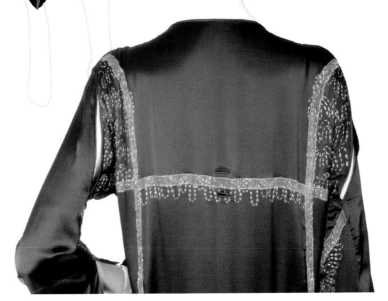

Early Innovations and Influences

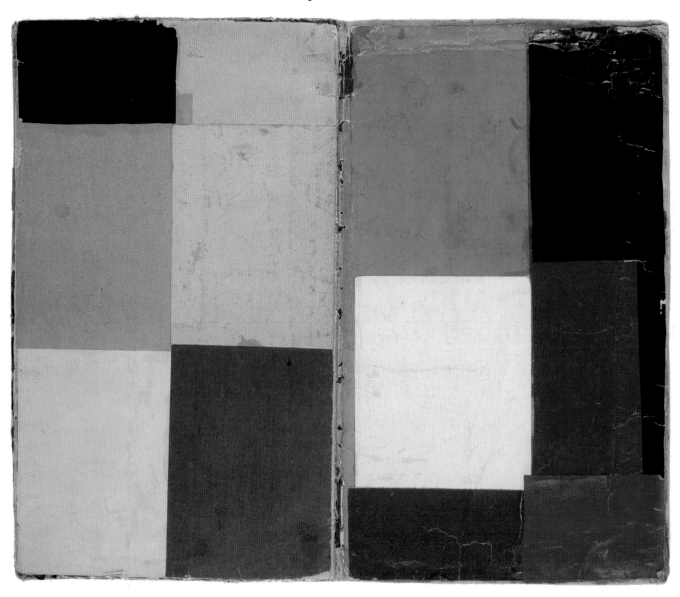

ABOVE Sonia Delaunay's 'simultaneous' colour contrasts on a painted surface. Artist, printmaker and fashion designer, Delaunay was a leader of the Orphism movement, an attempt to soften Cubism with lyrical colour.

As fashion and the female body freed itself from the constraints of the Edwardian stranglehold, new daring techniques sprung up. The avant-garde artists used bright geometric shapes printed directly onto the textile, creating a form of moving paintings. New ways of wrapping the body were created – the ancient craft of pleating was resurrected, and techniques such as cutting the dress along the bias produced new elastic drapes that moulded rather than bifurcated the female body.

Colour and textile design

In the years before the First World War new elements outside fashion influenced trends in a big way. The painter Sonia Delaunay covered fashion fabrics with patterns of colours in contrasting gradations – deep blues, black, white, yellow or green, or softer combinations of different browns and beiges. Her 'simultaneous' dresses with their geometric blocks of bright colour had an energy about them and were a kind of antifashion. Delaunay's embroidered coats (executed in *point du jour* using wool, cotton and silk), her *robes poèmes* (poem dresses) featuring lines of poetry beside swatches of bright colours, and her brightly embroidered beachwear were all dynamic visions of modernity.

An inventor of revolutionary fabrics, Mariano Fortuny devised vertical pleating, a process that he patented in 1909, whereby silk and cotton had an elastic quality and flowed over the contours of the female form. Pleats, often in the new 'painterly' colours such as eau de Nil, blues and soft reds, were twisted like skeins of yarn. He overpainted and dip-dyed again and again to achieve the desired shade. Silk cording was laced with heavy beads then handstitched along hems, seams and neckline to give weight to the dress. Fortuny combined his colour effects by stencilling and produced striking effects on heavy brocades and velvets, and incorporated textile patterns from East Asia and the Islamic world.

Bias cutting

With the bias cut Madame Vionnet rethought the relationship between fabric and flesh. She cut the fabric diagonally across the grain to produce a Grecianesque drape that seemed to spiral around the body. Reduced to their most basic lines, her dresses – often in silk and crepe de chine – were not so much fitted but fell in vertical folds that seemed to move with the body. With their clever simplicity and comfort of ease and movement, Vionnet's body-hugging dresses were of the modern age. They had no fastenings and required minimal underwear. She was also famous for her handkerchief points and the blouson dress, which was tied around the hips in a front bow.

Orientalism

During the 1910s fashion looked backwards to non-Western cultures. A craze for all things oriental was seen in the proliferation of Japanese prints and kimono-style dresses. Oriental embroideries and exotic colours, such as dark green, antique gold and rich reds, were juxtaposed with traditional pastels to create a new vibrant look. With Sergei Diaghilev's 1909 Ballets Russes and Poiret's 1912 Minaret collection, Eastern-influenced fashions swept in.

The Chanel suit

Radical in its understatement, the Chanel suit in jersey is more a way of life than an article of clothing. Chanel pared away fussy details and adapted male garments to create outfits that were feminine and untailored. With cardigan jackets and plain or pleated short skirts, plain and patterned wool jersey tops and horizontal stripes, her designs were the epitome of modern chic. Flannel blazers, delicately embroidered and with the famous saddle-style double belt, were worn with open-necked blouses and the sailor collar. Her clothes presaged sportswear – shown by her love of muted colours such as grey and beige.

LEFT Fortuny's famous Delphos gown, from 1907, a columnar dress of thin silk satin, loosely twisted and pleated, was draped from the shoulder and inspired by the chitons of ancient Greece.

FORTUNY HALLMARKS:

- Batwing sleeves laced along the top
- Hems weighted with Venetian glass or wooden beads
- Silk screening on seams and along edges of dresses to produce a showy effect
- Hand printing (*pochoir*) method used on cotton, velvet and silk
- Sleeveless Peplos and Delphos vertically pleated dresses, belted with a knotted cord
- Velvet garments, stencilled and overlaid with gold and silver
- Moorish capes and Persian jackets

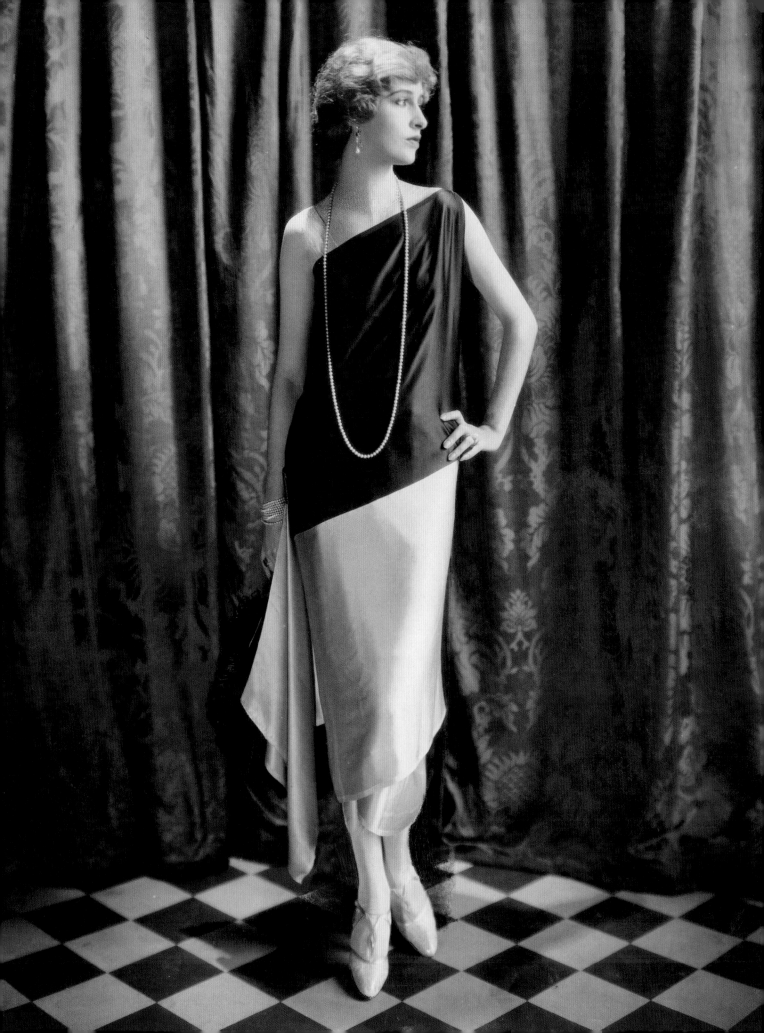

Modernism and Geometrics

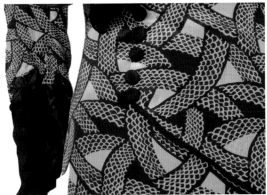

'God the machine' was the mantra of the modernist age. The turn of the century brought the automobile, the steam ship and the aeroplane. These were all innovations that had a tangible effect not only on the choice of fabrics, design and colours used, but also on the easy-to-wear fashions of the time. Designers created styles that catered to the cosmopolitan woman – 'Shipboard smartness' and 'Riviera chic', as *Vogue* dubbed them in 1926.

The flat, straight-up-and-down dresses of the 1920s were perfect for the stylized geometric-patterned prints that defined the modernist period. Influenced by the Cubist and Futurist art movements, their dynamic, uneven designs, straight lines, spirals, cones and zig-zags were all incorporated into the fashions of the day. Cubist abstract motifs were sewn on to dresses and evening coats. Horizontal stripes were juxtaposed with triangles on dresses, with the same pattern lining the coat. Embroidered circles and triangles in silver and gold thread brought to life the popular black evening dresses of the day, and diagonal patterns with shadings from black to grey produced amazing graphic designs from the prevailing Art Deco style.

Jean Patou's famous sweaters, with their Cubist-style blocks of contrasting colour in horizontal stripes inspired by the paintings of Picasso and Braque, were worn by the *beau monde*. Cubist pieces were all the rage, as were Egyptian-style motifs, with serpent designs, hieroglyphics and scarabs either appliquéd or embroidered on to day and evening dresses.

The modernist designers often concentrated on purifying form and cut: Vionnet, Lanvin and Chanel controlled the amount of ornamentation they used and, like the Cubists, were more interested in form and design. Lucien Lelong's *Ligne kynetique* was a range of severely tailored cloth dresses in two shades of jersey with a pared-down simple shape that suggested movement in the design.

Pleats and tucks were often executed as designs in themselves. Treated geometrically, there were

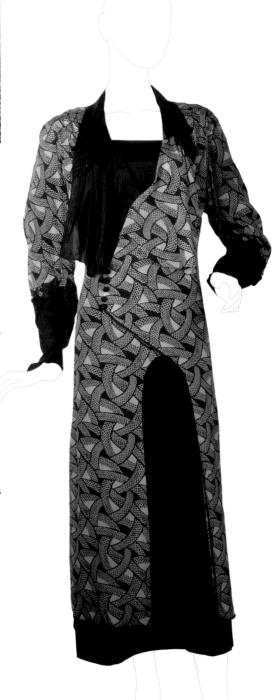

LEFT AND FAR LEFT A late 1920s silk serpentine-print dress. Although it is by an unknown designer, the graphic interlocking snake-like print and sharp curved lines that drape the form clearly reference modernism. Note the asymmetrical draped collar and the buttoned-waist detail.

OPPOSITE: Actress Marion Morehouse (the poet e. e. cummings's wife) models a one-shouldered bias-cut silk-satin sheath gown with a diagonally cut drop-bodice and slim skirt wrapped to form a two-layered hemline, by Callot Soeurs, 1924.

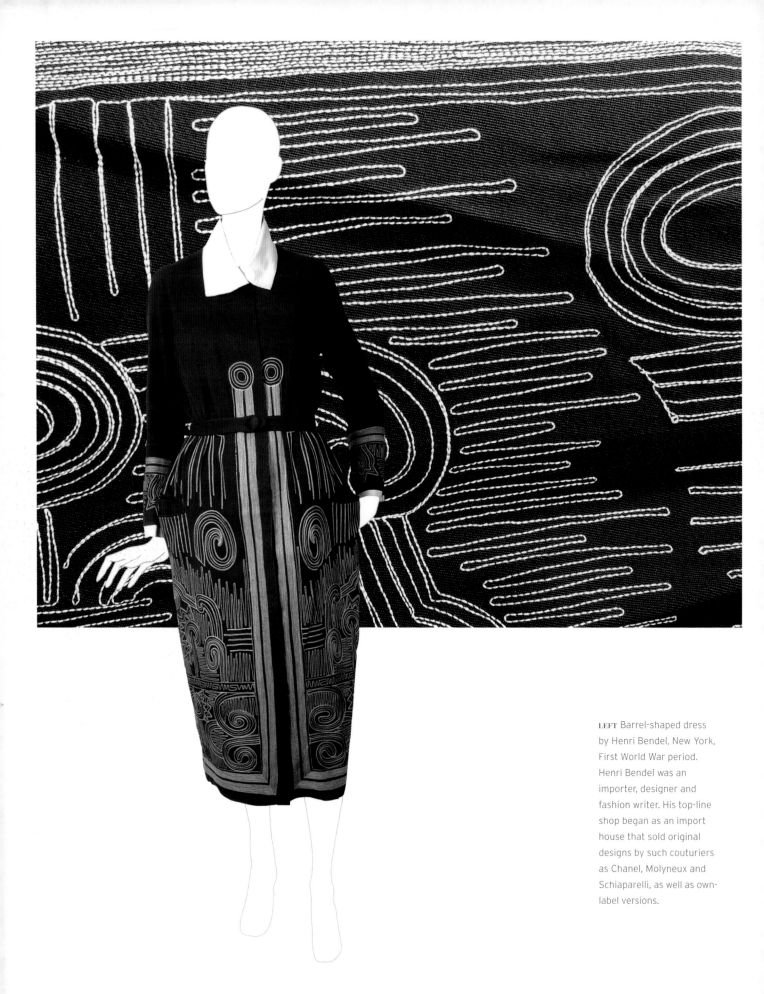

LEFT Barrel-shaped dress by Henri Bendel, New York, First World War period. Henri Bendel was an importer, designer and fashion writer. His top-line shop began as an import house that sold original designs by such couturiers as Chanel, Molyneux and Schiaparelli, as well as own-label versions.

perpendicular tucks in all directions – suits with horizontal pleats on the bodice and vertical pleating on the skirt were popular and contributed the modernist rectangular look.

The colour palette

Contrasting colours in the bold palette of the Fauviste painters was characteristic of the modernist look. Black and white was one of the smartest of colour schemes, and part of the avante-garde that dominated fashion at that time introduced neutral grey and beige. Other colour combinations – red and green; black, red and orange; and acid green and cerise pink – were popular Art Deco colours. Black was often used as a background for bright motifs – black taffeta dresses with red, green and mauve embroidery on collars and circular panels of embroidery on the skirt, for example. Contrasting hues of different browns and greys on a black background gave clothes a graphic look.

The influence of sportswear

'Sportswear has more to do than anything else with the evolution of the modern mode,' said *Vogue* in 1926 – and indeed the functional design of sports clothes was a perfect template for the casual sporting styles of the new age.

The nautical colours navy, red and white were incorporated into jersey tunics and sailor-style dresses with navy trimming. Knitwear, sporty cardigans and jumpers – lightweight and often made of cotton or spun silk, plain, striped and sometimes with decorative nautical motifs ,– were ultra-modern in feel. Jean Patou's sportswear, particularly his outfit for tennis champion Susanne Lenglen with its pleated shift dress and sleeveless buttoned-down sweater, was a prototype for the fashions to come.

RIGHT Silk white-and-navy dress with triangle detailing from the 1920s exhibits the fascination with clean modernist geometry .

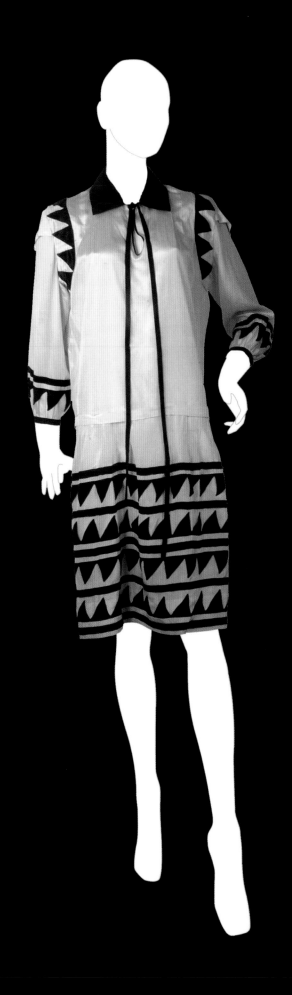

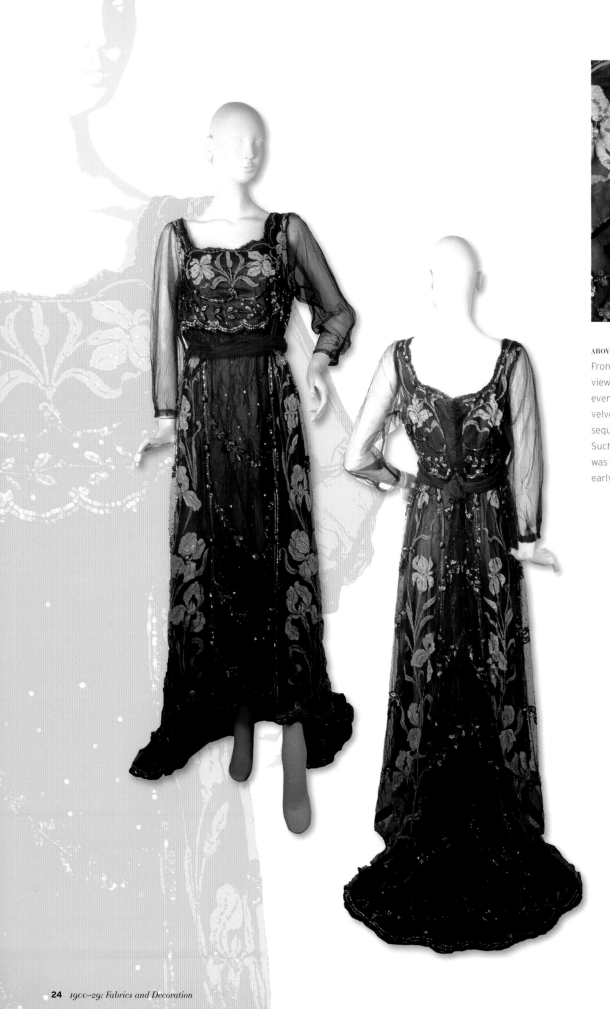

Fabrics and Decoration

The decorative arts and fashion fused during the 1920s to usher in a flamboyant look, and the simplicity of the cut and shape of the times was offset by elaborate surface decoration. Technical developments within the textile industry meant that new fabrics were being created, and mass-produced rayon dresses with the appearance of silk were popular for both daywear and eveningwear. Meyer artificial silks and woollens – Pelgram & Meyer was one of the pioneer silk mills in early century America – were available in a variety of weaves, colours and textures.

During the day, women would wear angular styles in practical materials like jersey, silk twill, mohair, kasha and rayon. Dresses in coarsely woven silk, jersey cardigans, lightweight tweeds and handwoven brocades were considered chic.

Fluttery evening frocks in flimsy materials like crepe satin and crepe georgette shimmered with diamanté. Dresses using the shiny side of the satin for the trimming and the dull side for the body section could be seen everywhere, and silk in combination with cotton was worn. Silver, gold and coloured laces were often combined with satin, lamé, taffeta, crepe de chine and georgette. Sumptuous lamé gowns of green and gold, worn with pearls and overlaid with thin lace, shone in the night, as did acid-green moire tubular frocks. Mariano Fortuny's handstencilled velvet coats and dresses woven with shimmering metallic thread were inspired by sixteenth-century velvets and his motifs and patterns reflected paintings of that period.

Surface decoration and trimmings

The tubular-shaped dresses of the day were an ideal surface for embroidery and other decoration. Appliqué, flocking, raised cord, metal and coloured thread, particularly gold and silver, were all seen in dresses following Art Deco styles. Silver embroidery livened up black chiffon dresses and embroidered bands were used to trim décolleté and bolero tops.

Paquin's gowns of green chiffon embroidered with pearls and gold threads on a Chinese design with bands of embroidery forming the dropped waist were seen on the pages of *Vogue*. Embroidery silks added glamour and diamanté embroidery for evening was said to be so 'brilliant' that the nightclubs hardly needed lighting. Beads were embroidered – creating motifs, lines or trimmings– on most eveningwear.

Oriental, Cubist and floral appliqué provided a decorative surface design technique, and gold and silver leather appliqué added dimension and texture to the background fabric. The beaded evening dress of the 'Roaring '20s' is the signature vintage garment. Designed to be 'brilliant', some dresses were completely covered in brightly coloured glass beads or genuine

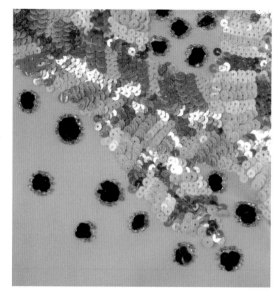

LEFT Sequins, beads and appliqué on a skirt from the 1920s. Sequins at this time were sometimes made of wax, and easily melted. In gowns you may find deterioration of the sequins where a dancing partner's hands would rest.

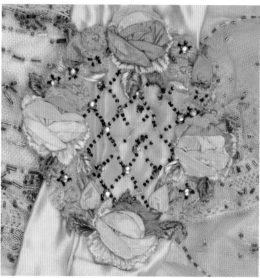

LEFT Ornate beadwork and with lace and flower appliqué on a satin bridal gown, 1905.

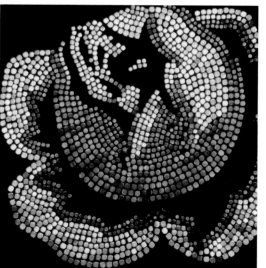

LEFT A 1928 Vionnet garment decorated with a stylized rose by the design house Lesage. Masterful shading is achieved by strategic use of subtly different colours. Lesage has been creating haute couture embroidery since 1924, and many designers have built a piece or a collection around a Lesage motif.

gems such as crystal and jet – black beads made from coral or glass. These could be sewn on to lightweight silk, rayon, crepe or chiffon to create a striking look.

White crepe georgette dresses with diamanté beads and pailettes were common. Black chiffon dresses with silver and gold beads were particularly spectacular, and whole skirts edged with crystal beads in the same colour or edged with rhinestone embroidery sparkled. The craze for sequins was a hallmark of the decade, as they reflected the light and could be overlapped to produce linear patterns.

Dresses were as diverse as everything else. White crepe de chine frocks were fringed with chatelaine and dresses with three-tiered fringing, the top layer of the fringe outlining the bolero top, created a swaying flounced shape. Wide fringed scarves were worn to give extra motion to the silhouette. Feathers were attached to the bodices and skirts of dresses and even featured as headgear.

Further ornamentation was evident in ruffles, sewn in even tiers and along the edges of skirts and jumpers. Bows were worn at the neck, hip and down the front and back of dresses, and lingerie touches at the neck and sleeves were popular. Leather – sometimes metallized – and fur trimmings on cuffs, collars and hems were key details. But for the ultra-glam woman, fur-lined and fur-trimmed gold lamé coats were a must.

Notable designers

Certain couturiers and designers of the period were notable for their expertise, not only in design but also for their use of embellishment. Known for her spectacular beading techniques and innovative surface embellishment, Lanvin's free-flowing ribbons at the neck or hip of the dress, petals and ruffles and delicate appliqué in pastel colours – especially Lanvin blue – and her elaborate thread embroideries were inspired by exotic travel and other elements.

Callot Soeurs' dresses in embroidered satin or velvet with Eastern motifs in kingfisher blue and black with gold and copper highlights were worn by society gals, as were their silver and gold lamé evening dresses and decorative dragon and paisley medallion motifs. The sisters – Gerber, Bertrand and Chanterelle, who formed the house in 1895 and who were authorities on antique lace – combined unusual materials such as rubberized gabardine or calf skin with gossamer silks worked with bands of gold lace or silk flowers.

Artist-designer Mary Monaci Galenga's Moyen Age teagown with a square or V-neck and tabard was a must-have of the time. Made of silk velvet or crepe de chine, the gown had panels of floating chiffon set into the side seams and was strewn with large Venetian glass millefiori beads. It also featured gold or silver stencilling in different tones and a variety of patterns.

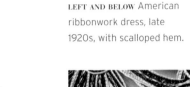

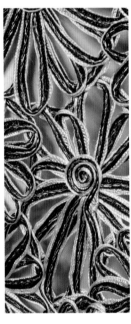

LEFT AND BELOW American ribbonwork dress, late 1920s, with scalloped hem.

OPPOSITE Mary Monaci Galenga stencilled crimson velvet, 1920s. Born in 1880, Galenga was a mentor of the Italian Futurists and developed the technique of stencilling gold onto velvet. A contemporary of Fortuny, by 1914 she was making clothes and textiles. Both Fortuny and Galenga were known for their Renaissance revival designs.

OPPOSITE INSET Fortuny seashell-stencil turquoise velvet, 1920s. His stencilled velvets have the look of antique frescoes, achieving multiple layers of pigment.

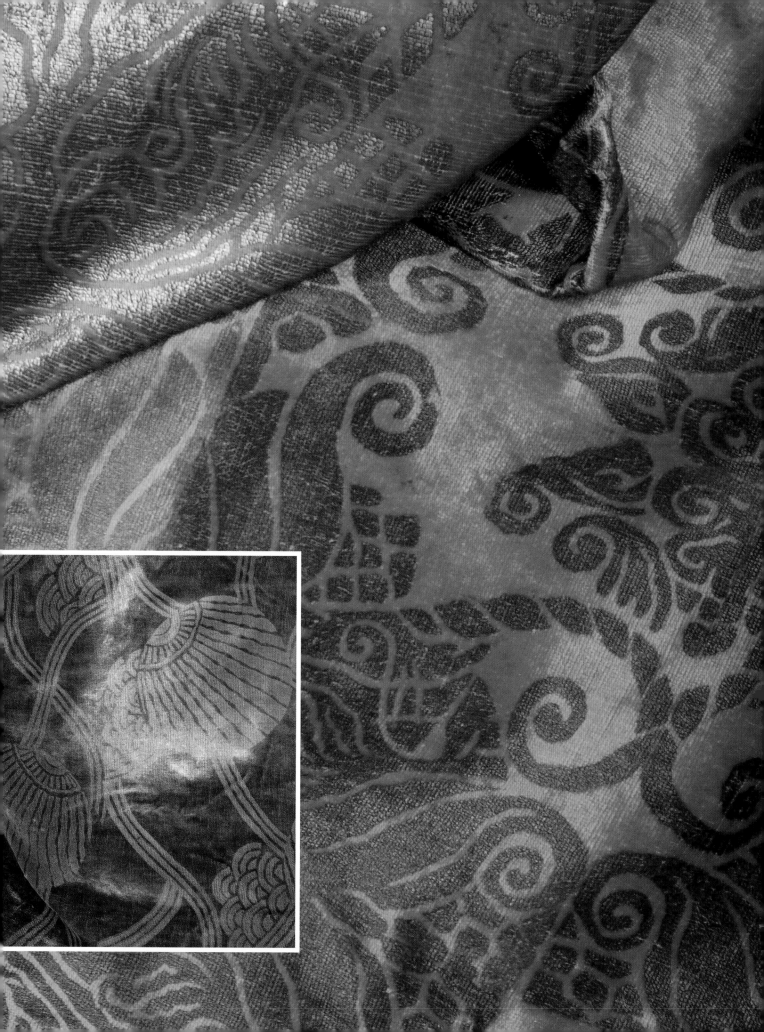

New Silhouettes

The fashions of the 1910s are the sartorial missing link between the *belle époque* (1890-1914) and the modern fashion of the 1920s. The Edwardian S-bend silhouette made way for the less restrictive empire line with raised waist (1908), followed by the dropped waist (1920s), where the waist and bosom simply disappeared.

The empire line and the hobble

By 1908 societal mores were beginning to relax and this could be seen in the changing silhouette of women's fashions. When Paul Poiret introduced his empire line in that same year, it was greeted with great enthusiasm. Characterized by the columnar silhouette and a slim skirt, his empire-style dresses were unprecedented. The waistline crept up from the waist to below the bosom, and the hemline rose slightly accordingly. With the waist no longer the focal point, the dresses were suspended from the shoulders, creating a linear form.

Loosely cut sleeves with crossed bodices were seen in evening dresses and the evening coats were based on simple wraps with batwing sleeves. These garments then became working surfaces, which the designers could use for their increasingly opulent styles. Fur trimmings were very popular and served as the new status signal.

Couturier Jacques Doucet's empire dresses were made of airy fabrics and had intricate floral details showing the influence of Art Nouveau's decorative language. Free-flowing with a simple construction, they were made in one piece and fell straight down which respected instead of bifurcated the natural form.

Paul Poiret introduced the hobble skirt in 1910 – a return to female imprisonment, as women's legs were clamped together in a skirt that was unfeasibly narrow from the knees to the ankles, causing women to walk like Japanese geishas. Yet it proved a short-lived trend – 'freedom' was the new buzz word.

The wartime crinoline

The long, clinging high-waisted dresses were swept away during the First World War when the chemise dress appeared. Pioneered by Lanvin, Worth and Paquin, the chemise was cut loose and full and belted under the bosom. Skirts rose suddenly to just above the ankle and filled out. More romantic in style, these new skirts were flared, and although they had layers of petticoats underneath – sometimes to crinoline proportions – they were easy to walk in.

The bodices of dresses were unfitted and the bust was flat. Women started to wear open-necked blouses that combined fashion and function, as everything was

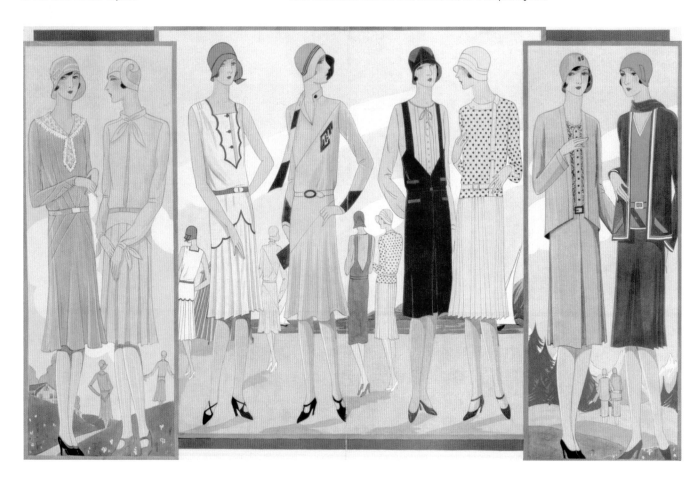

now loose and biased towards freedom of movement. They were simple and elegant, made in velvets for the afternoon and Charles Worth's tinted tulles and muslins for the evening.

There was a brief return to the barrel skirt in 1917 by couturiers such as Callot Soeurs, Doeuillet and Paquin. Cut wide over the hip, it had the pannier look – pulling the dress out at the hips – of a bygone age, sometimes with two or three gathered tiers.

Postwar fashions

After the war fashion did not quite know what direction it should take. The greater freedom women had enjoyed meant that fashion could not go backwards. Easy-to-wear elegance became the order of the day, although for the first half of the 1920s sudden changes of line or length of skirt were usual, and the hemline rose and fell in an erratic manner.

Coco Chanel and Jean Patou championed the shorter length with their forward-looking jersey suits and sporty style. Although in 1919 the hemline rose again and the look of the '20s flapper was nascent, most women still wore widish peg-top skirts and A-line styles – only slightly shorter than before. Jeanne Lanvin's new fluffed-up crinolines were the exception to the slimmer silhouette.

In 1920 an unprecedented mid-calf hemline came in at 7.5 cm (3 in) above the ankle and with dresses high-waisted. But twelve months later, hemlines dropped again, practically to the ankle. The longer skirts were circular in cut and dresses and tops were loosely belted to just below the natural waistline and above the hip. Eveningwear was still elaborately trimmed, with fringing all the rage.

From 1922 to 1924 hemlines were 10-13 cm (4-5 in) from the ankle and the focus was on a vertical silhouette – this was achieved by dropping the waistline dramatically to the hip and by vertically striped tunics or vertical pleats and tucks.

The two-piece came into fashion. This consisted of a blouse or jumper and skirt combination, the top completely unfitted and worn over the skirt to just below hip level, sometimes with a wide belt or sash. Along with ensemble dresses, which consisted of a matched dress and jacket, these were strong fashions, lasting throughout the 1920s. The bateau neckline – slashed straight from one shoulder to the other – was popular, as were scooped necks, V-necks, sailor collars and three-quarter-length sleeves.

'Paris agrees to disagree about the length of skirts,' said *Vogue* in 1923, as designers could not make up their mind how much leg to show. Some women loved Chanel's shorter skirt – a radical 22-25 cm (9-10 in) off the ground; others preferred Edward Molyneux's longer Egyptian sheaths that were almost ankle length.

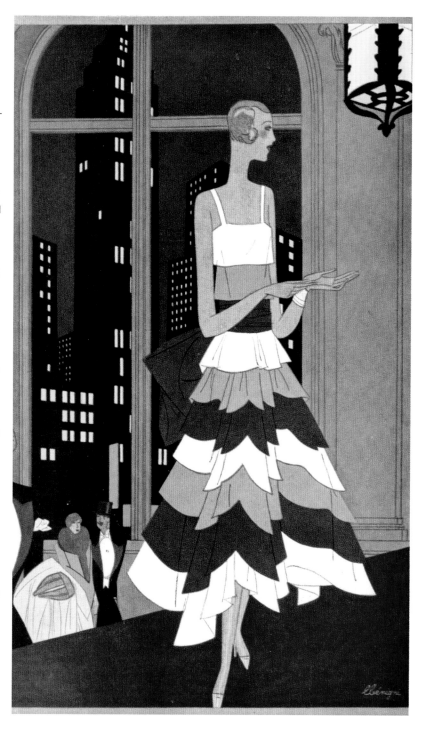

OPPOSITE Ladies 1920s daywear with dropped-waist dresses and pleated skirts with jackets, worn with cloche hats. The hemlines are high at just below the knee.

ABOVE Jeanne Lanvin fashion drawing, 1928, 'Under the Eyes of New York Skyscrapers', from *Femina* magazine.

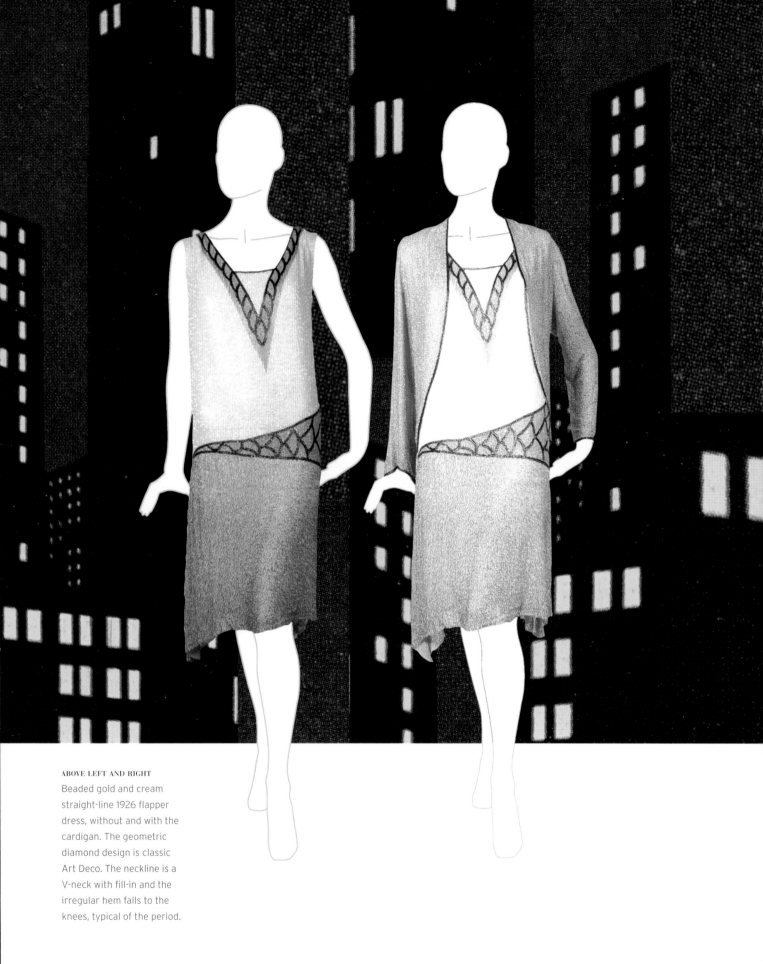

ABOVE LEFT AND RIGHT
Beaded gold and cream
straight-line 1926 flapper
dress, without and with the
cardigan. The geometric
diamond design is classic
Art Deco. The neckline is a
V-neck with fill-in and the
irregular hem falls to the
knees, typical of the period.

The Age of the Flapper

By 1924 the wise-cracking flappers were as much known for their reckless behaviour as for their style. Smoking and putting their make-up on in public, the bright young things drank and danced the Shimmy and the Bunny Hop in a frenzy of excitement. Taping up their breasts to get rid of unwanted curves, they looked youthful and boyish, and the new silhouette was slender, straight up and down like a board, and in fact became known as 'le garçonne'.

As if to herald the new mood, the waistline dropped dramatically in 1925 to below the hip, and by 1927 it had disappeared altogether and the hemline risen a scandalous 38 cm (15 in) to just below the knee. The flapper look was at its apogee and extremely short skirts were worn day and night. But hemlines crashed down along with Wall Street in 1929, just as waistlines and busts edged their way into fashion consciousness.

Flapper dresses were straight, loose and sleeveless, revealing a new body awareness. Arms were bare, and legs and backs were exposed for the first time, becoming new erogenous zones. The illusion of nudity was heightened by the use of diaphanous fabrics and little adornment. Beading was used to emphasize the see-through materials and catch the light, yet also highlighted the risqué nature of the outfits.

The short shift dress, which fell straight down from the shoulders and stopped above the knees, dominated the mid- to late 1920s. Ornamented with geometric and abstract designs, the chemise was often beaded with bands of glittering sequins.

For daywear the three-piece jersey suit was the cornerstone of female fashion: a blouse worn with a patterned or plain knitted sweater or a Chanel-style cardigan jacket with pockets was teamed with a narrow, short, pleated skirt. Day dresses were simple or decorated with details such as horizontal tucks, seaming or bias-cut panels and square boatnecks. Combinations of fabrics were used and two-tones,

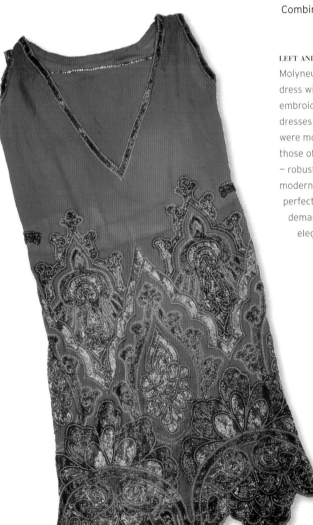

LEFT AND BELOW RIGHT
Molyneux orange silk 1925 dress with silver and gold embroidery. Even on flapper dresses Molyneux's designs were more minimalist than those of his contemporaries – robust fabrics, strong modernist motifs and a perfect cut made them demanding though utterly elegant pieces.

SIGNATURE FLAPPER ELEMENTS:

- Uneven split hems and handkerchief points that are longer at the back
- Egyptian- and Art-Deco-inspired motifs
- Visible seam decoration and double seams
- Diagonal lines and asymmetric trimmed necklines
- Pockets, buttons and belts
- Pleated panels on skirts and knife pleats
- Day dresses belted around the hips
- Low-cut necks and backs, with thin straps
- Narrow trailing scarves, sometimes attached to dresses

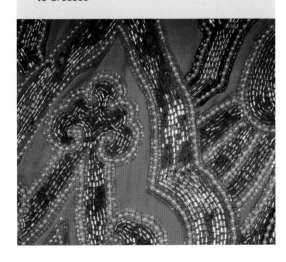

graded shades were popular, as were mannish suits, ties and small geometric prints.

A pioneer with Coco Chanel of the 'garçonne' look, Jean Patou designed sports ensembles with gradating stripes that could be worn with his geometric jumpers and cardigans on the Riviera. He designed beige three-piece jersey suits, dresses and wraps. His afternoon flapper-style crepe dresses had self-tied shoulder bows or decorative seams worked in zig-zags.

The bright young things wore trousers at home in the early evenings or at the beach. Loosely cut with drawstring or elasticated waists, they were sometimes called Oxford Bags and fastened at the side for modesty. Paquin's Chinese-printed satin pyjamas with embroidered satin jacket were all the rage.

The perfectly straight-line collarless coat that buttoned at the waist like a cardigan jacket and a high-collar coat with a sash at the waist maintained their popularity, as did the slightly circular coat with fur collar that wrapped over on the diagonal, fastening with a single loop and button at hip level.

Eveningwear

The modern social whirl of cabarets, fancy dress parties and dancing gave rise to more extravagant evening wear. And by 1928 Paris was determined to abandon the tubular dresses, and floating panels and Vionnet's bias-cut dresses, which followed the contours of the body, became popular. Draperies from the hips gave the illusion of length and fullness, and movement was added with attached panels or uneven hemlines. Chanel's black evening dresses with huge transparent draperies, Paquin's acid-green moiré dresses with a V-neck and bulk at the hip, and Molyneux's transparent printed dresses with full, scalloped skirts and arm draperies are all significant flapper styles.

Crystal-beaded waves with coral fish and lilac flamingos in lotus ponds were some of Molyneux's unconventional surface decoration on flapper dresses. He experimented with ostrich feathers and buttons resembling cigarette butts or lipsticks, and his beaded chemises are some of the most exquisite.

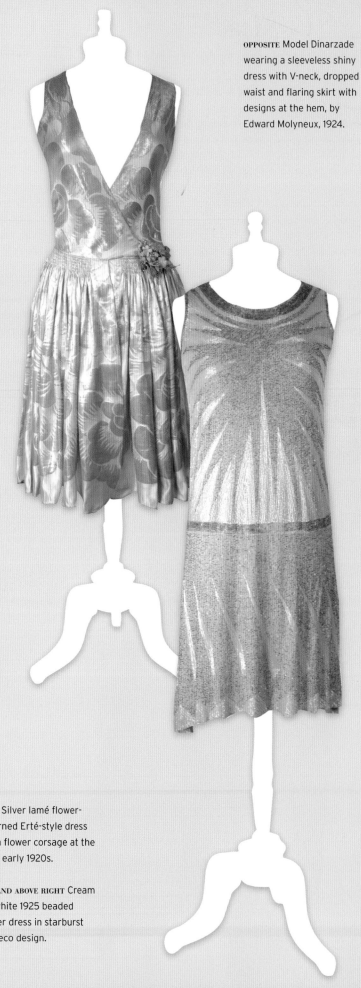

OPPOSITE Model Dinarzade wearing a sleeveless shiny dress with V-neck, dropped waist and flaring skirt with designs at the hem, by Edward Molyneux, 1924.

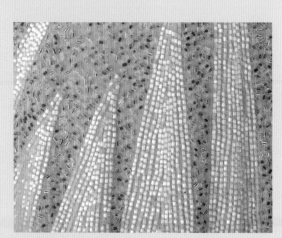

ABOVE Silver lamé flower-patterned Erté-style dress with a flower corsage at the waist, early 1920s.

LEFT AND ABOVE RIGHT Cream and white 1925 beaded flapper dress in starburst Art Deco design.

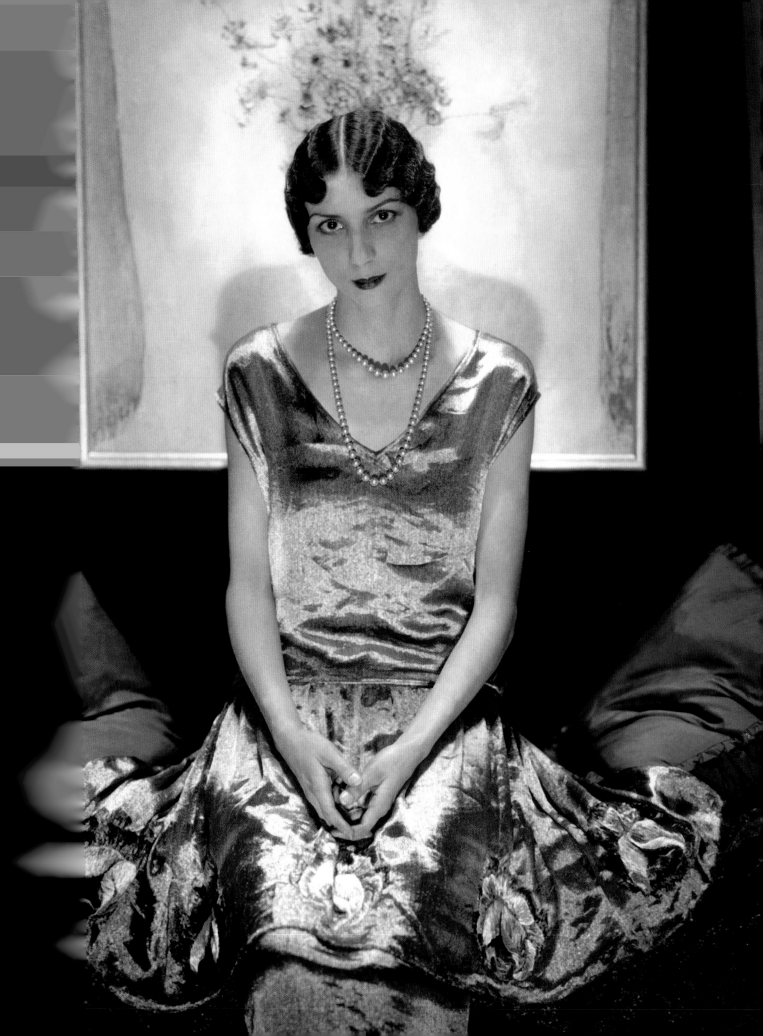

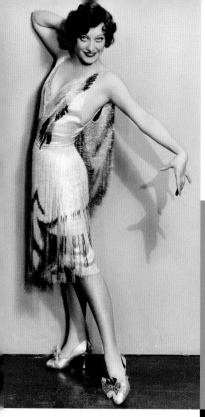

◀Beading and fringing
Evening dresses with sequins, feathers and other ornate surface decorations were characteristic of the period, as in this fringed flapper dress seen here modelled by Joan Crawford in the 1920s.

The sheath dress
The slinky sheath was made of chiffon, silk or crepe de chine, and clung to the female form from shoestring shoulder straps.

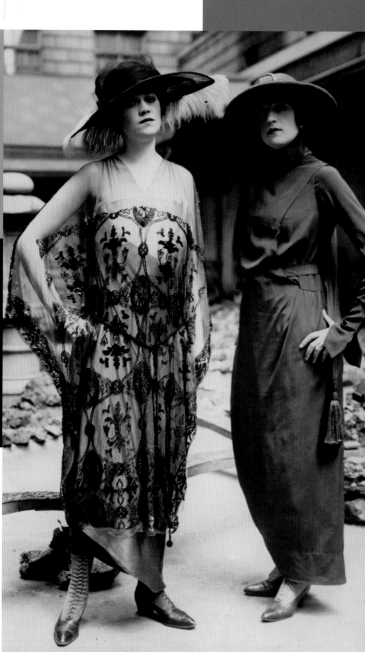

Key looks of the era
1900-1929

▼Geometrics
Sweeping bold curved patterns in deep colours that included dramatic red, black and blue appeared from 1910, along with other geometric patterns and Cubist motifs.

Edwardian blouses
The Edwardian blouse, made of lace with ruffles, or striped and purposeful, epitomized the dual femininity – both demure and assertive – of the times.

S-shaped corsets
The early-century corset created the idealized female form with a tiny waist – achieved through artificial distortion of the body.

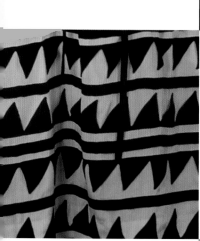

Style Russe
Chanel's early 1920s Russian style, attributed to her liaison with Russian Grand Duke Dmitri, consisted of tunic shapes, fur trimmings and embroideries. This look reflected the influx of Russians to Paris after the Revolution. 'Style Russe' would be revisited by many designers, as in Saint Laurent's 'Russian Revolution' in the mid-1970s.

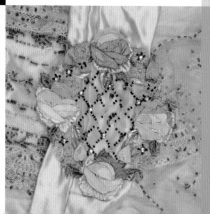

▲Hobble and kite dresses
After the emancipation from the strict *belle époque* silhouette, dresses became looser while the 'hobble', as created by Paul Poiret, was groundbreaking in developing the narrow, shorter hemline – an influence that can be seen in these kite dresses from 1918. Lace-up boots also came back into fashion during the years of the First World War.

Dropped waist

...urves and the hourglass figure ...ere out, and belts, sashes or ...es were worn around the hips. ...he waist disappeared to create ...he fashionable beanpole look ...eloved in the '20s, as typified ...the illustration from Mab ...atterns, April 1925, below.

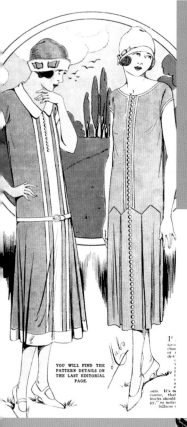

YOU WILL FIND THE PATTERN DETAILS ON THE LAST EDITORIAL PAGE.

Le Garçonne look

A new androgyny accompanied the flapper era, and women wore short hair and dresses that were straight, loose and revealed bare arms. The lithe, athletic, modern form was the new sexy look.

Velvets and furs

Fur coats, or coats trimmed in fur, were popular. Many had a single large button, or wrapped over, a shawl collar, wide cuffs and fell to the knees. Velvet was also used in jackets, wraps and dresses; the sumptuous material was part of the style of opulence and the luxury of Art Deco fashion.

▲ Kimono style

Japanese-style dresses were seen as very exotic and heralded a new form of beauty based on simplicity and oriental design. Many teagowns, like the 1925 dress above, had the square-cut sleeves and shape of the kimono.

▲ Bare backs and bias cuts

Cut on the bias, the new body-hugging dresses seemed to spiral round the body and moved with the wearer. Backless dresses, like the 1929 version above, with or without trains, began to make an appearance later in the 1920s.

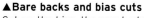

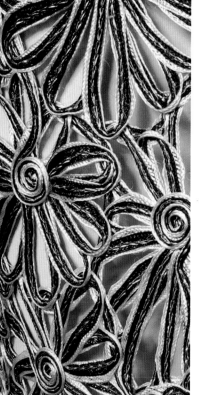

Sweaters

Silk or wool, and striped, plain or with *trompe l'oeil* motifs, the jumper was a key element in flapper style of the 1920s.

Trousers

Bright young things in the 1920s would wear silken pyjamas and sailor pants for early evening or as fashionable resort wear.

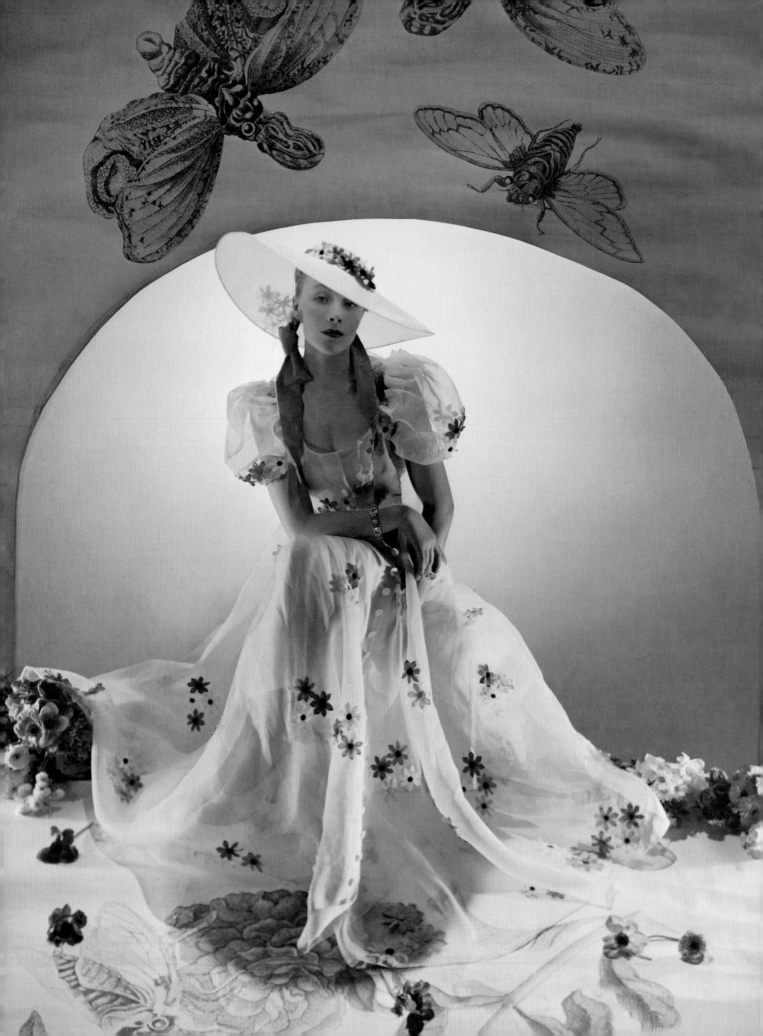

1930s

Epitomized by the elongated draped gowns worn by movie stars, the 1930s will for ever be remembered as the era of Hollywood glamour. Liberated from the corsets and cumbersome designs of previous years, women were now able to dress in a way that was both stylish and practical, while new fabrics encouraged designers to experiment with original looks.

Form was more important than detail and embellishment as designers focused on the silhouette. Unlike the boyish 1920s when breasts were strapped down and dresses were loose and boxy, clothes were cut to follow the lines of the body, showing off the female figure in a more provocative manner than ever before. Shoulders were bared in the first halterneck and backless gowns, and the bias-cut dress – pioneered by Parisian couturier Madeleine Vionnet – clung to every curve. Suits consisted of neat-fitting, waist-length jackets with skirts to mid-calf. Coco Chanel designed two-piece suits in wool jersey fabrics, which heralded a sportier look that became a surprise daywear hit.

However, many of these new trends were born of necessity. Coming between the two world wars and directly after the stock market crash of 1929, times were hard. The Great Depression meant that designers had to work with cheaper materials and ordinary women could no longer afford the sartorial excesses of previous decades. Even the wealthiest showed restraint in what they wore, while screen idols such as Katharine Hepburn and Bette Davis represented a glamour that most could only dream of.

Daywear Fashions

Until the 1930s daywear had often been more decorative than practical. But now, for the first time, women of all social backgrounds were beginning to lead busier and more productive lives and so clothes became easy to wear and unrestrictive. Although eveningwear had a strong element of escapist glamour, by day elegant and tidy clothes were key.

Money was tight, so women were no longer at liberty to indulge their every fashion fancy and had to find other ways to look smart. Clothes were mended instead of replaced and accessories played an important part. Costume jewellery, especially brooches, earrings and rings, was favoured as a cheaper alternative to the priceless gems that had previously been the required jewellery among the fashionable classes. Fine leather gloves in nubuck or lambskin also added an essential touch to daywear. Hats were worn at a fashionable tilt, and while the beret replaced the cloche hat, pillboxes also became popular and the turban emerged as one of the most glamorous accessories of the time.

As the decade progressed, function became more and more important, and by the time the Second World War had begun in 1939, simple clothes such as trousers, sweaters, classic shirtwaisters and low-heeled shoes were the staple of most women's wardrobes. Designers began to adapt the mood of their collections to more military-inspired, square-shouldered clothing, with skirts that hung just below the knee and often slightly longer at the back.

But this new liking for practical day clothes did not mean that fashion had lost its femininity – on the contrary, designers compensated by creating a more hourglass silhouette. Instead of sitting low on the hips as they had in the 1920s, waistlines returned to the natural waist, if not slightly higher, and were often cinched-in to create a more curvaceous figure. Necklines were lowered and frequently had wide scalloped edges and ruffled collars, while the jabot blouse – with its ornamental cascade of frills down the front – became hugely fashionable, as did the pussy-bow neckline.

Flamboyant floral and geometric prints were favourites for blouses and day dresses, while the most fashionable colours of the time were powder blue, maize, grey, navy, green, brown and red. Rose was popular among teenage girls, while black was generally reserved for eveningwear.

Accents were important, too: belts and sashes were wide, buttons were bold and silk flowers were substantial, yet always in proportion to the jacket or dress they were adorning.

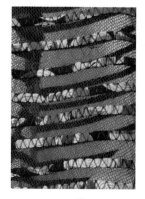

ABOVE AND LEFT Blouse with jabot collar and trumpet sleeves by Edward Molyneux, mid-1930s. The sleeves are worked with a rouleau detail of fabric, in which the material is rolled and applied to net, a typical 1930s technique.

PAGE 36 White organza 1938 bridesmaid's dress sprinkled with flowers by Jeanne Lanvin, worn with a wide-brimmed organza hat with streamers, in front of a backdrop of line drawings of moths.

OPPOSITE A 1932 illustration depicting 1930s day dresses by, from left to right, Goupy, Worth, Augustabernard and Schiaparelli.

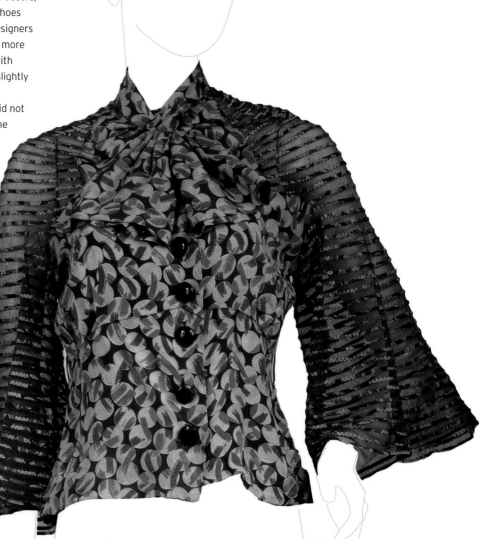

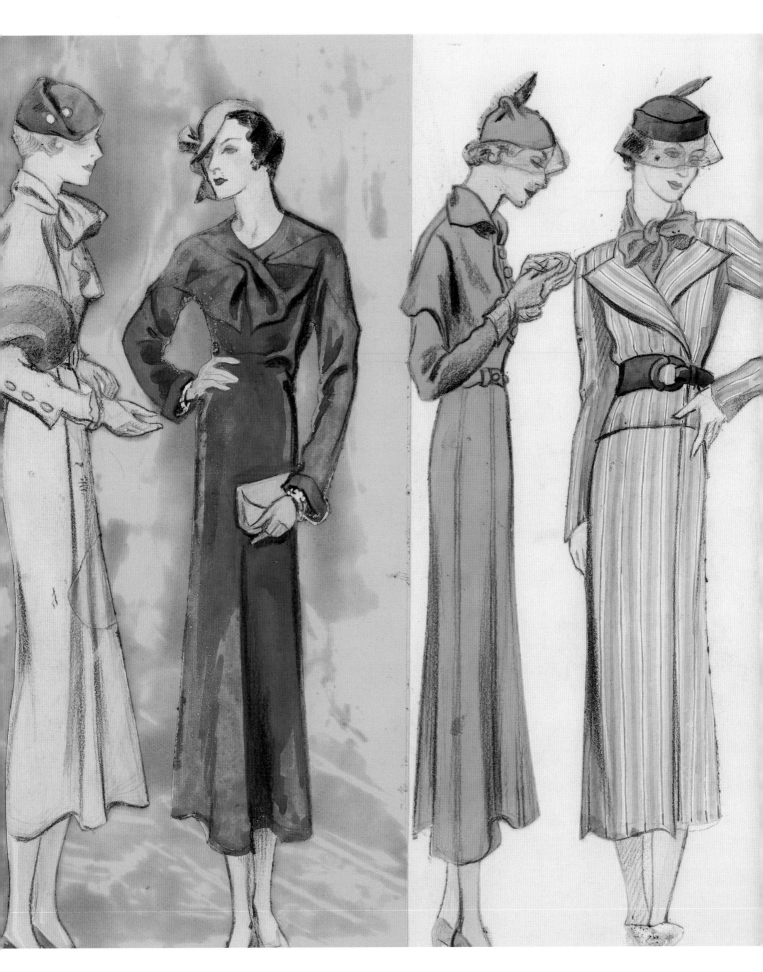

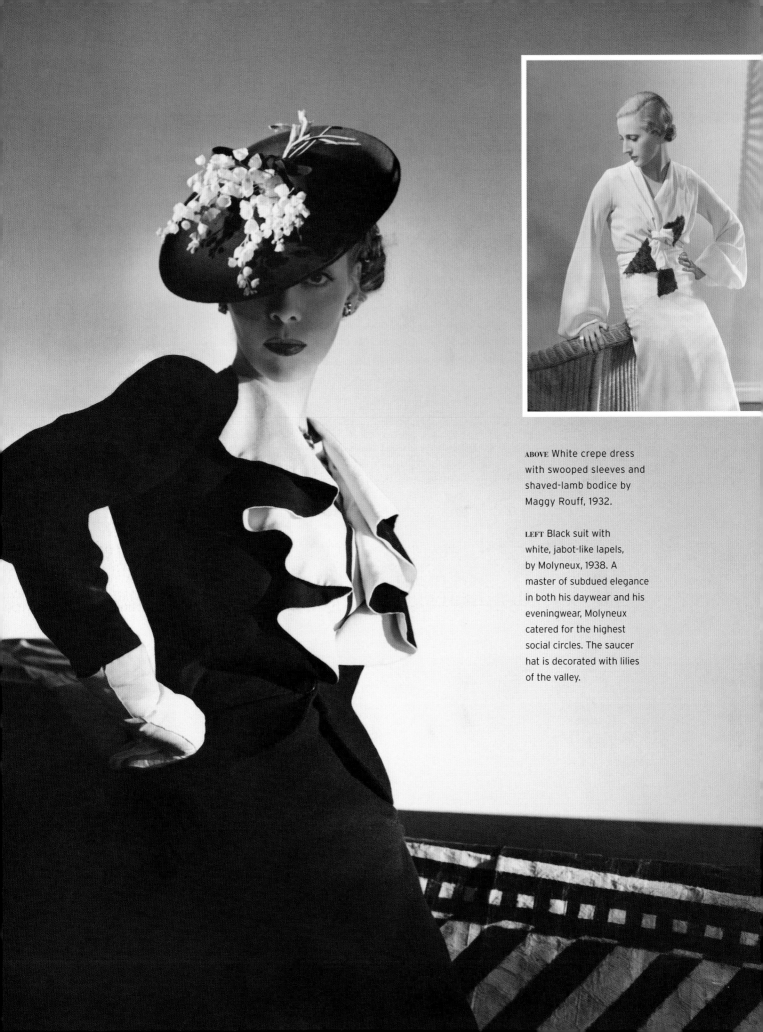

ABOVE White crepe dress with swooped sleeves and shaved-lamb bodice by Maggy Rouff, 1932.

LEFT Black suit with white, jabot-like lapels, by Molyneux, 1938. A master of subdued elegance in both his daywear and his eveningwear, Molyneux catered for the highest social circles. The saucer hat is decorated with lilies of the valley.

Day suits were revolutionized by Coco Chanel, who saw the affordable yet fashionable potential of wool jersey cloth. In America the Tirocchi sisters, who were loved for their afternoon dresses and eveningwear, also used wool jersey fabrics for suiting. The Tirocchis were the couturiers of choice for those who could afford the luxury of made-to-measure fashions. Creating one-off pieces for their customers, they – like Chanel – were fond of sports dressing. With the introduction of their wide-legged, pyjama-style trousers, they were trendsetters in the move towards softer and sportier tailoring, and reflected the more active lifestyle that women were embracing.

Health and fitness became an important aspect of daily life when, in 1930, Prunella Stack started the Women's League of Health and Beauty in Britain. Promoting the idea of a healthy mind and a healthy body, the League's motto was 'Movement Is Life'. Women began to enjoy a more outdoor life and sun-worshipping became a common leisure pursuit. Beach wraps, holdalls, soft hats and knitted bathing suits were all objects of desire for the summer season. Swimwear became briefer and more risqué as the backs were scooped out so that women could develop tanned backs to show off at night in backless gowns. In keeping with these new freedoms, corsets, although still available, were eschewed in favour of bras and girdles, while silk and rayon stockings began to replace woollen ones towards the end of the decade.

Living proof that fashion and an active life could go hand in hand, celebrated American aviator Amelia Earhart became as iconic a figure as any of the film stars of the time. Earhart always removed her goggles immediately upon landing and refused to don typical aviation gear. Instead, she wore elegantly tailored flying suits, silk neckscarves and wide-legged trousers, all of which spawned a multitude of high-fashion replicas.

As women became more interested in practical and accessible fashions, the brand name, ready-to-wear industry began to take off slowly. Off-the-peg clothing, available from department stores and mail-order catalogues such as Sears became popular ways for women to keep their wardrobes up to date. Parisian fashion was still the epitome of style for those who could afford it, but most women made their own clothes based on styles they saw in films and magazines.

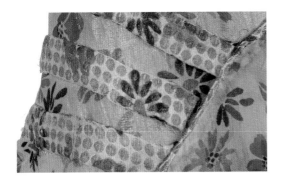

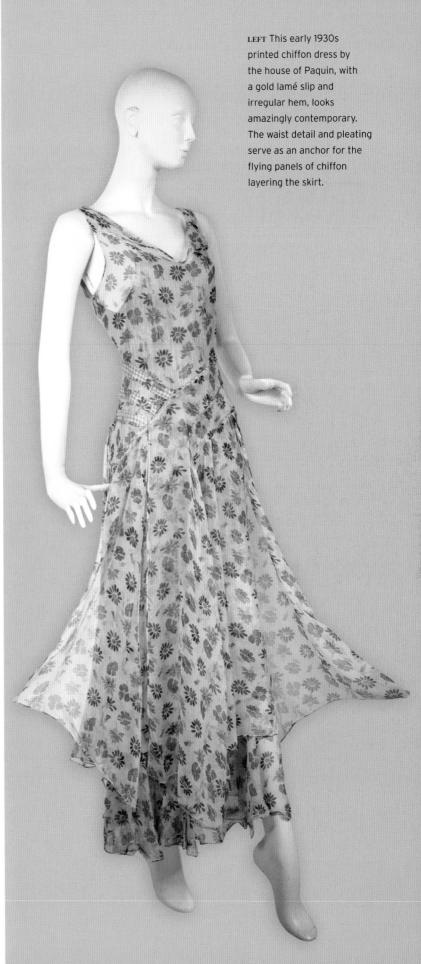

LEFT This early 1930s printed chiffon dress by the house of Paquin, with a gold lamé slip and irregular hem, looks amazingly contemporary. The waist detail and pleating serve as an anchor for the flying panels of chiffon layering the skirt.

Fabrics and Prints

Although the 1930s witnessed a great economic depression, it was still a period of industrial advances as machinery and techniques that were developed before, during and after the First World War, began to have an effect on everyday life.
Fashion benefited from many new inventions, such as zip fasteners and rayon – the first commercially used manmade fibre. In 1935 the DuPont de Nemours Company successfully synthesized nylon and this sparked a major trend for nylon stockings, which quickly replaced the woollen versions formerly worn. The arrival of these washable, easy-care fabrics was heavily marketed by manufacturers and was greeted with great excitement by fashion designers and housewives alike.

In the mood of financial restraint that characterized the decade, designers also began to experiment with fabrics previously not considered appropriate for mainstream dressmaking. In women's suiting Coco Chanel pioneered the use of cotton and wool jersey in women's suiting, a fabric that had previously been used predominantly for men's underwear. Her soft, fitted two-piece suits quickly became the toast of Parisian fashion and kickstarted the vogue for less formal attire. The emphasis now was on looking chic in a way that was not impractical for everyday life, and this was reflected not just in the materials used but also in the cut and patterns of the clothes themselves. But while these new fabrics took hold, soft crepe, chiffon and satin were still frequently used, and pure silk continued to be the most desirable fabric as it lent itself perfectly to the folds and drapes of 1930s couture.

Because of the numerous improvements in mass production techniques during the 1930s, a wider range of women had gained access to well-made and well-cut clothes. However, the advent of war in 1939 brought that temporarily to an end, preventing civilian access to clothing manufacturers for several years while much of the world focused on the war effort.

Fastenings
Originally known as the 'slide fastener', the zip had been invented as far back as 1893 but initially its potential was limited to being purely a shoe fastener. When it was finally adopted by the clothing industry in the 1930s, it became an instant hit in all areas of fashion design. A sales campaign was mounted for children's clothing, praising the zip for promoting self-reliance in youngsters because it made it possible for them to dress themselves. In 1937 the zip beat the button in the 'Battle of the Fly', when tailors raved over its usefulness in men's trousers.

The popularity of the fastener continued to grow during the 1930s and was quickly embraced by womenswear designers. Many designers including Elsa Schiaparelli even made a feature of it as an aesthetic detail, sometimes running it through the back of a dress or simply leaving it unconcealed. The predominance of zippers in manufactured clothing increased toward the end of the decade, primarily as side-closing fasteners.

Buttons too became part of surface decoration, with designers considering the fastening as part and parcel of the design. Schiaparelli created insect, flower and lip buttons, and others in Dalí-esque and whimsical shapes. By this point Bakelite plastic was cheap, fashionable and could be easily moulded; it was particularly well suited to Art Deco shapes. Black and brown Bakelite were the most common colours but lighter colours were developed during the 1930s. Lucite, a clear hard resin invented in 1931, was also used to make buttons during this period.

The new emphasis was on looking chic in a way that wasn't impractical for every day life and this was reflected not just in the fastenings and materials used, but also the cut and patterns of the clothes themselves.

Cutting techniques and dress patterns
The tricks of draping and intricate seaming first learnt in the 1920s were now applied to making dresses that clung to the body, creating the streamlined chic that characterized the decade. In addition, a new way of cutting fabric was invented by Parisian designer Madeleine Vionnet. Her bias-cut technique meant that, for the first time, women wore clothes that clung flirtatiously to their figure and showed off their body in a more naturalistic way than ever before. At the same time, necklines were lowered while torsos were sensuously moulded beneath squared shoulders. For evening the bared back became the new erotic zone, replacing the legs of the 1920s.

OPPOSITE A selection of print textiles exhibiting the fascination with Art Deco – the two left top and bottom are earlier than the two right top and bottom. The lower right is a souvenir shirt from the maiden voyage of the Queen Mary, 1936.

FEATURES OF 1930S PRINTS:
- Designs printed on silk, rayon and crinkle crepe
- Bold lines and patterns of the prevailing Art Deco style
- Graphic designs and lettering, polka-dots and hand-drawn circles, bold florals
- Contrasting colours and bright shades to emphasize print
- Picture prints, such as cars, animals or popular objects
- Influences from Cubism and artists such as Picasso and Man Ray

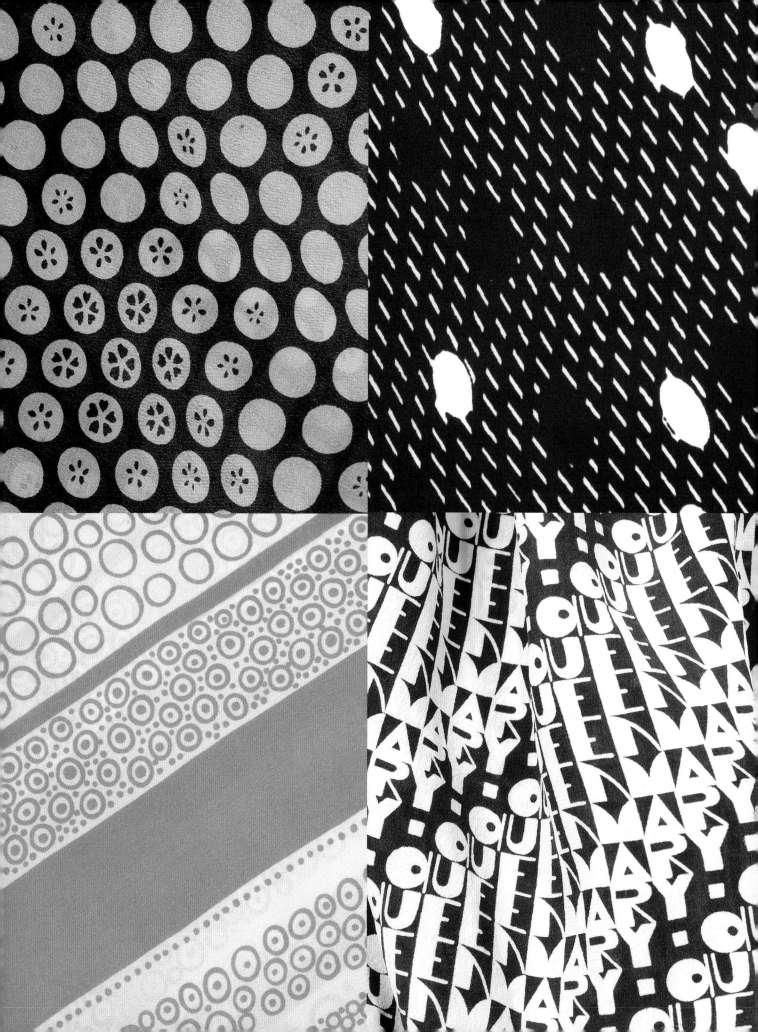

At the beginning of the decade, hemlines dropped dramatically to the ankle and they remained there until the end of the 1930s. Skirts were designed with great detail. Upper-skirt yokes appeared for the first time, designed in a V-shape and extending from one hip to the centre of the yoke then continuing to the opposite hip. Layered and ruffled looks appeared on skirts, sometimes in tiers. The skirt bottom was often full, with pleats or gathers. Soft gathers replaced darts, dress waists returned to the natural waistline and moderately full skirts accentuated a small waist and minimized the hips. Dress bodices were designed with inset pieces and yokes that provided extra interest. Necklines received dramatic attention by designers, often with wide scallop-edged or ruffled collars. Arms also took on a new importance as designers experimented with new shapes such as voluminous puffed or flared sleeves.

Prints and surface decoration

As a continuation of the Art Deco styles popular in the 1920s, embroidery and appliqué continued to be favoured as a decorative touch on cardigans, blouses and dresses. These designs were often highly detailed, featuring small-scale floral motifs and more animated subjects such as show-horses, kittens and cars. Metallic lamé became a fashionable yarn for eveningwear and was used as often as a detail in embroidery as it was throughout an entire piece of cloth. Textile design in general became more interesting as polka-dots, geometric patterns and colourful prints became de rigueur.

There was a great cross-fertilization of visual ideas from such artists as Salvador Dalí, Jean Cocteau, Alberto Giacometti and Marcel Vertes, whose work influenced not just print and textile designs, but embroidery and jewellery.

Furs and trimmings

During this era fur of all kinds was worn extensively in winter – both by day and at night. Fur capes, coats, stoles, wraps, accessories and trimmings completed women's outfits. Pelts in demand were sable, mink, chinchilla, Persian lamb and silver fox.

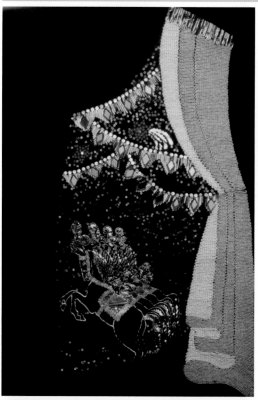

RIGHT Embroidery sample by Lesage, created for Elsa Schiaparelli's Circus collection – the perfect marriage of a master embroiderer and a visionary couturier.

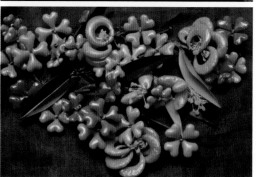

RIGHT 1936 Schiaparelli garment with a mad profusion of beaded decoration by the design house Lesage.

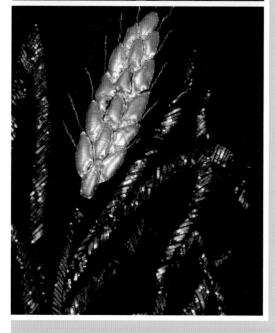

RIGHT Embroidery detail from a 1930s evening jacket. The unusual corn motif in raised gold leather is typical of the decorative avant-garde style of Elsa Schiaparelli.

OPPOSITE Rayon dresses designed by Lucien Lelong, from a fashion plate from *Femina* magazine, 1935. Rayon was the decade's most prominent fabric achievement, providing the feel of silk in an easy-care material.

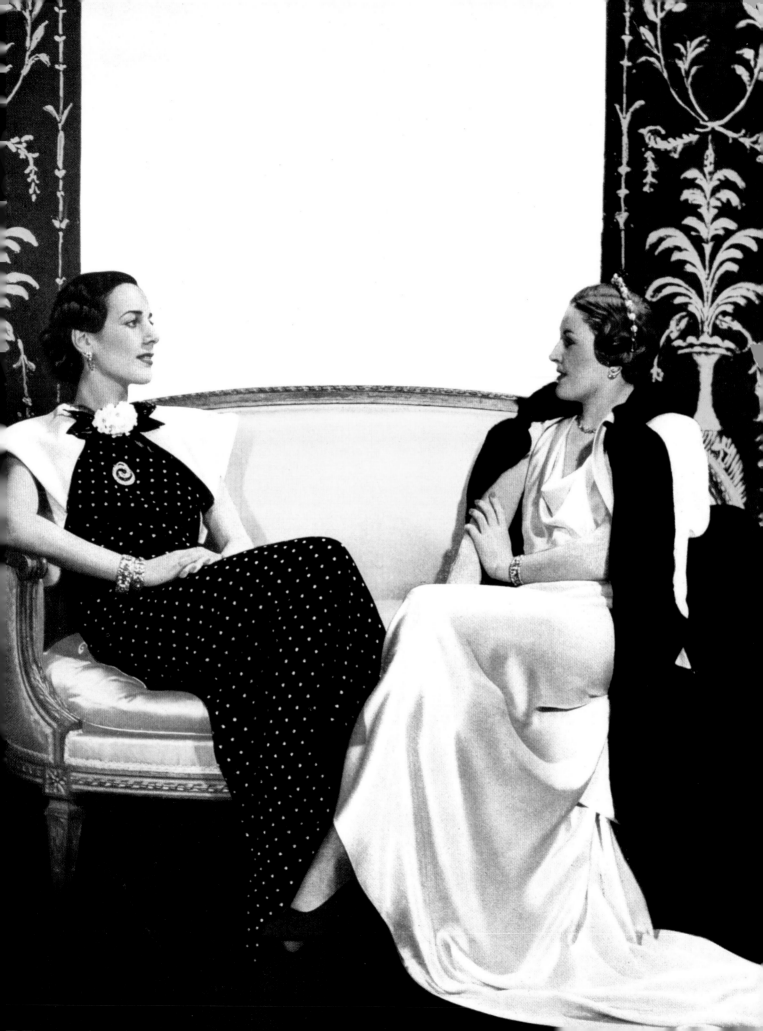

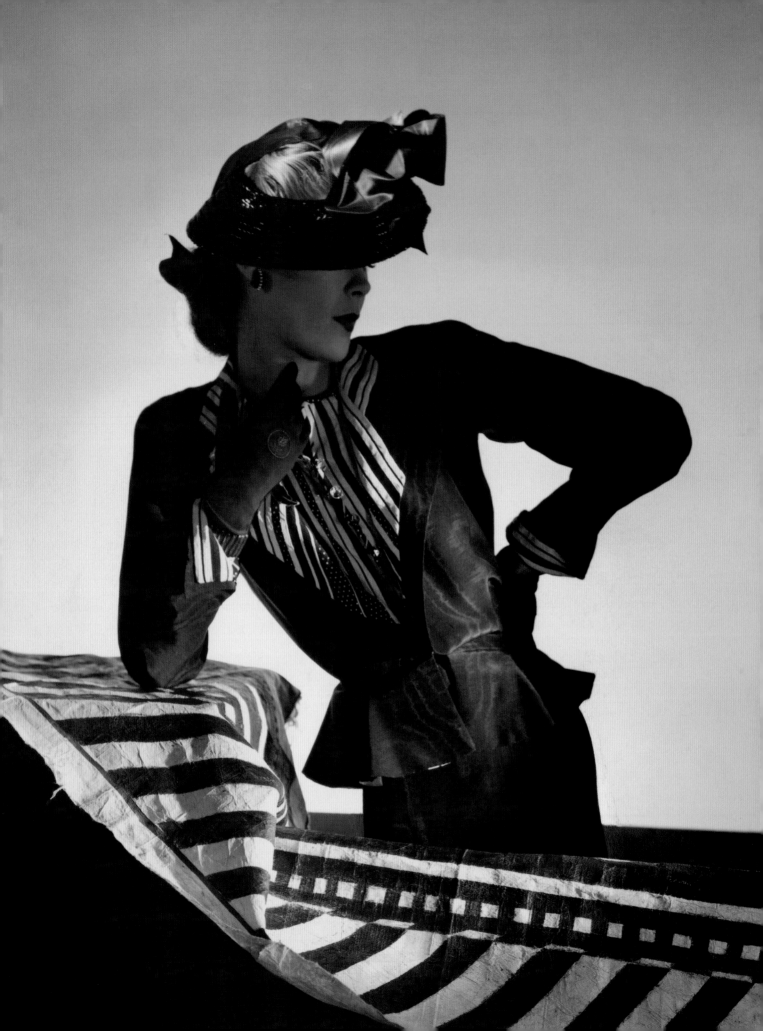

Elsa Schiaparelli and Coco Chanel

Arguably the two most important designers of the 1930s, Elsa Schiaparelli (1896–1973) and Coco Chanel (1883–1971) could not have been more different. Schiaparelli created high-octane, almost shocking clothes in bright colours and with groundbreaking textile designs and an exaggerated silhouette. Chanel designed easy-to-wear clothes in a palette of black, white and beige. With such opposing aesthetic values, it is hard to imagine that these couturiers could have thrived alongside each other in Paris during the same decade. And yet, while Chanel remains one of the most successful luxury goods brands of all times whereas Schiaparelli is much less well known, during the 1930s the two were the greatest of rivals.

Barely 1.5 m (5 ft) tall, Schiaparelli had always been told that she was ugly. Her garments were high-waisted, broad-shouldered and designed to elongate the figure – an aesthetic evidently formed to suit her own sartorial tastes and requirements. Chanel on the other hand owed a certain amount of her success to her good looks. The embodiment of her brand with her slim, boyish figure, cropped hair and tanned skin, she became an ideal to a generation of women.

Ten years older than Schiaparelli, Chanel rose to professional distinction against far greater odds. Her mother died when she was six years old and the rest of her childhood was spent in an orphanage. During a brief career as a concert-hall singer, Gabrielle – as she was originally called – adopted the name Coco. It was during this time that she became a mistress to a wealthy English industrialist whose connections and financial backing enabled her to open her own millinery shop in 1910.

Born in Rome, Schiaparelli came from a family of monied intellectuals. Her father was a scholar in Islamic and Arabic studies and her uncle a renowned astronomer – the influences from her upbringing were regularly apparent in her work, not least in her winter 1938–9 Lucky Stars collection.

The different backgrounds of these two designers were reflected constantly in their philosophy towards their work. Chanel regarded couture as a profession while Schiaparelli always insisted that it was an art. A close friend of Picasso and the Surrealist artists Dalí and Man Ray, Elsa was a firm fixture on the early twentieth-century international arts scene and a book of her poetry was published in 1911. She even managed to bridge the gap between fashion and literature by inventing poetic names for the specific colours she used in her collections – shocking pink was introduced in 1937 while other colour names, which have became part of our everyday language, include royal blue, wheat yellow and ice blue.

OPPOSITE Black moire suit with a crepe black-and-white stripe blouse, by Chanel, and a black straw hat with a ribbon chou, 1938.

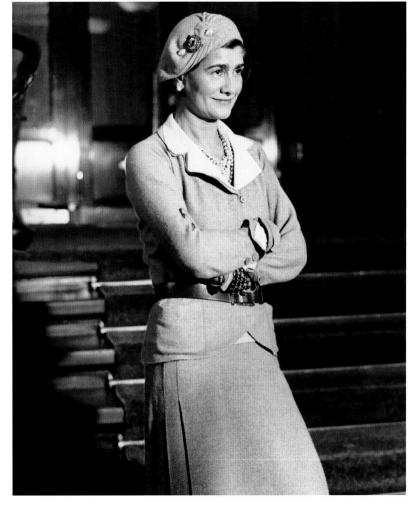

RIGHT Gabrielle 'Coco' Chanel in suit and beret, 1930s. Her unique style of menswear-influenced sporty clothing was meant for modern, active women like her.

Coco Chanel's legacy could not be more evident today as Karl Lagerfeld, creative director at Chanel since her death, continues to plunder the fashion house's archives, working strictly with her vision in mind. Aside from her iconic Chanel No 5 perfume, the wool jersey suit is perhaps one of her most famous innovations. Comfort was key to her designs and she is credited with revolutionizing fashion – liberating women from their restrictive corsets and introducing them to a freer, more casual elegance. In stark contrast to the clothing seen in her youth, Chanel said that she wanted to give women 'the possibility to laugh and eat without necessarily having to faint'. For Schiaparelli, however, comfort and practicality were secondary to fashion. She famously said, 'Never fit a dress to the body but train the body to fit the dress.'

While Schiaparelli and most other international fashion houses continued to create ankle-length sheath dresses, Chanel seemed uninterested in the more formal etiquette of fashion; her designs were largely limited to daytime or sportswear dresses and suits that inevitably reached mid-calf in length. Rather than creating the long, bias-cut evening gowns popularized by Hollywood movie stars, she preferred designing more versatile two-piece cocktail suits, which allowed the wearer to go elegantly from early evening to late night soirée without having to change outfits.

For Schiaparelli, it was the *trompe l'oeuil* 'bow' knitted sweaters that effectively launched her career. Her later innovations included the use of zips as decorative elements, a backless evening gown with a pleated, bustle-like compartment for stashing a flask, and a fabric print composed of newspaper clippings. Her customers needed plenty of confidence as her clothes were definitely designed to stand out.

Perhaps one of the best examples of her use of colour and textiles is a floor-length, harlequin-patterned wool felt coat from her 1939 Commedia dell'Arte collection. Composed of graduated lozenges of primary colours plus black and white,

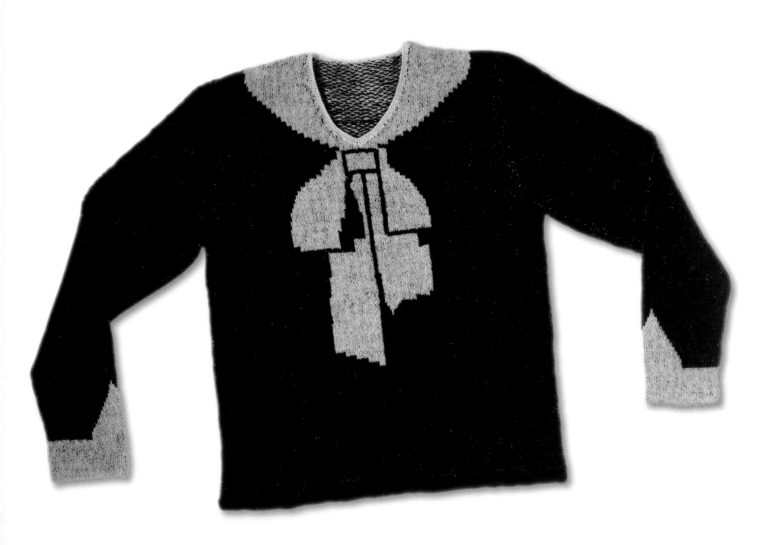

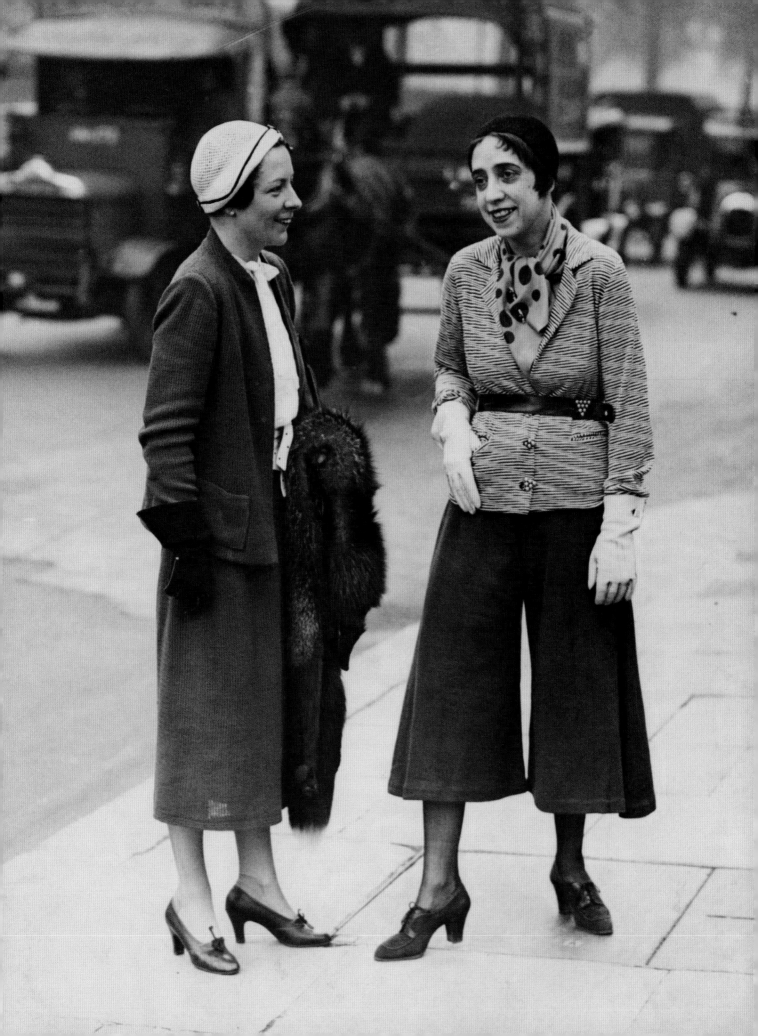

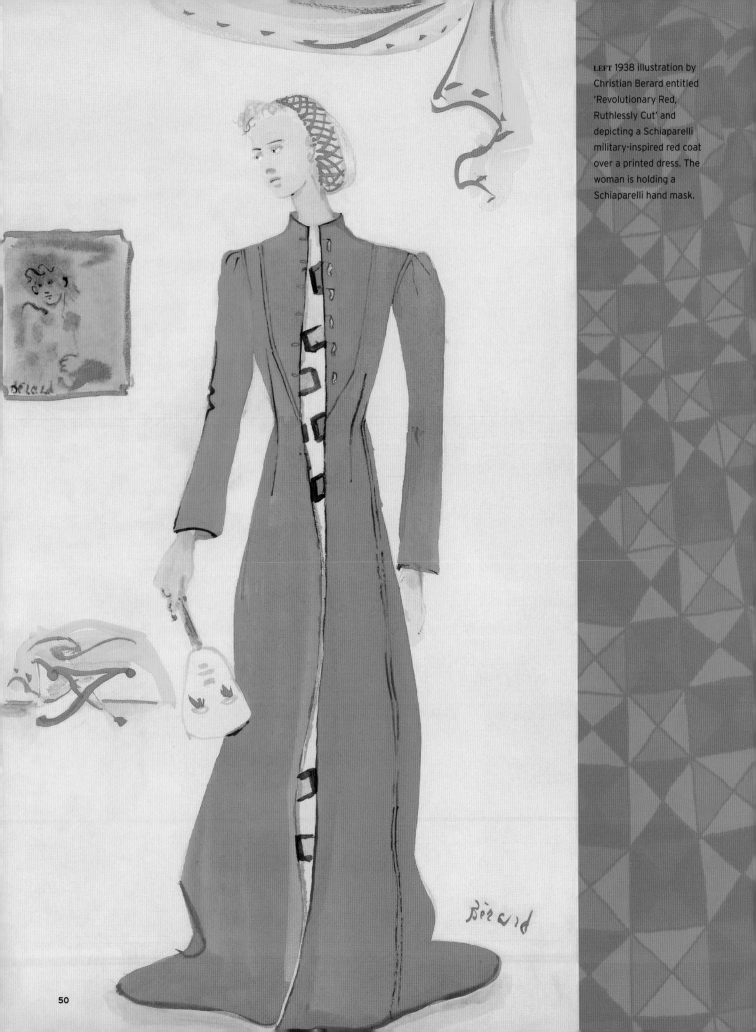

LEFT 1938 illustration by Christian Berard entitled 'Revolutionary Red, Ruthlessly Cut' and depicting a Schiaparelli military-inspired red coat over a printed dress. The woman is holding a Schiaparelli hand mask.

the faceted patchwork is strongly reminiscent of Man Ray's Cubist painting *Le Beaux Temps*, of the same year. The garish use of colour and geometric design could not have been further from Chanel's 'sophisticated' tastes.

By the early 1930s Chanel's reputation had grown enormously and in 1931 she was paid a million dollars by MGM boss Samuel Goldwyn to dress the female stars of many of his motion pictures, including Katharine Hepburn, Grace Kelly and Elizabeth Taylor. Schiaparelli created clothing for many stage productions and films, among them costumes for Mae West in *Every Day's a Holiday* (1937) and Zsa Zsa Gabor in *Moulin Rouge* (1952). Among her regular clients were the Duchess of Windsor, Marlene Dietrich and Katharine Hepburn.

The Second World War marked the end of Elsa Schiaparelli's business. She retired from fashion, dying in 1973. Coco continued to run her business until her death in 1971, in her residential suite at the Ritz in Paris.

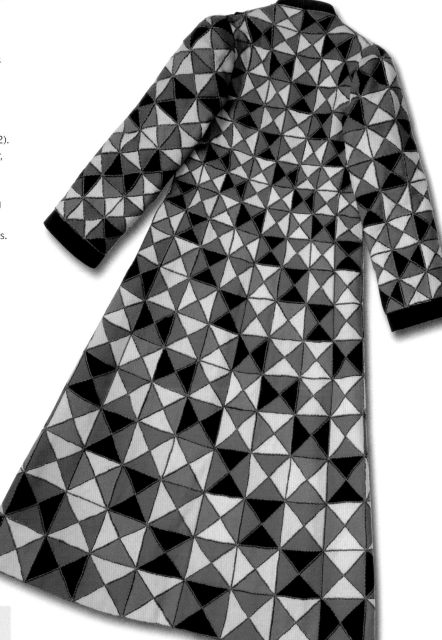

ABOVE Floor-length, harlequin wool felt coat from Schiaparelli's 1939 Commedia dell'Arte collection. The striking faceted patchwork is strongly reminiscent of the Cubist painting *Le Beaux Temps*, by Man Ray.

SIGNATURE SCHIAPARELLI ELEMENTS:

- ❖ High waistlines
- ❖ Shoulder pads and broad shoulders
- ❖ Exaggerated silhouettes, including small bustles
- ❖ Bright colours, such as shocking pink and royal blue
- ❖ *Trompe l'oeil* knits
- ❖ Zippers as decorative elements
- ❖ Long-line bias-cut dresses
- ❖ Backless evening gowns
- ❖ Geometric and Picasso-inspired patterns

Evening Glamour

While Paris couturiers of the 1930s were the driving force behind changing trends, the era is perhaps best exemplified by the Hollywood film stars who brought their clothes to life. Actresses such as Marlene Dietrich, Joan Crawford and Barbara Stanwyck epitomized the look with their penchant for elongated bias-cut, halter-neck gowns in shimmering silk fabrics. During this time of economic crisis, when even some of couture's wealthiest customers were forced to rein in their shopping habits, Hollywood became the ultimate showcase for a designer's work.

Depression-weary audiences flocked in record numbers to the cinema, hungry for some much-needed glamour and escapism. And although some of the films of the time took on a tone of gritty realism, the leading ladies remained relentlessly stylish and groomed to perfection. Inside these movie theatres existed a world of opulence that most of the audience could only dream of – and the costumes worn had almost as much pulling power as the stars themselves.

Fashion and film joined hands as the same designers who dressed the stars for their red carpet appearances were also called upon to create costumes for the films they starred in. At Paramount Studios costume designer Travis Banton brought understated glamour and elegance to actresses such as Mae West and Carole Lombard with his beautifully cut suits and bias-cut dresses. Meanwhile, Gilbert Adrian, head of costume at MGM, is widely credited with creating the signature looks of the studio's major stars including Greta Garbo and Jean Harlow. The broad-shouldered suits in which he dressed Joan Crawford became hugely fashionable and the puff-sleeved dress that she wore in the 1933 film *Letty Lyndon* sent female members of the audience rushing to their sewing machines to create their own versions of the look.

This was a time before the term 'fashion stylist' had even been invented and Adrian's role in introducing stars to designers was of fundamental importance. Although Madeleine Vionnet is said to have invented the bias cut and Elsa Schiaparelli – who designed clothes for more than 30 films – was credited with inventing padded shoulders, it was Adrian who had the awareness to bring these high-fashion looks to the silver screen. In so doing, he created the style that dominated American fashion during the 1930s. Referring to the suits she wore in some of her films, Joan Crawford praised his emphasis on simplicity and his ability to make a dramatic point through clever costume choices.

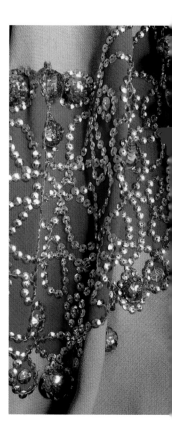

ABOVE AND LEFT Green 1939 crepe de chine dress by Jeanne Lanvin, with tie neckline and heavily embroidered balloon sleeves. The dress features typical Lanvin elements – a long slim silhouette and intricate embellishment in the form of both embroidery and appliqué.

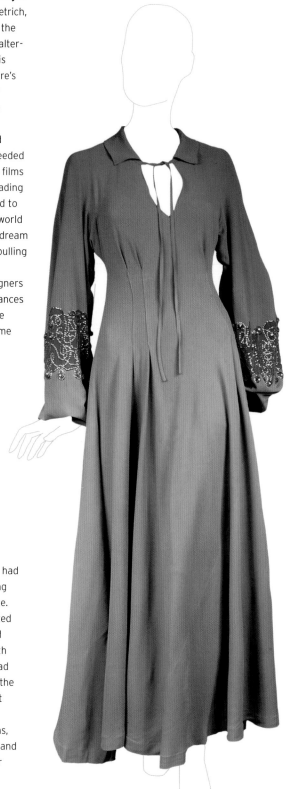

OPPOSITE Crepe dresses by Lucien Lelong, 1935.

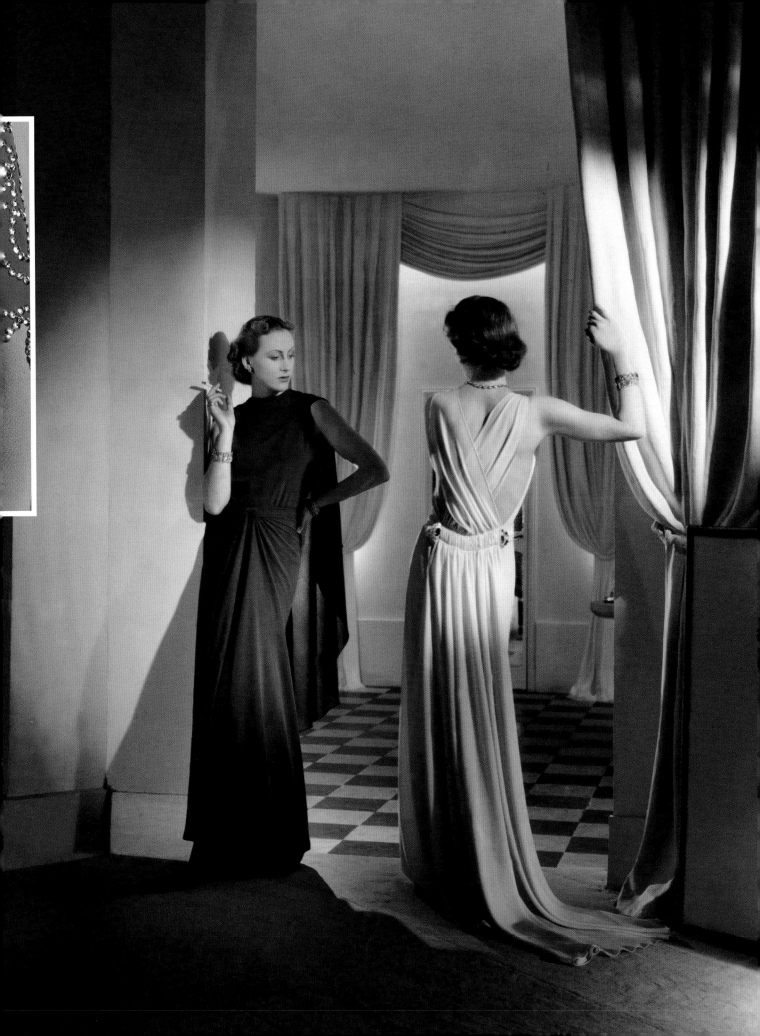

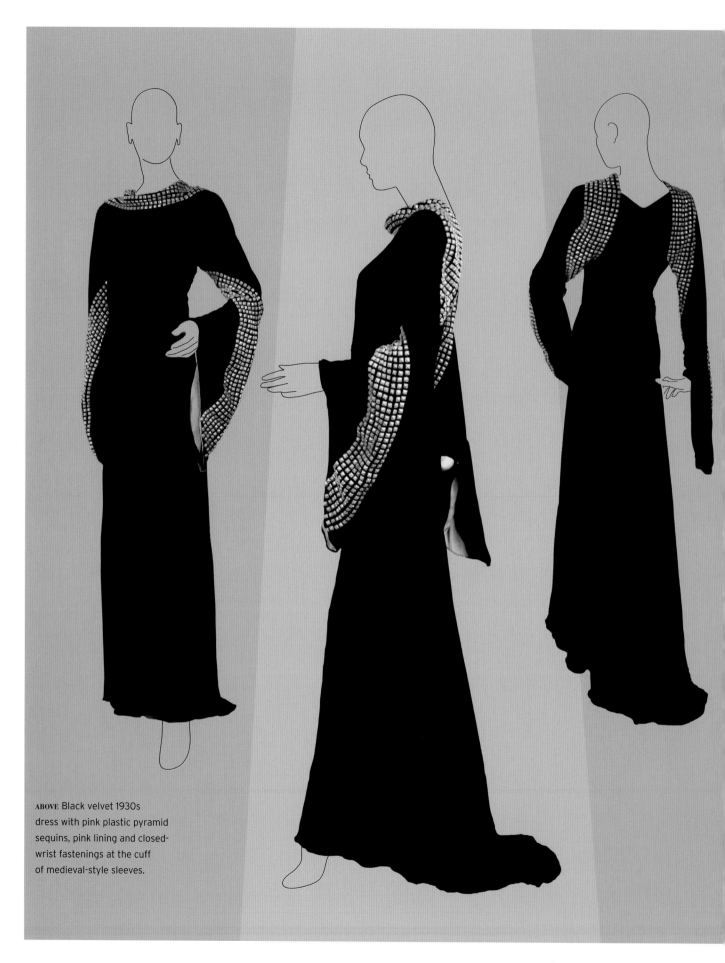

ABOVE Black velvet 1930s
dress with pink plastic pyramid
sequins, pink lining and closed-
wrist fastenings at the cuff
of medieval-style sleeves.

Adrian's understanding of light and shadow ensured that the clothes looked as good on black-and-white film as they did in the flesh. A master of form and structure, he had an impeccable eye for perfectly cut clothes and held Parisian couture in the greatest esteem. It was Gilbert who, in 1931, persuaded MGM boss Samuel Goldwyn to pay Coco Chanel a staggering million dollars to provide clothes for the studio's major stars.

But although Gilbert was an undeniably powerful figure in both film and fashion, he nevertheless had rigid guidelines to adhere to when dressing his stars. Bound by what was known as the Hayes Code, costume designers were strictly censored on what they could allow an actress to show. Following the titillating and scandalous films of the 1920s, the 1930s saw a return to modesty and prudishness and too much cleavage on display was considered obscene. In order to get around these rules, actresses removed their bras and wore slinky, draped dresses which clung to the body without revealing too much bare flesh. While the conservatives could not complain, the female form was now visible in a more provocative way than ever. And while the cleavage was kept under wraps, designers created dresses to unveil alternative androgynous zones. The halterneck evening gown made its fashion debut and – as long as the belly button was covered up – bare midriff top and skirt combinations enjoyed a brief spell of popularity.

While intricate beading, appliqué and encrusted jewels were often used as features on the sleeve or waistline or as a detail around the back or neckline, for the most part the evening gowns of the 1930s were exquisite by virtue of their simplicity. Gowns were perfectly cut to create the illusion of a long and slender silhouette, often with elongated flared sleeves and exaggerated trains at the back. Fur of all kinds was seen as highly desirable and was worn everywhere by all who could afford it. Wraps and capes were frequently teamed with full-length silk satin evening gloves.

In contrast to the riotous 1920s, the new aesthetic was sophisticated and elegant and it was not just film stars who put high fashion in the spotlight. Royalty were equally revered and images of the Duke and Duchess of Windsor, Princess Marina and the Duchess of York (later Queen Elizabeth, consort of George VI) also filled newsreels and newspapers. The clothes they chose to wear were as much of a talking point as in more recent

RIGHT Black wool coat with ermine fur collar by French label Jenny, 1938.

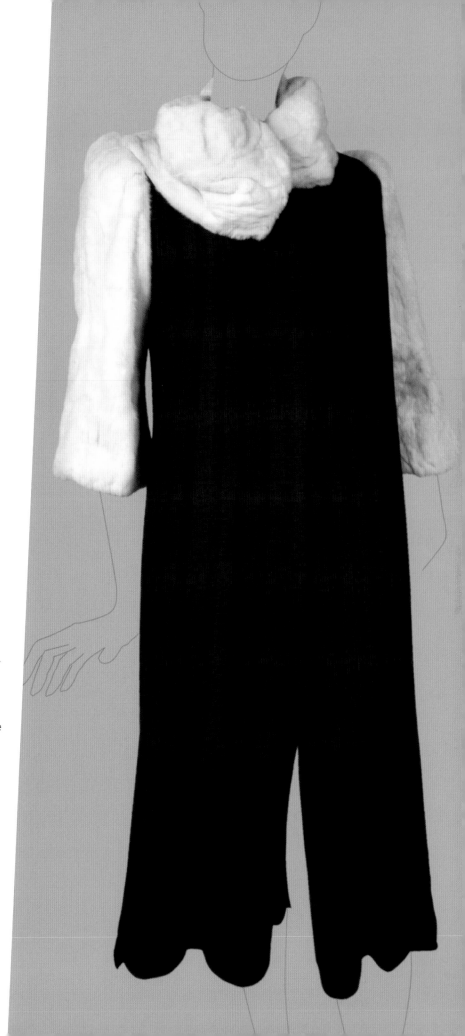

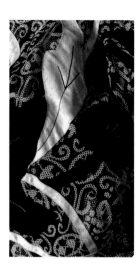

ABOVE AND RIGHT Net appliqué late 1930s dress with lime underslip and short balloon sleeves, by Jeanne Lanvin.

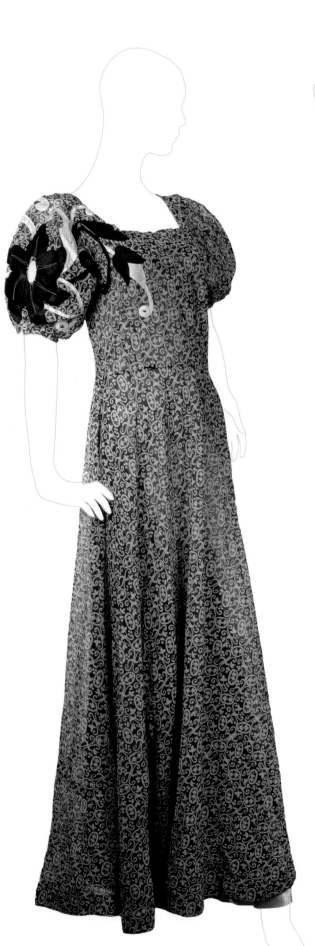

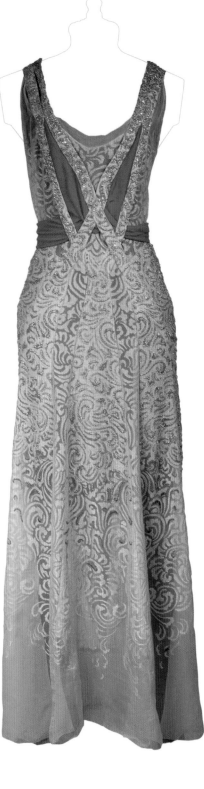

LEFT AND BELOW Front
and back views of a
1930s Paquin chiffon
evening gown with an
embroidered pattern of
silver beading sequins.
The scarlet crepe inserts
are a striking colour accent
and have been cleverly
combined with the straps
to create tie-backs that
define the waist.

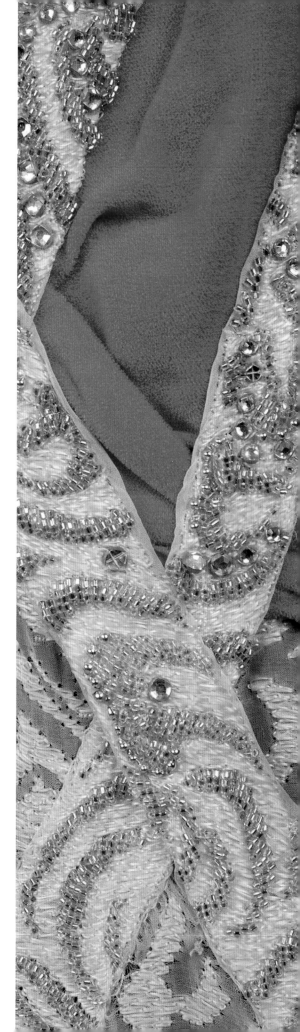

years with modern royals such as Diana, Princess of Wales. *Life* magazine featured a story on the Mainbocher blue wedding dress worn by the divorced Mrs Wallis Simpson, who married the Duke of Windsor in 1937, and the garment won enormous international admiration. Smaller clothing companies such as Bonwit Teller of Fifth Avenue, New York, which sold a copy for a tenth of the price, immediately produced it in short-sleeve versions. Within six months the 'Wally' dress was available for even less at the Lord & Taylor department store, and finally a mere $8.90 could buy one at Klein's Cash & Carry in New York.

By the 1930s countless fashion houses had come to prominence and their designs were widely emulated. British-born designer Edward Molyneux, the epitome of cool elegance, became known as 'the man to whom a woman would turn if she wanted to look absolutely right without being utterly predictable'. His clothes can usually be recognized by their understated elegance and he generally designed evening dresses in a discreet colour palette of black, navy, grey and beige.

Augusta Bernard, who styled her name as one word for her label, Augustabernard, was another fashion designer to enjoy notable success during the decade. She made slim bias-cut evening dresses in pale moonlit colours. Although based in Paris, Bernard had a large American clientele who found that her simple dresses were an exquisite backdrop for their expensive jewellery.

These designers belonged to an eminent band of Parisian couturiers that also included Louise Boulanger, Cristobal Balenciaga, Robert Piguet and Madeleine Vionnet, all of whom managed to a greater or lesser extent to survive during the difficult years between the First and Second World Wars. As well as serving the social elite of their day, many of these designers became icons in their own right and – no matter what their background – found themselves mingling with stars, aristocracy and royalty.

Perhaps more than any other era in fashion, the eveningwear styles from the 1930s continue to directly influence eveningwear designs popular today. The elongated gowns, halter-neck dresses and the draped cowl neckline so frequently seen on the red carpet today owe a great debt to the 1930s. Designers such as John Galliano, Valentino and Julien Macdonald continue to reference this decade – when Hollywood glamour was born.

▼Bias-cut gowns

Fabric was cut on the diagonal, allowing dresses to cling naturally to the body. Introduced by Madeleine Vionnet, this was one of the most significant elements of 1930s fashion. Below a black velvet dress trimmed in ermine and a white crepe and panne velvet dress, both by Vionnet, circa 1930.

▶Skirts with wedge-cut pleats

Fitted at the hip with yokes, skirts often featured wedge-cut pleats giving a fullness to the hemline, which ended at mid-calf. The fashion pictured here also exhibits other classic 1930s styles: hat and gloves, neckline bow and fur stole.

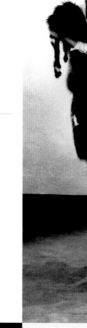

Rayon

The first commercially used man-made fabric was available in several different finishes and was quickly exploited by designers keen to experiment with new textiles.

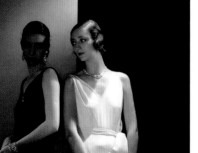

Key looks of the decade

1930s

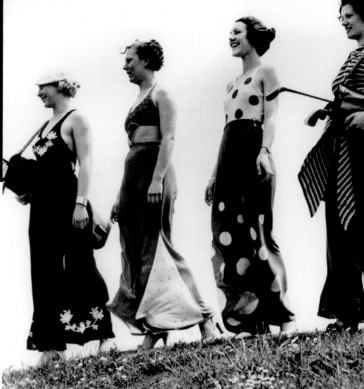

Jabot blouse

Decorative frills cascaded from the collar down the front of the blouse or dress, becoming a popular style, particularly for daywear.

▶Sportswear influences

Tailoring took on a sportier feel Coco Chanel pioneered the use of soft wool jersey fabrics for women's suiting. More women engaged in outdoor activities and such athletics as golfing. Here four women play golf wearing beach pyjamas in 1935.

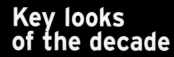

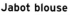

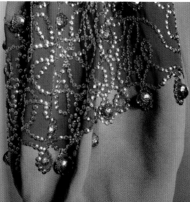

▼Bias-cut gowns

◀Flared sleeves

Narrow-fitting at the shoulder, blouses featured sleeves which widened towards the wrist. These were often exaggerated and elongated on evening gowns.

Costume jewellery

Often made in enamel and glass, costume jewellery such as brooches, bracelets and beaded necklaces were a fashionable and affordable new look.

Narrow suits worn with a hat and gloves

Slim-fitting tailored suits were a practical look for daywear and were teamed with gloves and hats of various styles.

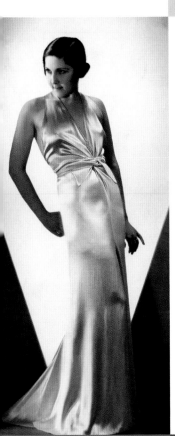

Zips

Slide fasteners were a welcomed new invention, which quickly replaced buttons in many areas of fashion. Some designers, such as Schiaparelli, even made features of this metal fastening.

◀Halterneck backless evening gowns

Backs became the new erogenous zone as designers draped fabric around the neck, leaving shoulders and backs on show, as seen here in a 1935 satin version.

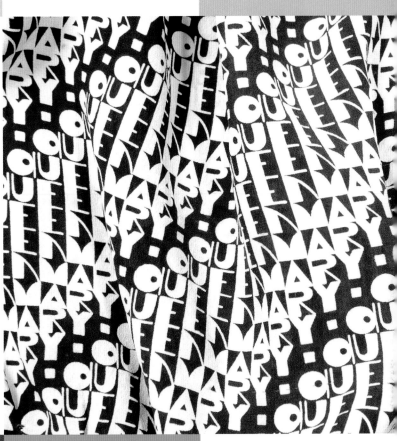

▲Art Deco patterns

Characterized by symmetrical geometric patterns, Art Deco prints were a left-over trend from the 1920s and were regularly seen on dresses, blouses and scarves.

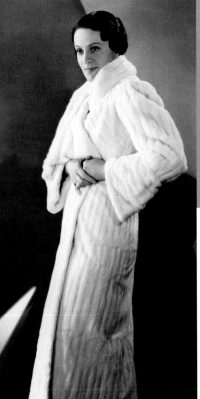

◀Fur

Worn day and night, fur creations of all types were popular luxury items. Capes, coats, stoles and wraps were made using pelts of ermine, fox, mink and chinchilla. This ermine version from 1935 has a draped collar.

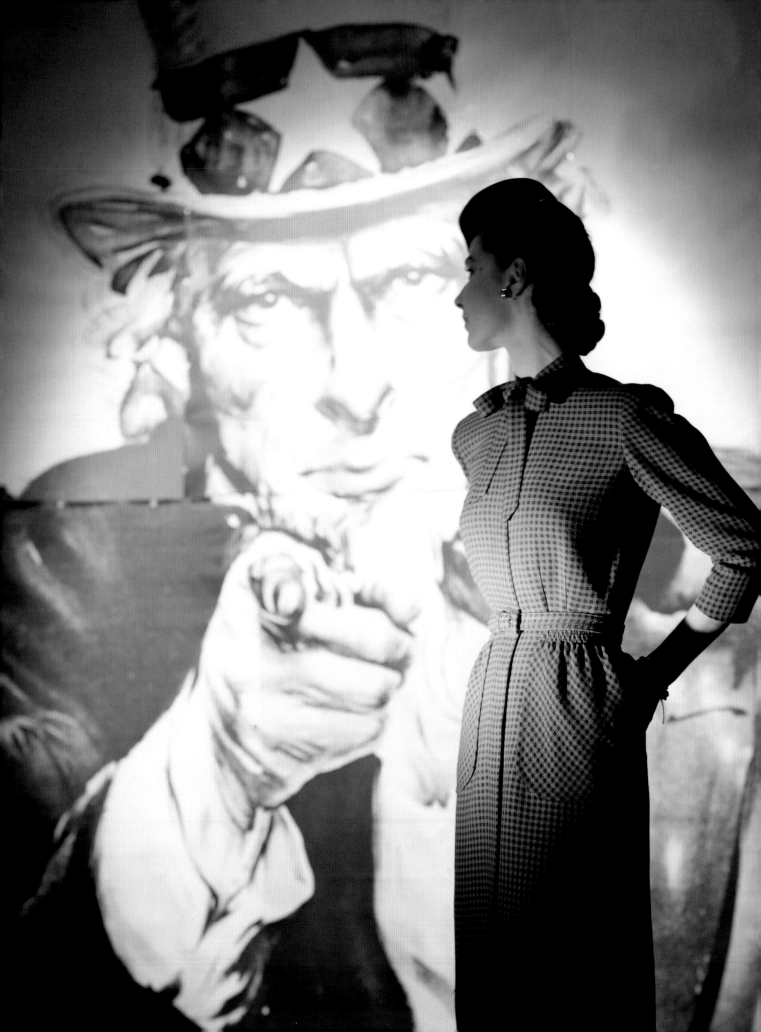

1940s

Social trends dictate fashion. Nowhere is this more evident than in the 1940s. With the outbreak of war, things changed very quickly. There were shortages of everything and civilian life was taken over and transformed. The conscription of women in Europe and America changed the female role and brought the woman out of the home to be directed in war work. Materials like silk and wool were needed for the war effort, factories were used for parachutes and other war supplies, so many of the 1940s vintage clothes are made out of rayon, synthetic jersey and other manmade fabrics. In 1941 clothing rationing came in and the government Utility scheme forbade the use of trimmings and certain materials as fashion was subject to government decree. The nonfashion fashion of the war years resulted in a conservative and military style, yet the tailoring was magnificent – outfits had to last several seasons. British couture was still being made, but only for export to procure much-needed dollars for armaments. France lost its position at the apex of fashion in 1940 under German occupation and did not regain its undisputed leadership until the liberation in 1944 when its couture collection was splendid. Meanwhile, America looked to its own designers to create fashions; the functional and easy American ready-to-wear was born with brightly coloured playsuits in materials like gingham, cotton and denim. After the war, the direction of fashion was slow to change, especially where rationing was still in place. The American softened silhouette presaged the dramatic New Look unveiled in 1947 by Christian Dior and the mood changed irrevocably.

The Wartime Silhouette

Il faut 'skimp' pour etre chic', – you must skimp to be chic – declared _Vogue_ in October 1941, referring to the tight, short-skirted silhouette that was ushered in that year and welcomed with horror by the public. Suddenly the flirty fullness of the 1930s curvy female gave way to an angular, hard silhouette that, as _Vogue_ declared in the same year, 'would be brutally unbecoming unless women kept their figures'. Driven by the wartime economy, the sculptural silhouette was the result of government rationing. The stiff tailoring, economy of cut, nipped-in waist and narrow skirts produced a slim shape that de-emphasized the female curves and made the form appear slender yet mannish. Elaboration was out and pared-down elegance was the order of the day. The silhouette therefore, inadvertently gave the illusion of brisk competence. And with its 'sensible' image, 'beauty' was not part of the wartime aesthetic. _Vogue_ said in 1942 that it looked, 'Sharp, cold and even bold'.

The ladies' suit

The drab uniformity of the war years was mirrored in the severe military-cut suit, which formed the bedrock of wartime fashion. Women wore clothes that were cut along the lines of the uniforms worn by men. Monochrome colours such as air-force blue and flag red were used, as these reduced wastage. Military influences were everywhere, from half-belts like those on uniform great coats to the padded-shoulder severity of wartime jackets. _Vogue_ called it 'couture austerity'. Driven by necessity rather than by desire, restrictions on materials resulted in a silhouette that became refined and unadorned. Indeed, it was unpatriotic to be concerned with flounces and fripperies.

The suit was cut in a straight mannish style – often refashioned from the existing male suit – with sharp-edged shoulder pads to give women a brisk no-nonsense air, in keeping with their role as key wartime workers. Boxy, with wide shoulders and barely nipped in waists, the jackets were short, at 63.5 cm (25 in) or less in length. Single-breasted and often unlined in order to comply with fabric restrictions, they were, however, tailored and well made as they had to last several seasons. If they were lined, it was often with rayon. To save material, cuffs and patch pockets were banned in America as part of a 'no fabric on fabric' rule. Sometimes jacket sleeves were cropped short to reveal the blouse underneath and belts buckled at the back to leave the front smooth. The buttons, restricted to three or less, were often covered in the corresponding suit material.

As wool was impossible to come by, new materials like jersey wool, thick heavy rayon and crepe took their place. Despite what seems like an era of drab uniformity, a lot of the 1940s non-Utility suits have clever detailing. Clever panelling, set in different ways, in corded material for example, and crenellated yokes, added a dash of variety to the standard fare. Soft velveteen suits were fashionable and had gored skirts, accompanied by an unlined cardigan or jacket with a blouse feel. The outfit was completed with platform heels, often in cork or wood.

After the war, the female silhouette, while remaining slim, started to show changes. A softer line was creeping in with jackets losing the military cut. Gathered and curved-in waistlines, scalloped shoulders and gathered sleeves were seen in the Sears catalogue in 1946 and _Vogue_ featured Parisian suits with hip-draped skirts and coat frocks with stand-up collars.

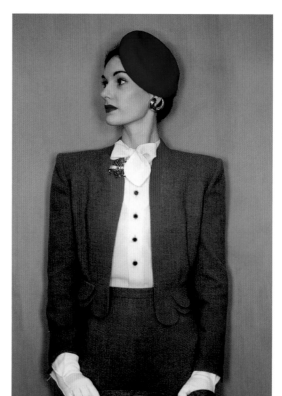

PAGE 60 Red checked dress in spun rayon, 1943. Two staples of the time, rayon and gingham, are used in this 1940s dress with three-quarter-length sleeves, necktie bow and hip pockets. The model stands in front of an Uncle Sam recruitment poster for the US armed forces.

LEFT Grey wool suit with red trim by American label Foxbrownie, 1944. Foxbrownie (or Fox-Brownie, as it is sometimes seen) was formed in 1937 by designer Stella Brownie and partner William Fox.

RIGHT Model wearing a Vogue pattern by Pierre Balmain, 1949. By this point in the decade, a more nipped-in hourglass shape was emerging. Balmain set up on his own in 1945, and designed elegant, feminine daywear, reaching his zenith with luxurious gowns and costumes for Hollywood starlets.

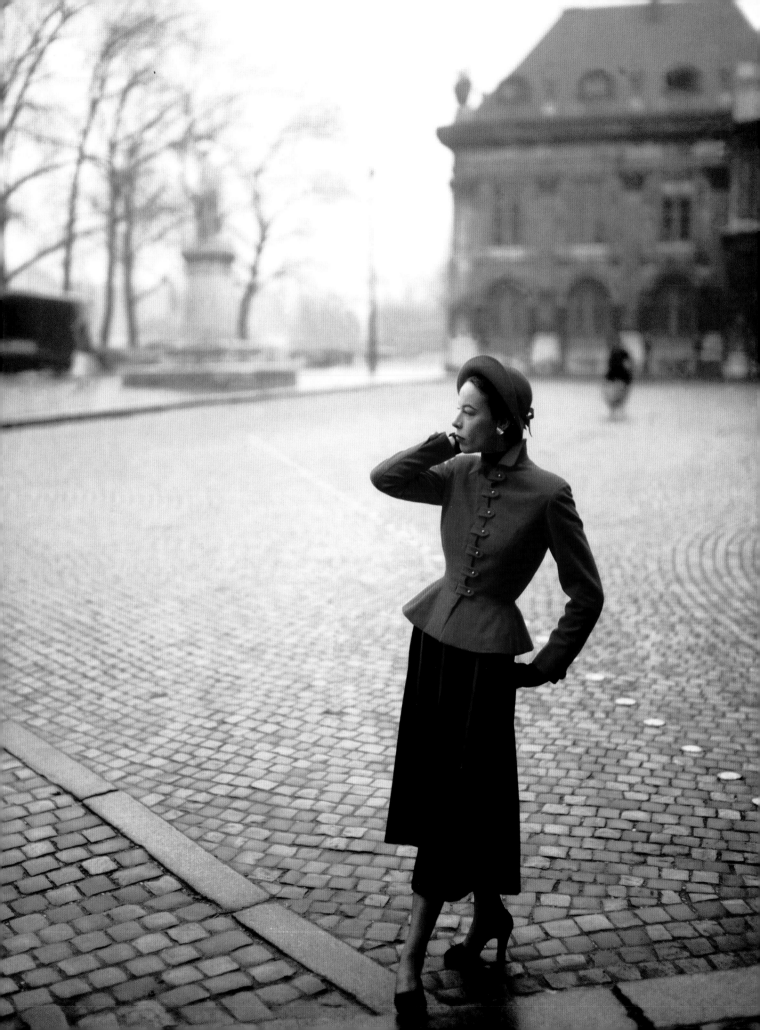

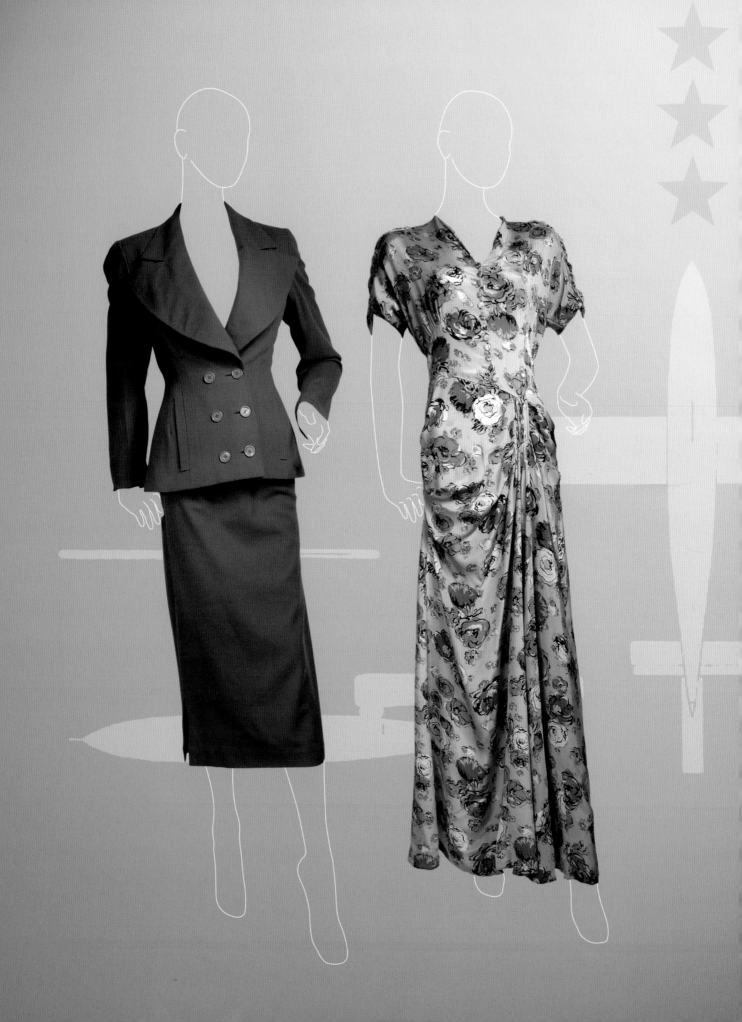

Blouses and sweaters

Rationing kept blouses simple and short, often in plain colours. A simple breast pocket was permitted. Yet no blouse was considered fashionable without the shoulder pad – these knife-edge bits of rubbery material were a predominant feature of the decade. Peasant blouses with gathered bodices were popular, and after the war blouses became more diaphanous with colourful prints, deeper necklines and bows.

For sweaters, *Vogue* declared that basic simplicity and surface decoration was the trend. Indeed, sweaters were a big fashion in the war years, partly because they were so versatile and warm. To counteract the restrictive mood, they were often highly decorated in sequins and beads that bestowed outfits with much-needed razzmatazz and glitz.

Skirts and trousers

No wider than 180–203 cm (72–80 in) and with hems no deeper than 5 mm (2 in), the skirt epitomized the restrictions of wartime clothing. Flounces and ruffles were out and a strict not-below-the-knee length was official. Tailored and narrow over the hips, the skirt had a casual and no-nonsense look, often with a front and black pleat to save material, or simply pleatless. As the decade wore on, American women were seen in fuller dirndl skirts that twirled round as they danced to the big band sound.

After the war, skirts were longer and slimmer – although even during the war, women had been letting their hems down. Despite rationing in Britain until 1949, the female silhouette changed and coupon clothing featured lightly gathered skirts with soft unpressed pleats and a subtle flair. These were often made in rayon or dirndl and were perfect for dancing. Knife-edge pleats came in and other skirts had discreet padding and a floating softness to the cut. As the waist grew smaller, *Vogue* featured exercises to achieve 'tiny waists'.

Wartime occupations required practical dress and fitted flannel trousers, especially in grey, were popular. Casual slacks were worn during the day as part of a sartorial economy drive to save on afternoon dresses.

Day-to-evening dresses

The pared-down military silhouette was echoed in the standardized dresses of the war years. Tailored and made on restricted lines, they featured shoulder pads, stitchbox pleats at the front and back of the skirt, buttons to the waist, and a slim belt. They had narrow revers collars with collars and cuffs sometimes in contrasting colours. As rationing took hold, designers made use of the fact that women would probably be able to afford only one dress, so jacket dresses with smooth lines were introduced. *Vogue* called them the 'war-wise dress', as they were so adaptable to wartime conditions, looking smart from morning right through the evening.

Bodices were often tight-fitting, buttoned to a low waist and with a gathered or pleated skirt. Decorative rayon dresses in pretty colourful prints with draping and shirred fronts were worn in the daytime, sometimes with a soft crossover bodice. Mexican prints were popular and loved for their exotic colour, giving a touch of drama to the otherwise drab uniformity of the day. As material restrictions gained ground, sleeves were shortened and the cap sleeve was introduced – sometimes slashed to give ease of movement. Particularly popular were dolman and three-quarter-length sleeves.

The manufacture of metal zippers was severely hit by the war, and consequently the zipless dress was a hit. All stitching, seaming and buttons were for use and not for decoration, and in America turn-up cuffs, double yokes and sashes were banned.

After the war, a deep rounded neckline became a popular feature and dresses had a drapier, fuller-skirted feel that extended below the knee. The waist grew smaller and pleats were widely in evidence.

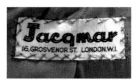

ABOVE The British Jacqmar label. A fabric manufacturer, Jacqmar was known for producing propaganda prints during the war years

OPPOSITE LEFT Air-force blue 1940s Jacqmar day suit, with strong military detailing at the shoulderline.

OPPOSITE RIGHT Yellow 1940s crepe dress. Note the draping at the waist and the classic '40s-style cap sleeves, here gathered to fall from the shoulder.

SIGNATURE 1940S DETAILS:

- Flyfronts on jackets that emphasized their straight cut
- Flap pockets on jackets
- Bolero jackets
- Narrow revers collars on jackets and flyaway revers on blouses and dresses
- Dolman sleeves
- Tiny kick pleats to soften the straight skirt
- Crossover bodices on dresses and blouses
- Suits piped with velvet or grosgrain
- Pussy-cat bows on blouses and dresses
- Shirring on bodices and skirts
- Sparkling buttons on plain cardigan jackets

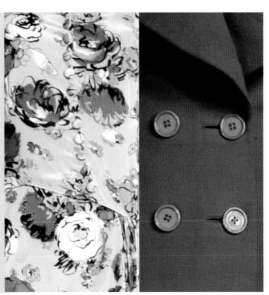

FAR LEFT Most daywear was in conservative colours, though many dresses and blouses were made in bright floral and naturalistic prints, as here.

LEFT Ladies' suit jackets were often double-breasted with high or rounded revers.

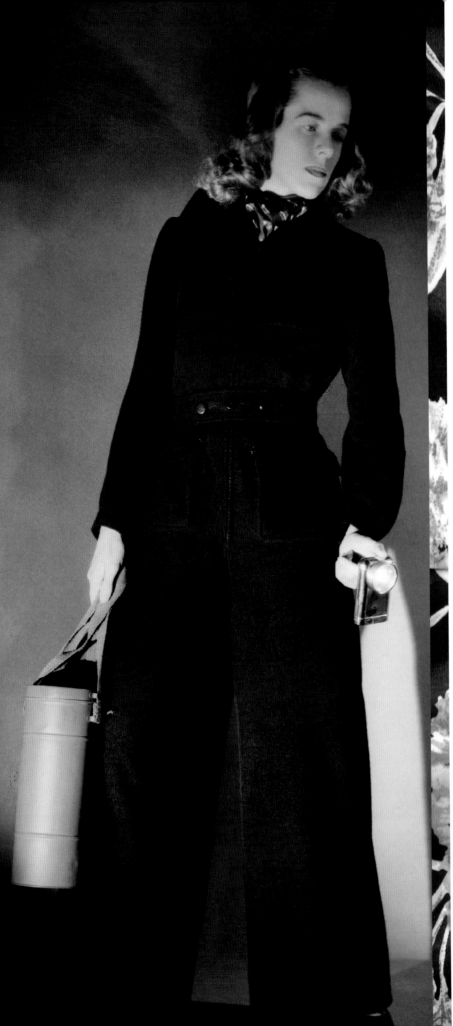

Utility Clothing

The Utility suit in England, the Victory suit of America, and Everyman's clothing in Germany were all the foundations of the cloth and clothing schemes that were introduced in Europe and America during the war. The aim was to restrict style and simplify design to save material and labour. In the US, designers such as Tina Leser and Claire McCardell (under Townley Frocks) created uncluttered, inexpensive ready-to-wear that reflected the fabric scarcities of the time.

In Britain, the Board of Trade worked with a number of leading designers to produce the kind of fashions that fitted the framework of the clothing orders. The group included Norman Hartnell, Bianca Mosca and Hardy Amies, who designed a range of 34 Utility designs all bearing the now famous CC41 label. The collection contained four basic items; a coat, suit, afternoon dress and suit dress for the office. Hartnell designed some of the best-known Utility suits and dresses for Berkertex in Bond Street. Using leading designer names was a way of making prototype garments more attractive. And with their individual 'signature', these items became sought after by the fashion conscious of the decade. A Mosca dress advertised in *Vogue* July 1942 has buttons inscribed 'Austerity Bianca Mosca'. Standards of manufacture were controlled and the public demanded long-wearing, well-made clothes. Wonderful tailoring and double stitching make 1940s vintage among the best.

Siren suits

When the siren went, women reached for their 'Utility' siren suit. An all-in-one garment, it was the original jumpsuit. It had a quick-zippered front and was not only practical but warm. Elsa Schiaparelli designed a beautiful one in silk with large slouch pockets and Digby Morton showed zipped and hooded siren suits in tartan Viyella. Over the siren suit, people would wear the kangaroo cloak coat – so called for its large pockets.

Dollar couture

The couture houses shut down during the war to make way for munitions, but Britain continued to promote designs and fabrics abroad, such as Harris tweed, to procure much-needed dollars. Designers such as Hartnell, Molyneux and others created beautiful dramatic couture pieces that were exempt from austerity and featured the long-barred dressmaking details. There was much play of colour and design in the British collections; *Vogue* wrote in 1946, 'Mushroom pinks, yellows and bright greens. Floral and narrative prints on crepe and silk. A soft feminine feel with sloping shoulders, rounded hips, easy bloused fit... much hip swathing and skirts drawn back in modified bustles... raglan sleeves, softly tailored suits, draped evening gowns in embroidered chiffon and daytime dresses often with floral and narrative prints.'

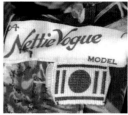

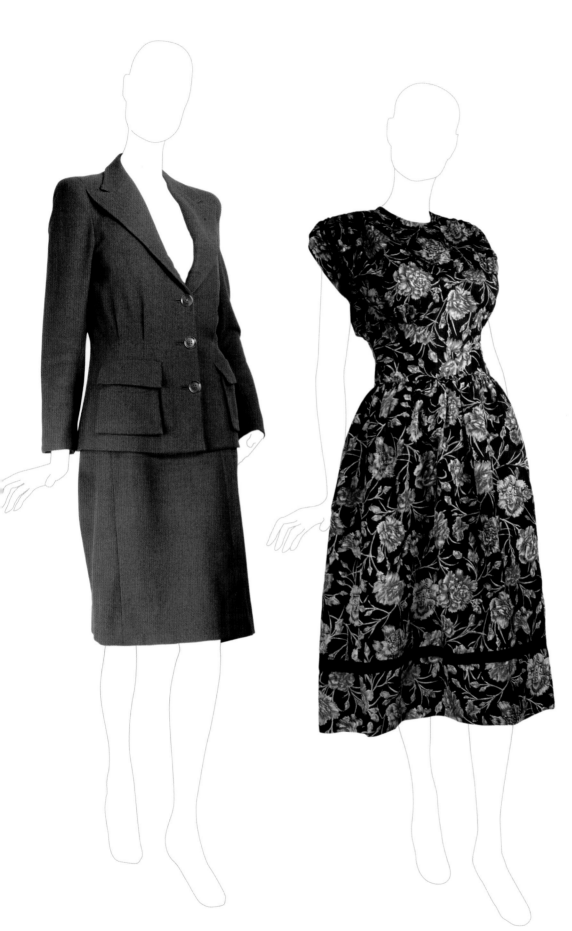

FAR LEFT Norman Hartnell brown 1940s Utility suit. Hartnell made well-tailored suits and coats in woollens and tweeds, but was most lauded for his elaborately embroidered and sequinned evening gowns. Utility designs followed the square-shouldered and short-skirted fashions of the war era but adhered to strict regulations for using minimal cloth. Buttons were limited to three and turn-back cuffs were forbidden.

LEFT Black floral 1940s Utility dress for luxury export only.

OPPOSITE Schiaparelli's air raid jumpsuit. The garment was easy to remove and had zippered pockets for valuables, making it ideal for wearing in air raid shelters.

Colours and Textiles

During the war years, women would walk down the street in Britain and America in outfits coordinated in the colours of the American flag and the Union Jack – red, white and blue. Names such as air-force blue, army tan, flag red and cadet blue all enforced the notion of patriotism and made the wearer feel they were helping the war effort.

Drab colours were the rule in the early 1940s as dyes were diverted to help the cause. Blues, browns, greens and black were all part of wartime understatement. Necessity became fashion. *Vogue* showed suits and dresses in soft beige, green and grey flannel. In the magazine's famous 'economy portfolio', it advised the reader how to 'Brighten up a brown suit with a red bolero or soften with a soft blue hat... Wear your grey suit with a red tie printed blue and a dramatic red belt.'

Naturalistic colours like salad and bottle green were popular and plain rayon dresses in dark colours were given dramatic relief with the clever use of shirring and draping. Despite a uniform drabness, colour did filter through in the form of exotica. Ochre yellows, terracotta reds and clay tones came from Mexico. These were often used to liven up dresses and suits, especially those made out of black – often using blackout material; a typical example might be an ochre bolero top over a black evening dress. After the war, the colour palette changed to reflect the lightness of mood. Roses and pale blues swept in, as 'grey turned to gay'. Shirtdresses were being worn in lively colours like yellows and chartreuse, and patterns became more whimsical and less heavy in nature.

Rayon was the dominant fabric of the decade and was used from coupon to couture. Practical and economical, it was the perfect stand-in for silk and flax, in severe shortage. It had the appearance of silk, it was noncrush and did not shrink or stretch. Made in two weights, the heavier linen variety for suits and the lighter crepe rayon for dresses, it was double-faced and looked elegant enough for eveningwear, which was often made in the new Celanese-printed crepe.

Linen was another material used extensively for the war. Reserved for the export couture market, wonderful evening dresses and suits can be found in 1940s linen. In Britain traditional cotton could not be used, as it came from India, so Scottish linen replaced it. Linen details date from the late 1940s and were part of the move to 'cheer people up'. Appliqué surface design techniques were much in evidence. Flowered appliqué was pretty and added dimension to otherwise plain linen or rayon outfits.

Because wool was in very short supply, as it was used for uniforms and blankets for the soldiers, wool blends were introduced, along with fabrics made out of recycled wool and rayon versions of the material. Synthetic jersey was a fashionable substitute and used to create the ubiquitous jersey shift. Velveteen and corduroy became the new materials for suits and dresses. Other fabrics that were not needed for the war effort, such as net, taffeta and faille, were used for evening dresses.

Prints and patterns

Great play was made with prints, using them cleverly with their own accent. Close bands of dots or other motifs, for instance, outlined yokes and pockets. Homey geometric designs, based on the plaids of the pioneering cowboy, were taken up in the war. Part of the frontier fashion, plaid and gingham were used to make romper suits, shirtdresses and eveningwear. Icons of popular culture and cosy domesticity, regional scenes and even cactuses and pink thimbles made their way on to clothes and were part of the trend for narrative fashion.

RIGHT Deep green wide-neck knit dress by Hattie Carnegie, 1943. Carnegie's designs were always youthful and chic and her hallmarks were exquisite workmanship and fabrics. Galanos, Norell, Trigère and McCardell all worked for her at one time or another.

BELOW Felt appliqué flowers decorate a 1940s American-made skirt.

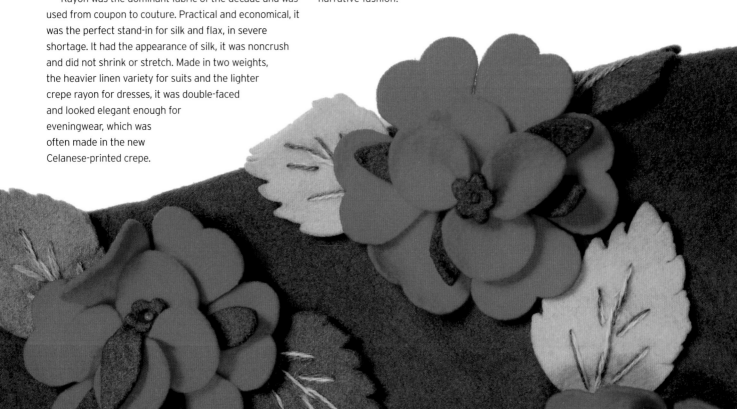

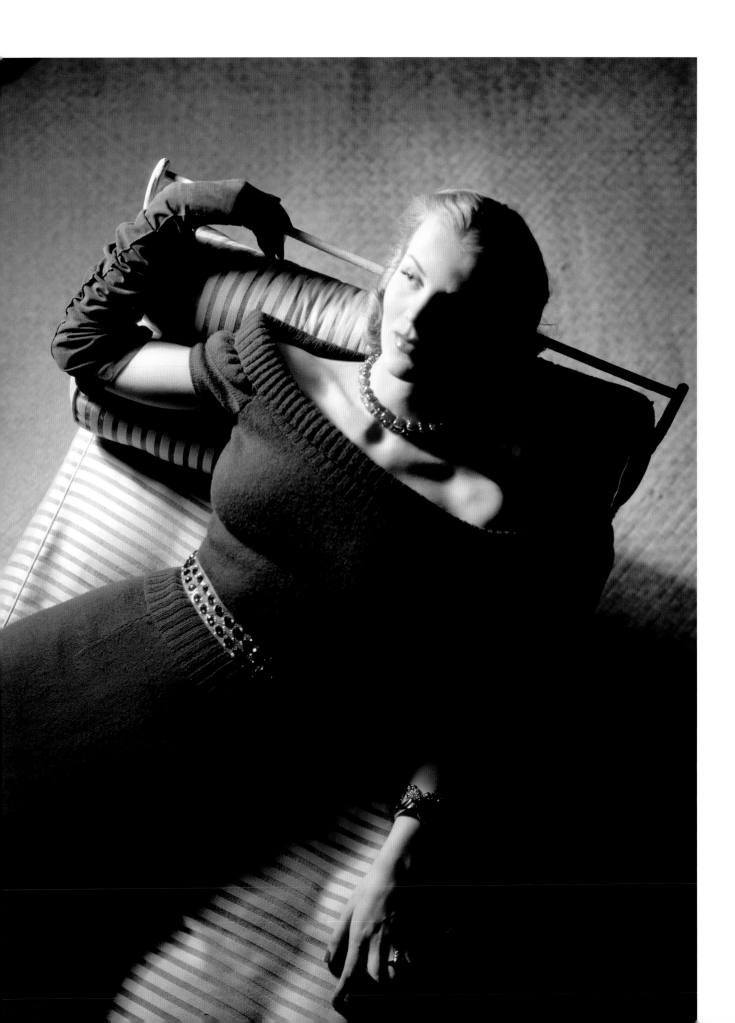

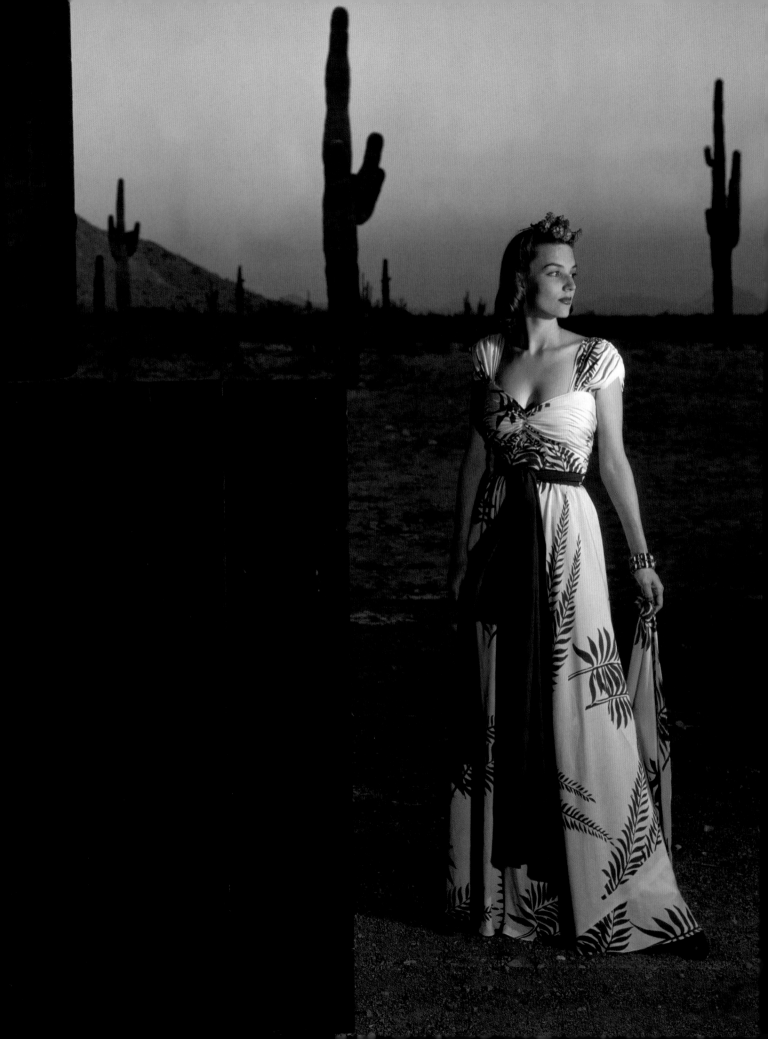

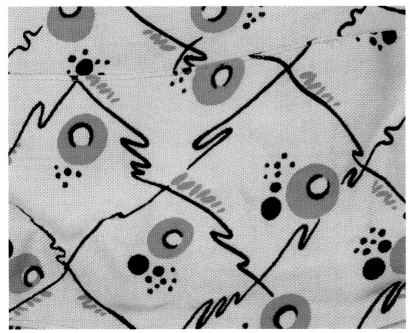

Garden prints in salad green with cabbage roses or ferns were seen on cotton chintzes and rayons, and exemplified the naturalistic theme that permeated the early part of the decade. After the war, designs became bolder and bigger and presaged the geometric abstract explosion of the 1950s. Amoebic shapes became popular, as did abstract designs of floating harps and roses in a sea of musical notes.

Patriotic and propaganda prints

Military motifs such as battleships and aeroplanes shoot across monotone prints, and sailors and tropical islands were other popular motifs featured in the Sears catalogue of 1941. Stars and stripes, checks and dots were the mainstay of '40s print design. In 1942 a range of prints were made up into clothes by designer Bianca Mosca to be worn by prominent women for propaganda purposes. 'Dig for Victory' and 'Happy Landing' were some of the most popular mottoes. Material printed with maps and flags were made into dresses and shirts and worn with pride.

Hawaiian and ethnic influences

In California, Hawaiian prints and island motifs on sarong dresses and halter dresses were worn, especially with the trend for resortwear growing. In particular, designer Tina Leser managed to turn fabric shortages to her advantage. She cleverly fused the exotic design of island fabrics with quintessential Americana style and produced brightly patterned play clothes. She used Hawaiian, Tahitian and Mexican fabrics, as well as prints adapted from kimono silks, and turned them into wrap skirts, sarong-style dresses and cotton playsuits. A hand-woven blanket was transformed into a strapless dress and long narrow pants made out of oriental fabrics were chic.

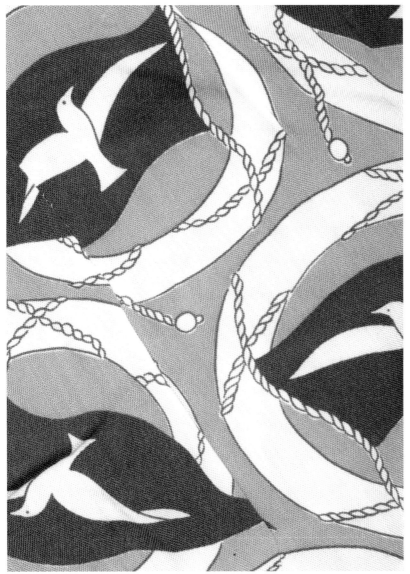

LEFT TOP AND BOTTOM
Postwar linens featured vibrant colours and patterns that lifted the mood after the war years. Above is a pink circle amoebic pattern on a turquoise field; below a seagull print. Silk was rare during wartime due to the disruption to shipping from India, and Irish linen was a useful alternative.

OPPOSITE: Celanese rayon cactus green gown, 1941. The model is standing by a barn door in Midwest America at dusk; her dress is indicative of the frontier fashions and natural leaf and plant motifs of the time.

The Emergence of American Style

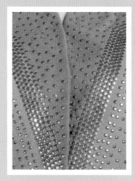

ABOVE Detail from a Fred A Block suit, opposite. The American company was known for its fabulous 1940s jewellery, made with enamels, gold metals, clear plastics and rhinestones.

With the occupation of Paris in 1940, France was cut off from the rest of the world and America lost its sartorial direction. Until then, department stores like Lord and Taylor and A T Stewart copied and diluted Parisian couture designs, then sold them at a cheaper price thanks to mass production. New York found itself cast adrift and a unique challenge presented itself. Add to the mix the clothing rationing in 1942 – the War Production Board put severe restrictions on the use of wool and the amount of yardage that could be used in garments with its Regulation L-85 – and America was left to create its own style.

The Victory suit

The dominant style through to 1946 was the American Utility suit, which – while echoing the austerity lines of the British Utility suit – was far less grim. The severely cut suit was, in fact, attributed to costume designer Gilbert Adrian who designed the austere look during the 1930s for Joan Crawford when he wanted to emphasize her authority and independence. In 1941 when he set up his ready-to-wear business, he emboldened his designs and gave women the broad-shouldered geometric suit with its three-dimensional tailoring and design detailing that accentuated the bust and waist. Self-piping ties at the fronts of jackets replaced hard-to-come-by buttons and sleeves were narrow. Adrian Originals suits and evening gowns were so popular that they were rationed to two per customer at his Beverly Hills store.

Ready-to-wear separates

Top of the line ready-to-wear American designers such as Jo Copeland, Vera Maxwell, Norman Norell and Claire McCardell all became household names and designed mix-and-match separates for the real woman. Unadorned and uncluttered, ready-to-wear styles avoided padding, corsetry and built-in bras and instead followed the natural line of the body. Classic items such as the tailored shirtwaist dress made of gabardine, the drawstring-waisted dress and the narrow synthetic jersey shift dress were easy to wear and elegant. Bright sporty plaids, checks and stripes were often used in daywear and eveningwear and halternecks were worn with culottes and flat pumps.

The trend of peasant-inspired clothes was important during the war years. Designers used prints handwoven in places like Mexico and Hawaii. Women wore peasant skirts with blouses with signature drawstring necklines and puffed sleeves. Louella Ballerino's famous peasant dresses with her bold prints and wide, bright stripes are coveted vintage items.

Claire McCardell was perhaps the most influential originator of the American casual style. Forerunner of Calvin Klein, she liked simple uncomplicated designs in

ABOVE AND BELOW Jacket and button detail from a purple 1940s Lilli Ann peplum jacket. The American label, founded in 1933 by Adolph Schuman, was known for its bold colours, coats and dresses, and tailored details. Schuman developed close relationships with French and Italian textile mills after the war.

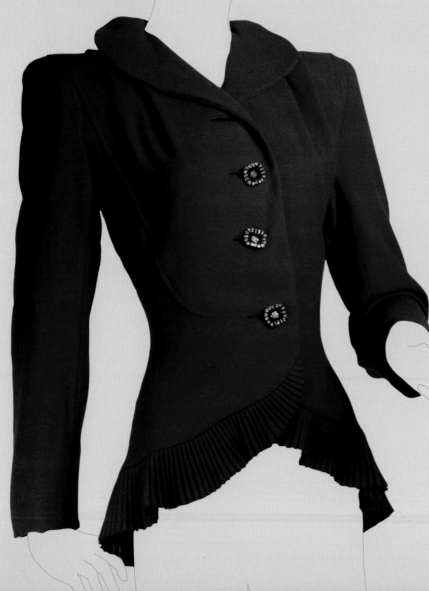

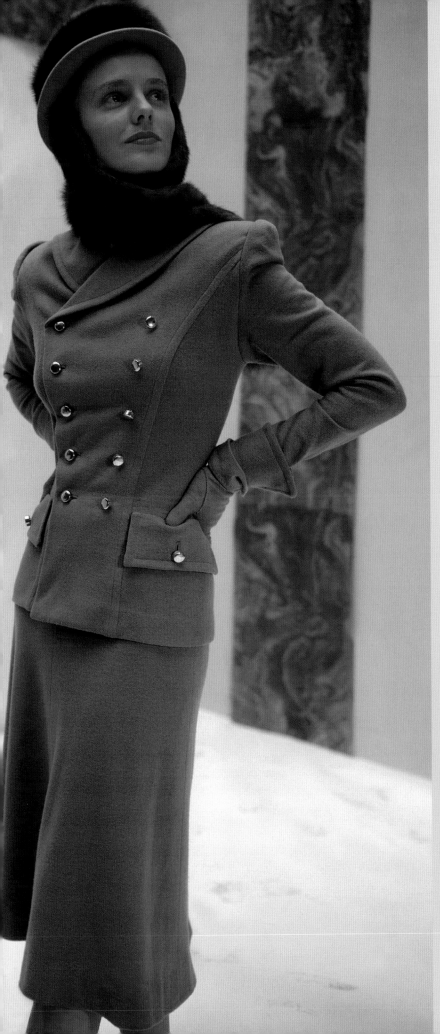

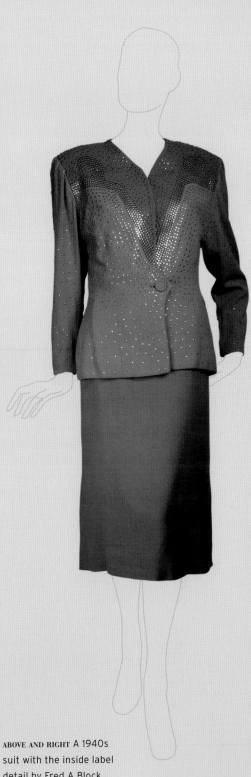

ABOVE AND RIGHT A 1940s
suit with the inside label
detail by Fred A Block.
Block produced typically
American-styled tailored
suits in the 1940s, often
featuring studded
patterns, as here.

LEFT Steel-grey double-
breasted fitted suit by
Manhattan designer
Larry Aldrich, 1946.

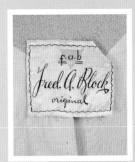

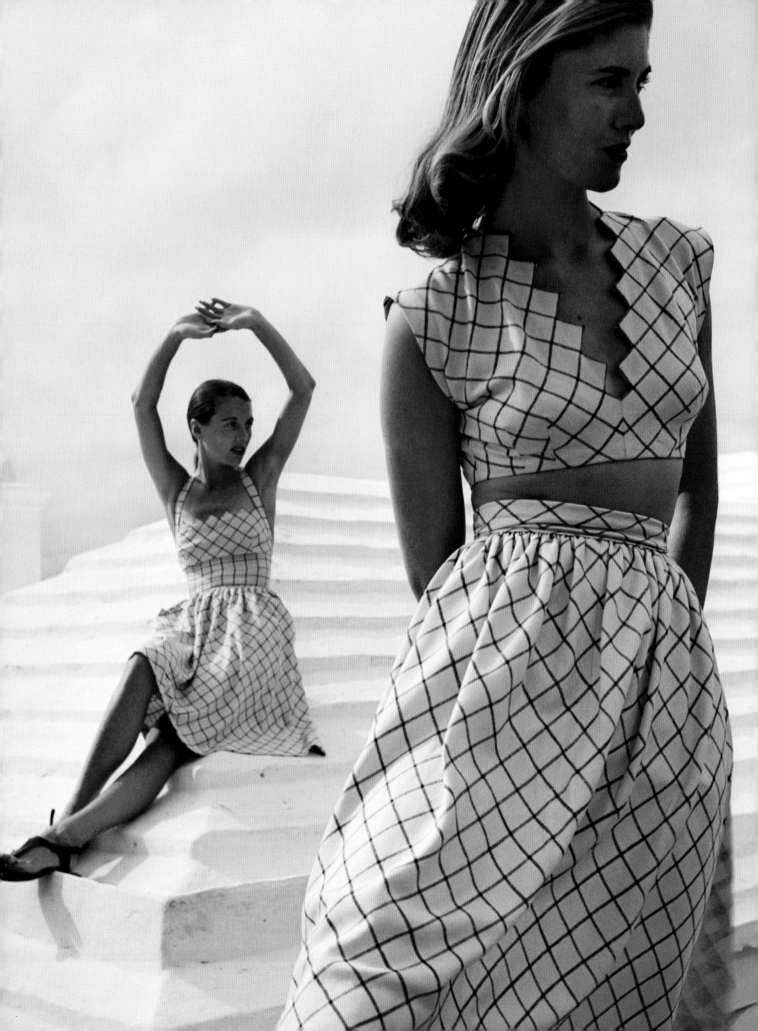

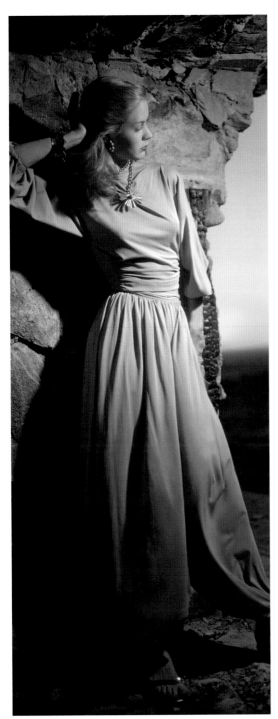

not least, her sundresses, with the famous spaghetti straps that crisscrossed repeatedly to form a halterback, were considered the height of chic, especially when worn with the ballet pumps she introduced to the consumer.

LEFT Claire McCardell's Arabian Nights trouser set in grey rayon jersey, 1946, shows her simple chic styling and feminine shape.

Classic sportswear

During the war, America was forced to use its own materials and techniques. One main inspiration was sportswear that had started in the 1930s on the college campuses and the relaxed West Coast. Worn by the stars, the look had trickled down to the department stores. Designers showed weekend wardrobes with mix-and-match pieces, such as jackets that could be worn with slacks, or over cardigans or pre-dinner dresses. Wool ribbed sweaters over white polo shirts, and crisp neat slacks, shorts and buttoned-down skirts, were modelled by young, healthy-looking models. The lines were created by such Californian manufacturers as Fay Foster, Koret, Jantzen and Cole of California.

Pat Premo golf dresses and Koret's top-stitched pleated skirts were all quality-made sportswear designs. Often in two-tone plaids, they looked crisp and smart. The Californian sundress in cool white cotton and backless 'sunshiners' in gingham with flutter ruffles and edged in ricrac were worn by younger women, and the pinafore dress with fitted bodice and gathered waist, as seen in the Sears catalogue, was both cute and practical. The bare-waist playsuit with its bra-esque top and brief short skirt with front buttons or side zip and underpanties with snug legs was created in the 1940s and the midriff was born – not to shock but to save on material! They were loved by Hollywood starlets who wore them when posing for such publications as *Life* magazine. Swimwear was glamorous and alluring in the 1940s. Inspired by Hollywood pin-ups like Betty Grable, flattering one-pieces were often made of gold and silver Lastex. Sculpted with built-in boning, elasticized nylon and featuring shirring and draping used in eveningwear, these flattering items clung in the right places and minimized the flaws of the wayward female figure. Pareos, pyjama pants, pirate shorts and wrap skirts were all sold to coordinate with and, more crucially, to cover up the new brief styles.

Hollywood glamour

Hollywood lost its glamour in the 1940s and was not exempt from L-85 regulations. Gritty realism films set an example by showing actresses like Bette Davis and Joan Crawford in suits, skirts, sweaters and slacks. The Hollywood western gave America frontier fashion – fringing on jackets and shirts, and denim detailing were commonplace. Frontier pants with front panelling and topstitching were popular with stylish women and fitted in with their growing independence. Blue jeans, made sexy by a young Marilyn Monroe, were specially cut for the feminine figure with side openings at the cuff, as these were more ladylike.

unsophisticated fabrics, such as chambray, cotton jersey, denim and mattress ticking. She incorporated the functionality of sportswear and experimented with pattern and cut to create great trouser suits with graph-paper checks (a McCardell trademark) and long shorts in jersey wool with streamlined hooded sweaters. When her monastic dress was brought out, *Vogue* heralded it a triumph. Loosely fitted and shaped like a voluminous tent, it created a soft shape when belted. Women loved her popover dress, a simple wrapover design often with a dramatic belt, and they queued up to buy her playclothes in denim with white topstitching. Last but

OPPOSITE Summer dresses with the trademark graph-paper check by Claire McCardell, 1946. Her midriff-baring designs heralded a new relaxed style that was made for leisure activities. She used fabrics such as jersey, denim and cotton to produce her sportswear-influenced classics.

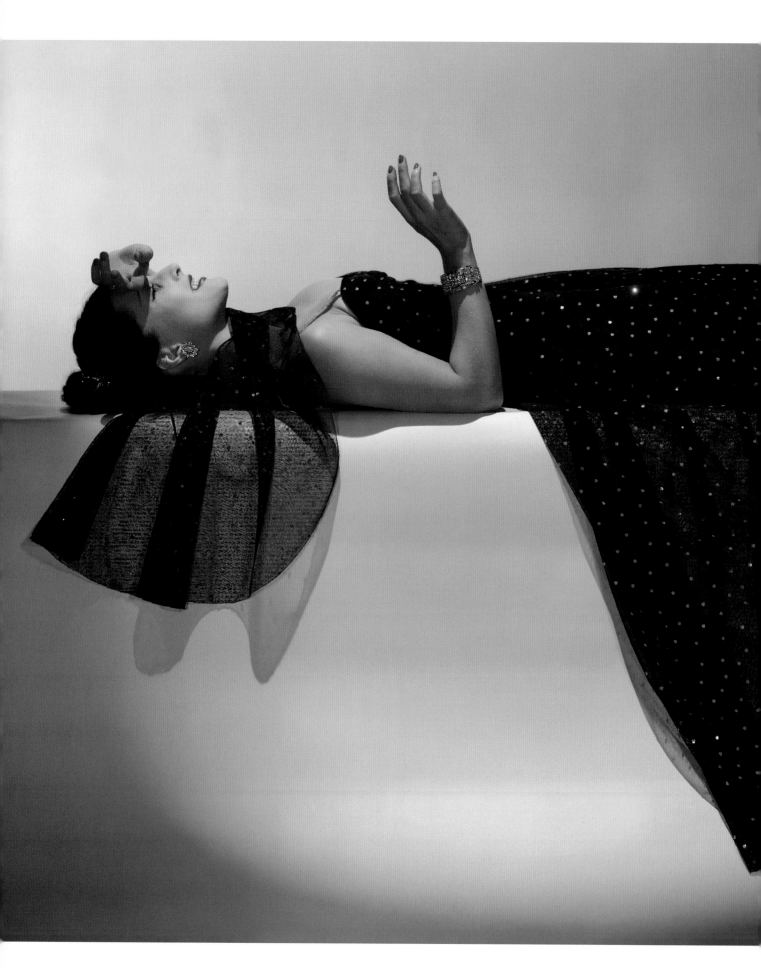

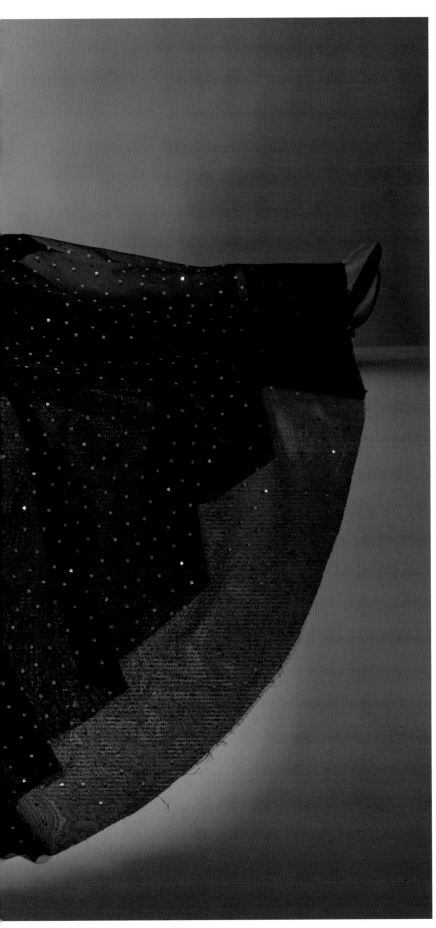

Eveningwear

Despite the wartime devastation, civilization reasserted itself during the evening. Extensive drapery and dazzle created the much-needed illusion of glamour and was in stark contrast to prosaic daywear. Dinner suits were popular and often comprised long plain dresses that could be worn with or without sparkly jackets. Shorter evening dresses with draped bodices and low-slung sarong skirts were worn to save materials, yet still managed to look sophisticated. By mid-decade the little black cocktail dress was considered a vital part of any woman's wardrobe.

Sequins were not rationed and seemed to be sewn on everything, long or short. Jewelled bodices and glass starring provided welcome glitter on otherwise plain dresses, and jewelled capes were thrown over to glitter in the dark. Evening dresses often had to be made out of undyed material (called 'greige goods').

The column shift dress

The slim body-conscious lines that were set in the 1930s were followed in the '40s, and the tubular shift evening dress inspired by Greek statuary was much in evidence. In a bid to save material, this style was used in many guises from dinner suits to opulent gowns. Adrian's columnar evening gowns, embroidered with gold beak and Greek bands, circa 1945, is one such example. Dresses based on the toga and the pleated chiffon in rayon crepe were all features of the decade.

While silk had been the preferred choice in the 1930s, now that other fabrics had to be used crepe and rayon became favourites. Rayon, with its silk-like quality, yet much cheaper and unrationed, was draped and shirred to form fluid dresses that maintained that 1930s 'poured in' look. Side-draped, side-buttoned, simple dresses made out of black rayon were particularly popular. Shirred bodices and front-bodice drapery are characteristic of the period. Short bolero jackets were worn over sheath dresses with draped crossover bodices in two different colours.

Capes and cutaway jackets made out of taffeta and net covered up the plain dresses and were part of the wartime trend of mixing and matching to create more outfits. The strapless evening gown showed off the female sloping shoulderline and was much in evidence – it saved material and was elegant to boot.

LEFT Star sequin-studded midnight blue rayon and net evening dress and cape by Hattie Carnegie, 1945. Sequins were much-used as there were no wartime restrictions on them.

Export couture gowns

While Britain made do and mended, the couture evening gowns were exuberant and luxurious. Reserved for export, they escaped austerity rules and designers indulged their fantasies in these feminine creations, such as beautiful taffeta shawls over moulded tubes of satin or jersey and black velvet bodices with plunging necklines. Hip drapery caught in bustles added to the flamboyant feel of the couture evening wear, especially when topped off with wildly bouffant sleeves. Eveningwear was often sculpted and seemed to envelop the wearer.

The Molyneux export collections are particularly of note and featured beautiful floor-length gowns with complicated embroidery and luxury fabrics. The designer's black full-length gown in slipper satin with pink bertha and hem and weighted with roses had dropped shoulders and oodles of fabric.

Elsa Schiaparelli's love of colour, high drama and sartorial frivolity all coincided in her close-fitting mermaid dresses: these flared at the bottom and accompanied by hip-length capes in gaudy colours with her signature fantasy embroidery. Her bustle dresses appeared in many fabrics in 1939, and her exuberant evening gowns are coveted items. In 1941 Schiaparelli left for New York where she remained until the war was over. Schiaparelli's house remained open throughout the war and produced collections, although they were not created by the designer herself. Her early wartime designs were made before she departed for America.

Americana and American designers

New York was a haven for couture and glamour. The American halfway-hem ballet skirts in such fabrics as mousseline with tiny waists and full skirts presaged the New Look and were not available in Europe. Hattie Carnegie's little black cocktail dress was worn by women all over the country.

In America materials like gingham and cotton were being used in evening dresses. Gilbert Adrian employed gingham and Pennsylvania Dutch motifs in his Dolley Madison ballgowns made in organdy and patterned with patchwork quilt designs. Claire McCardell's simple halterneck evening dresses made out of gingham cotton looked simple and unbourgeois. Gingham was also used frequently by Anglo-American Charles James, head of costume at Metro Goldwyn Mayer (MGM) from 1928–41, and who famously used gingham to dress Judy Garland as Dorothy in *The Wizard of Oz* (1939), and later in his wool gingham suits.

James elevated dressmaking into an art form. His ballgowns are sartorial sculptures with asymmetric shapes that were made in such unforgiving fabrics as velvet, heavy satin and faille. His full intricately shaped skirts over understructures were classically elegant. He disliked printed fabric and would create dresses using several different types of material all in the same colour range. His colour combinations were unusual – such as

orange and rose, black and aubergine. His sculptural approach to eveningwear is reflected in a series of dresses he made during the 1940s that became known as 'Charlies'. A dressmaker of consummate skill, he was awarded a Coty for his 'magical use of colour and artistic mastery of drapery'.

Other coveted couturiers of the period include the Russian-born American Valentina Sanina, who favoured couture clothes that looked effortless and understated and operated a small house known as Valentina Gowns. Known for her floor-gracing silk jersey gowns and her bolero evening creations, Valentina was a meticulous designer with an eye for the dramatic. Norman Norell's evening gowns were striking in their simplicity, and he favoured a revealing round neckline that he would offset with jewelled buttons or pussy-cat bows. His prolific use of sequins and beads – often covering entire garments is testament to his admitted love of the 1920s, as was his use of the straight up-and-down silhouette. Jo Copeland's, grand evening gowns are a collector's dream. She worked with pure silks, rayon and wools and loved asymmetric cascading ruffles, trumpet-flaring skirts and wide side draperies.

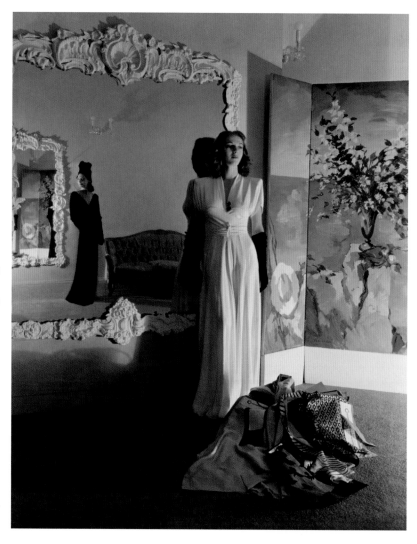

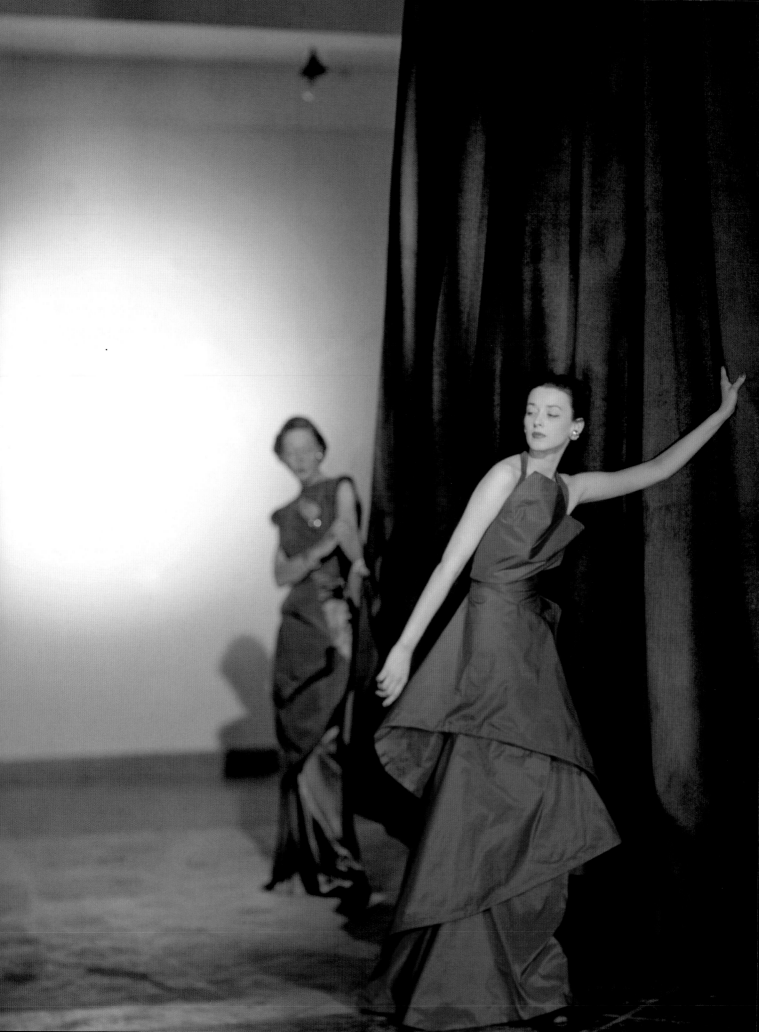

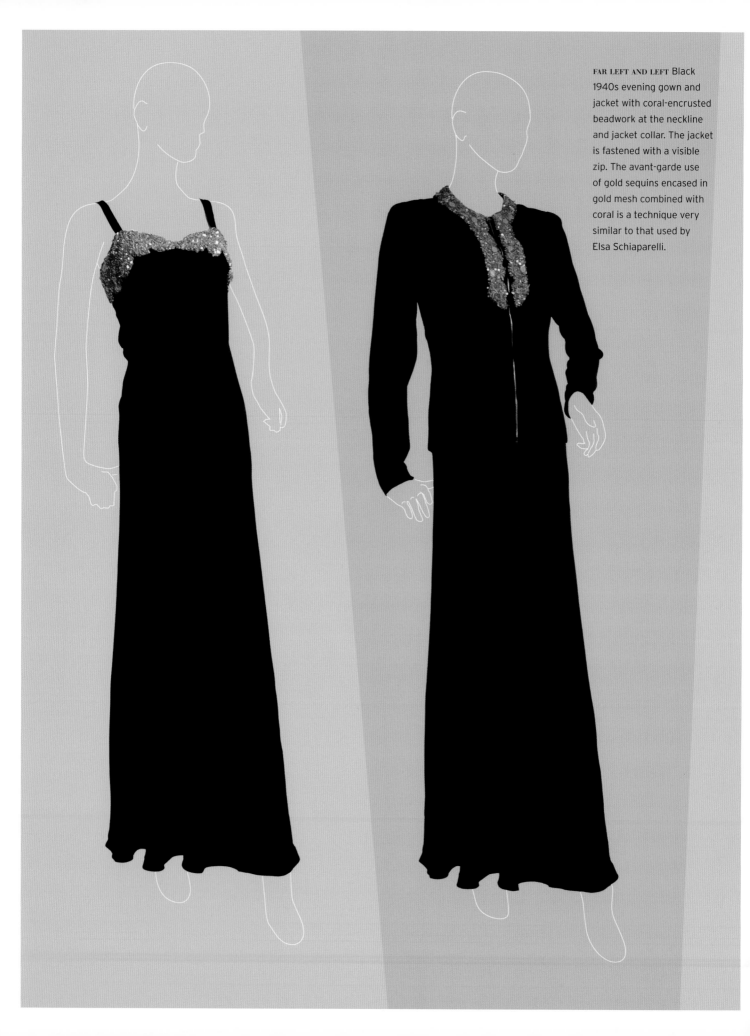

FAR LEFT AND LEFT Black 1940s evening gown and jacket with coral-encrusted beadwork at the neckline and jacket collar. The jacket is fastened with a visible zip. The avant-garde use of gold sequins encased in gold mesh combined with coral is a technique very similar to that used by Elsa Schiaparelli.

Surface decoration on eveningwear

The early years of the 1940s were characterized by an ornate look that was left over from the extravagant 1930s. As the wartime restrictions bit hard, surface decoration was replaced by clever shirring, tucking and appliqué. Beaded dresses were fashionable throughout the decade, and sequins were the queen of the evening as these were not restricted by the wartime effort; all-over beading is a characteristic of '40s eveningwear. Gold palettes and black sequins livened up dresses and bead embroidery, often in the shape of jewellery, gave glamour to the pared-down styles. Postwar luxury was a welcome respite and the Paris Collections featured full-blown evening gowns in taffeta and satin with lace trims and even silver fox on the hems of capes and coats.

Postwar eveningwear

After the war, eveningwear took on a softer, more feminine feel. The postwar silhouette with its rounded shoulders and gathered skirts was reiterated in the evening gowns that showed a much tinier waist and more flounce. Romantic, satin gowns of rayon net flared below a slim waistline, and showed bows, flounces and low-cut necklines with ruching and puffed sleeves. These elements were influenced by the Southern belle, glamorized in films *Gone with the Wind* (1939) and *Meet Me In St Louis* (1944).

This romantic femininity that harked back to the pre-war period was ironically to appear in a flurry of net taffeta in 1947, when Christian Dior's New Look burst on the scene. His evening dresses were so whale-boned and petticoated that they could stand unaided. The tiny waistline was achieved only by wearing a *guêpière* – a type of corset – and the yards of tulle made women look like meringues. The sloping shoulders and deep plunging neckline showed off the rounded female body once again and the wartime silhouette had gone for good.

DECORATIVE ELEMENTS OF THE 1940S:

- Jet, bugle and glass beadwork and bead-embroidered waistbands
- Sparkling and covered buttons used as decorative elements in themselves
- Sequins and beads that simulated jewellery
- Appliqué and pique appliqué
- Grecian bands of gold and silver embroidery
- Satin roses on bodice fronts and hems weighted with roses
- Double puffed peplums and giant back bows made of taffeta and silk
- Pleated lace collars and demure eyelet ruffles
- Fur pompons on dinner jacket sleeves
- Silk and moire sashes on tulle gowns
- Laced V-necked bodices

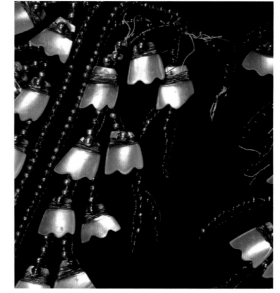

RIGHT Mother-of-pearl beadwork adorning the front of an early 1940s Molyneux bolero evening jacket. This piece was probably created while the French couture houses were still in full operation – prior to 1942.

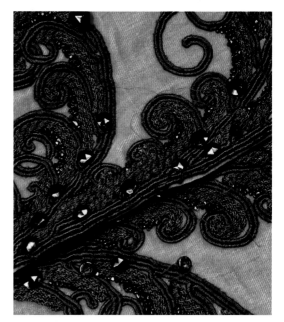

RIGHT Pink velvet 1940s evening jacket with black frogging and beads by Stassner.

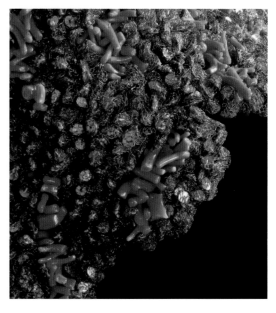

RIGHT Detail of the coral and gold sequins encased in mesh on the evening gown pictured opposite.

▼ Slacks

All styles of slacks, especially pioneer pants, became popular as women got used to wearing trousers at work. Here actress Lilli Palmer is shown in 1946 wearing her man-tailored grey gabardine slacks, along with a beige suede jacket.

▶ Sequins and beads

Not rationed by the war, sequins were sewn on dresses, jackets and shawls to add sparkle to daywear and eveningwear. This 1945 white crepe gown, covered with bugle beads, and with dolman sleeves is by New York costume designer Kiviette.

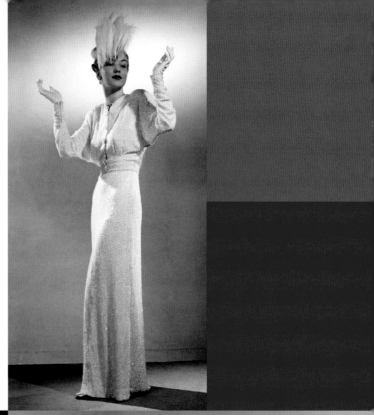

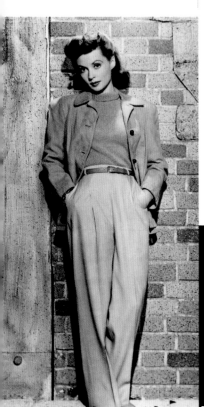

Utility suit

Clothing by law. Designed along tailored lines in military-style boxy jacket and narrow, short skirt, they were most often made in blues, blacks and browns.

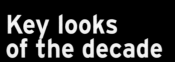

Key looks of the decade

1940s

▶ Trench coats

Military styling was evident in jackets and coats during the war years; here a red wool belted trench coat, lined in black rabbit, is by Traina-Norell, 1943. Bell-shaped coats with large collars were also popular.

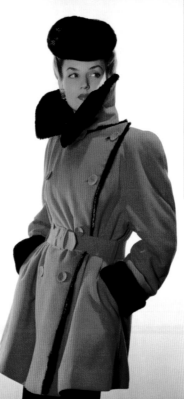

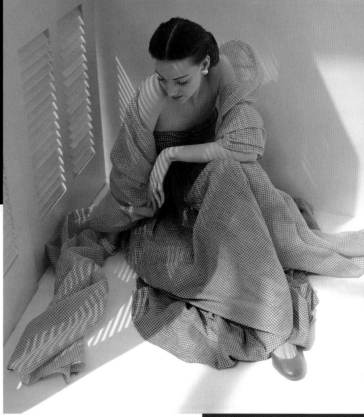

▲ Gingham

America's favourite fabric. Shirtdresses and pinafores all had a fresh new look in gingham, which became popular during the war years. This 1947 blue gingham dress is worn with a red gingham scarf and red kid shoes.

ture eveningwear

...ctured couture gowns in
...n featured elaborate detailing
... were made in unforgiving
...ics like velvet, and heavy
...n and faille. Greek-inspired
...ath dresses based on the toga
...le use of pleated chiffon in
...n crepe and greige.

...astic dress

...sely fitted and shaped like a
...minous tent, the dress was
...n a soft shape when belted.

Peasant dress

Exotic handwoven printed
skirts and off-the-shoulder
blouses with drawstring
necklines and puffed sleeves
were popularized, partly due
to the success of the Brazilian
bombshell, Carmen Miranda.

▶Bolero jacket

Short and emphasizing the
waist, with padded shoulders and
shirring, the bolero was often worn
over strapless evening dresses.
Here a navy bolero is worn with a
white blouse and red skirt – classic
patriotic colours – in 1942.

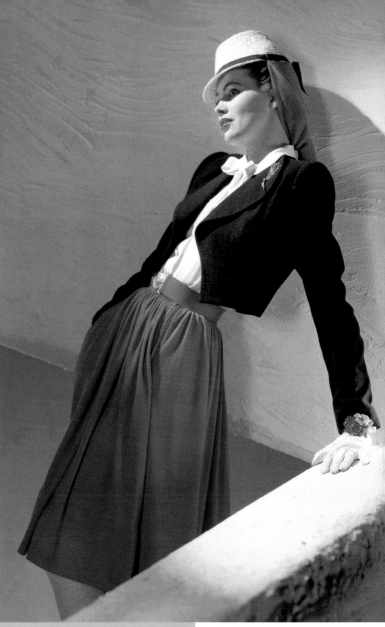

...sey shift dress

...ple and elegant, the shift was
...ortish unstructured design in
...thetic jersey, which was made
...ular by New York designers,
...h as Norman Norell.

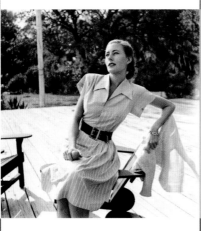

Rayon print dress

Pretty for daytime wear in the
new noncrease rayon fabric,
dresses exhibited colourful prints,
often with shirring and draping
on the bodice or waist.

▲Sportswear and beach

Summer dresses and midriff-
baring tops with matching shorts
were influenced by outdoor
athletics, as in this 1946 day
dress by Claire McCardell.

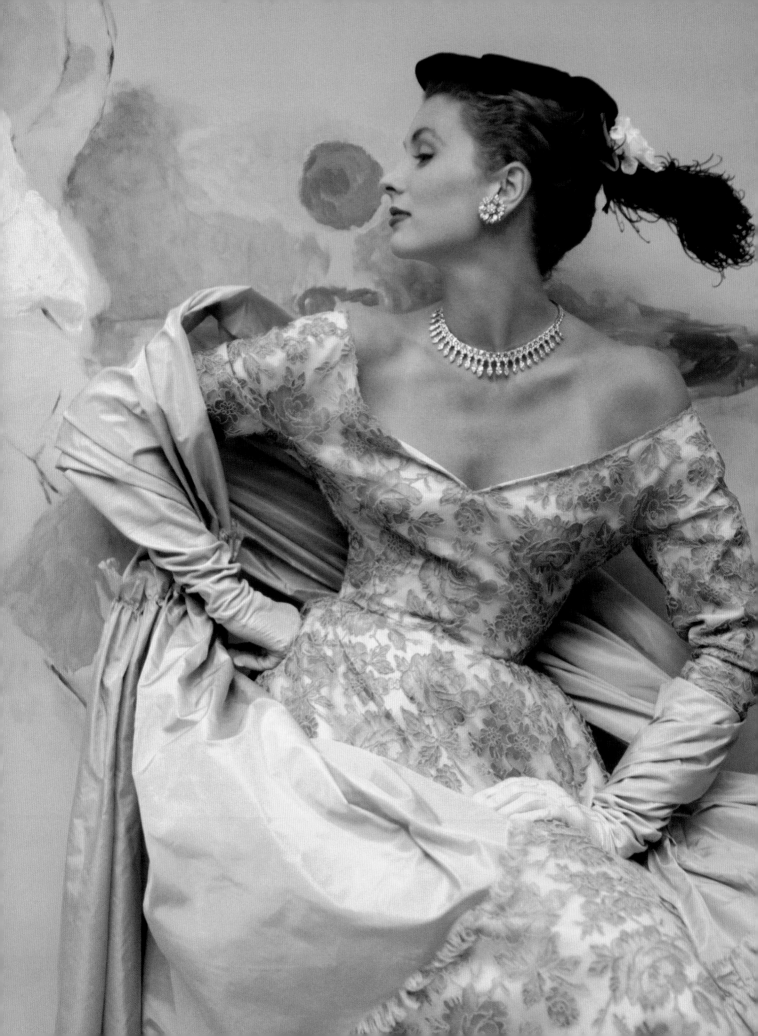

1950s

The 1950s kicked off with a feeling of hope and euphoria following the conclusion of the Second World War, and the generally rapturous applause that had greeted Dior's New Look in 1947. In Great Britain the government promised to 'Make Britain Great Again', and immediately set to work on the Festival of Britain exhibition that took place on the South Bank of the Thames in 1951. There was a significantly optimistic outlook for the world in general, and that included the fashion industry. After years of hardship and drudgery, when women had worn sexless, utilitarian work garments (and when there were fewer men around to impress), there was an understandable desire to dress up in luxurious feminine clothes. While Britain itself was almost bankrupt and rationing dragged on until 1954, the sheer extravagance of Dior's New Look seemed to point to a future of confidence and prosperity, something that everyone aspired to. Dior's designs were to dominate, but not everyone was thrilled; for some Dior seemed out of tune with postwar Europe and a symbol of luxury, extravagance – some of his skirts required 18 m (20 yards) of material – and privilege that many hoped the war had destroyed. Times had definitely changed. For all the hardships and tragedies that women had dealt with during the war, it had in fact been a time of liberation and equality. Hundreds of young women had been freed from the domesticity of housework and sent out to work as land girls, driving ambulances or in munitions factories. The idea that fashion now intended them to revert to a romantic notion of femininity with a padded bosom and nipped-in waist, was something many were not prepared for.

Fit or Flounce Silhouettes

**The 1950s was the last decade when Paris still
dominated worldwide fashion. Dior was unstoppable,
and he remained influential until his death in 1957;
alongside him were other great designers determined
to succeed.** Cristobal Balenciaga, Jacques Fath and
Hubert de Givenchy were all leading names of the era,
but the clock was ticking and as the decade unfolded
there were signs that the elitism of haute couture was
starting to lose its dominance. The decade was a
transitional one that moved from the austerity of
the 1940s to the prosperity of the 1960s; in fact, the
dividing line was becoming clearer by 1956 with the
increasing influence of the teenager youth culture in
America, and the identification of the young as a
separate consumer group.

The decade will be remembered mainly for two
contrasting silhouettes, although there were myriad
alternative shapes (not all of which were hugely
successful) that flourished briefly and then
disappeared. The great full skirt that swirled and
sashayed and the slim pencil tubular skirt that fell
to the knee were quintessential silhouettes, and
both placed great emphasis on the narrowness of
the waist. After the miserable war years, women were
eager to embrace the femininity. Strategic padding
and structured underwear did much to improve a less-
than-perfect body, so that Dior's extreme silhouette of

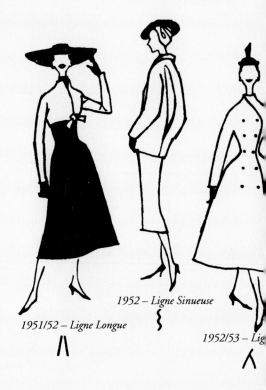

1951/52 – Ligne Longue

1952 – Ligne Sinueuse

1952/53 – Lig

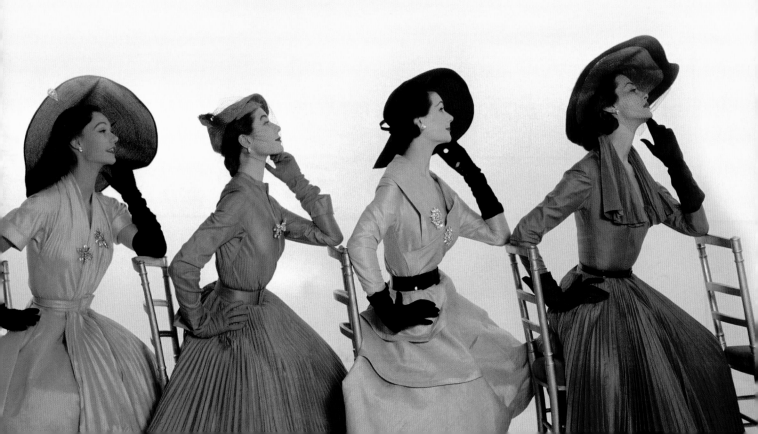

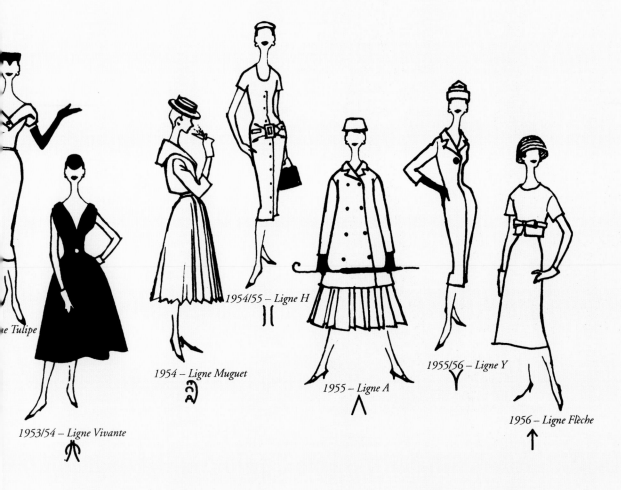

ne Tulipe

1954/55 – Ligne H

1954 – Ligne Muguet

1953/54 – Ligne Vivante

1955 – Ligne A

1955/56 – Ligne Y

1956 – Ligne Flèche

nipped-in waist and swirling mid-calf skirt could look fabulous on everyone. The nylon all-in-one corselet gave a waspish waist, pulled in the hips and shunted the breasts upwards and outwards to give a perfect hourglass figure, as seen in Anita Ekberg in Fellini's *La Dolce Vita*. Fashion was still dictating rigid and uncomfortable dress codes, and women continued to fall into line as they wanted to appear alluring and sophisticated.

Women everywhere fell in love with the glamorous clothes of the time, chronicled as the 'fashion-conscious '50s'. An elegant appearance required the correct accessories, and smart women were still expected to wear hats, gloves and matching shoes and handbag to be considered well dressed. Although functionality and simplicity were increasingly prevalent in daywear (easy separates and sporty slacks reflected an increased interest in athletics), eveningwear was dramatically show-stopping, with long gloves, high heels and drop earrings essential to complete the look. Hair was worn high on the head, in variations of a Dusty Springfield beehive, or cut short to the face in a gamine Jean Seberg crop.

Dior's hourglass figure was not the only silhouette of the decade though, and he himself experimented with many other shapes; almost every Dior collection saw the introduction of a new silhouette – the Princess line, the A-line, the H-line and the S-line all followed each other in quick succession. Dior's invention of the A-line was quite simply a dress that fell from fitted shoulders outwards towards the hem and used stiffened fabric to create the shape. The A-line and the H-line were offering women even more choice and another set of vastly contrasting shapes were hailed as the latest look.

The waistline started to fluctuate, changes in length and line came in quick succession, and women were expected to keep up with many innovative directions. Skirts ranged from voluminous fullness through neat tailored pleats to snug slimline pencils. The Sack, Princess, Tulip and Trapeze lines were all to come and go before the end of the decade, as designers seemed to waver between very structured clothes that could almost support themselves and clothes that were much more fluid and relied on the female body to provide form and shape.

ABOVE Almost every Christian Dior collection of the decade featured a new silhouette, though all kept a narrow waist and a below-knee hemline.

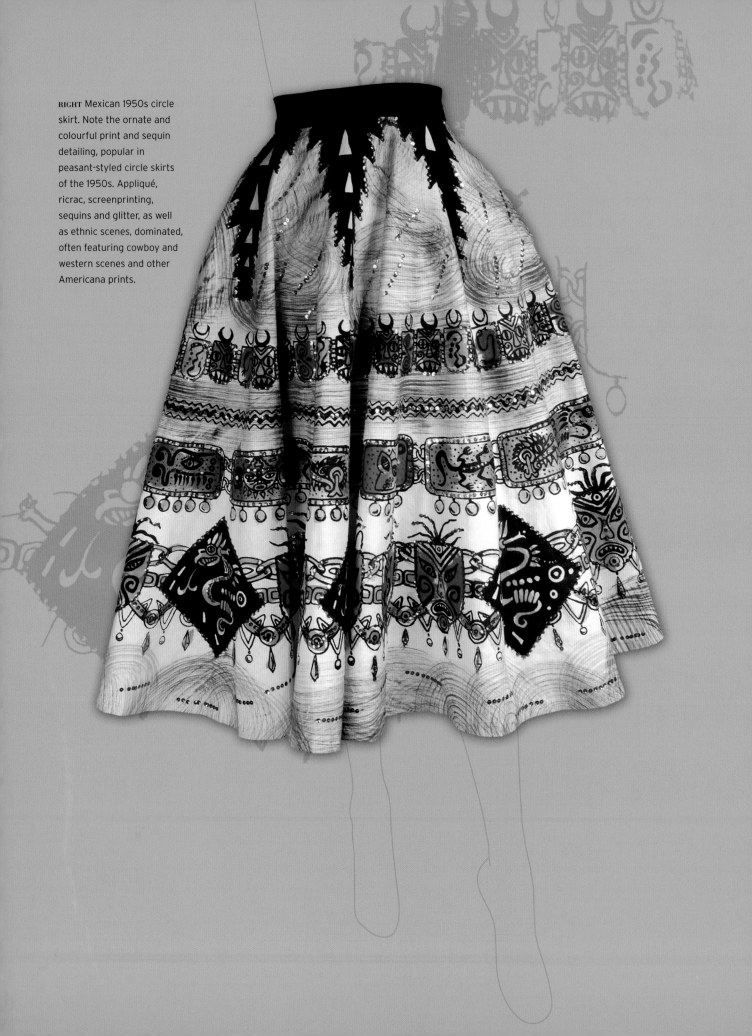

RIGHT Mexican 1950s circle skirt. Note the ornate and colourful print and sequin detailing, popular in peasant-styled circle skirts of the 1950s. Appliqué, ricrac, screenprinting, sequins and glitter, as well as ethnic scenes, dominated, often featuring cowboy and western scenes and other Americana prints.

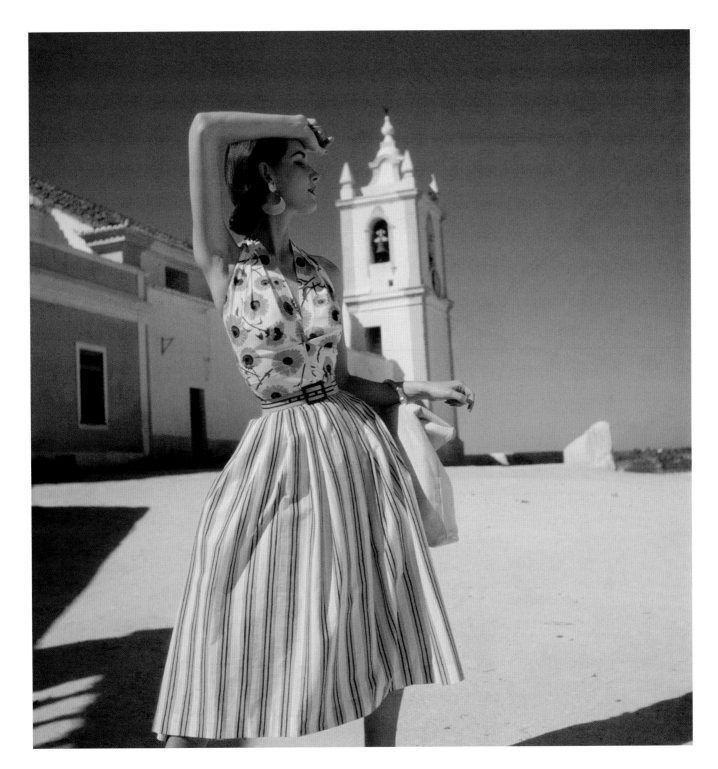

A more relaxed attitude

Other designers began to nurture the lifestyle changes that were taking place across the globe and encouraged women to develop a more relaxed attitude to clothing, with designs that were less formal and allowed more freedom of movement.

A master of undulating line, Jacques Fath came to prominence in the postwar period, with a less structured approach than either Cristobal Balenciaga or Christian Dior. The first Frenchman to design for the American ready-to-wear market, under Joseph Halpert, he catered

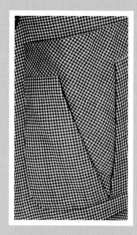

ABOVE AND RIGHT Dogstooth 1950s suit by Charles Worth, in a classic fitted shape. The house of Worth was known for innovative sleeve variations and trimmings, as seen here in the unusual three-quarter pleated sleeve and, above, the pleating detailing in the pocket.

for high society and the Hollywood set with his showy elegance and asymmetrical necklines that drew attention to the breasts. Daring to use such vibrant colour combinations as green and blue, his daywear and eveningwear were also noted for their diagonal lines and panels that were designed to enhance the female form. He set up his own ready-to-wear line in Paris just before his tragic, early death in 1954 from leukaemia.

Hubert de Givenchy was another leading name who had studied with Jacques Fath in the 1940s and then left to set up his own couture house in 1952. He became known for structured minimalist clothing, and was the first to design a collection of separates. Givenchy went on to create the Sack dress, and the funnel-collared coat. His success in designing beautiful understated clothes for Audrey Hepburn in the movie *Sabrina* in 1954 led to a collaboration between the actress and the house of Givenchy that lasted for over 40 years. In 1957 Givenchy started the trend for straighter shift-like dresses that had no waist at all by inventing his Sack dress. It was almost formless in shape, and although women could still look elegant by the addition of jewellery or a hat, it was a revolutionary breakthrough as it freed them from the restrictive clothing to which they had become accustomed. The Sack was to have lasting influence as it became the springboard for Mary Quant's early tunic dresses that launched her meteoric rise from the tail end of the 1950s into the explosive '60s.

Crossovers from couture to ready-to-wear

Ranging from casual wear to formal evening gowns, ready-to-wear took off after the war. Many designers never revealed their full names on the garment labels, instead collaborating with others. In Britain the Irish-born Digby Morton, though prominent in the Utility schemes of the 1940s (see pages 66–7), was a postwar ready-to-wear designer who found favour in the American market. Under the name Reldan-Digby, Morton introduced ready-made clothes to the British public that happened to have a couture appeal, as well as a collection of separates that were successful in both America and Britain. For his wearable tailoring, Morton used traditional fabrics, but in less conventional colourways. His clever cutting and stitching lines gave new life to the traditional tweed suit.

Another Irish-born designer and traditionalist in the use of Irish wools and tweeds who found success

OPPOSITE Tailored ready-to-wear suits, 1953. The narrow fitted silhouette made the hips look slim and the legs longer.

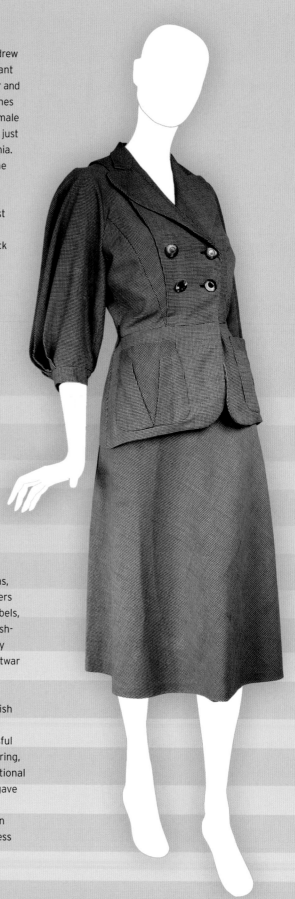

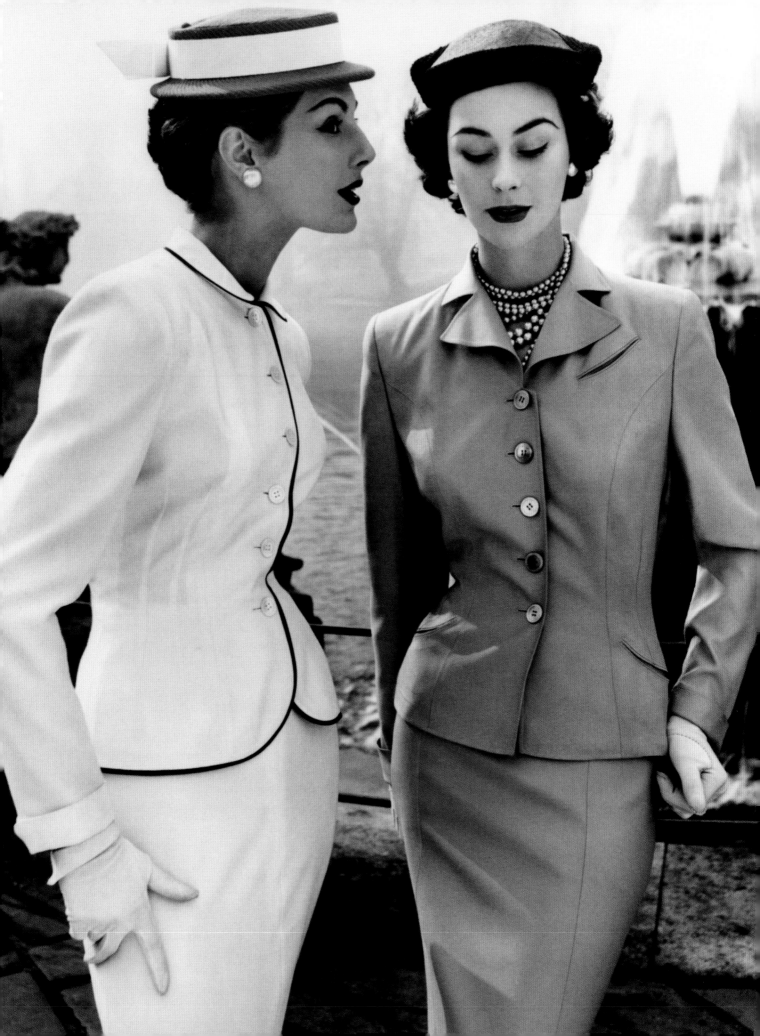

The burgeoning youth market

By mid-decade, all the major French fashion houses had started to diversify. Product lines such as shoes, jewellery, leather goods and of course perfume were being licensed around the world, and small boutiques full of prêt-à-porter (ready-to-wear) collections were appearing in major cities. Existing manufacturing businesses like Maison Weill and Lempereur (the first to use a young Brigitte Bardot to model its range) started to look for talented young designers to create their own style of clothes for the burgeoning youth market. Up-and-coming designers like Daniel Hechter, Emmanuelle Khanh and Jean Charles de Castelbajac were contracted to such companies as Lempereur and Pierre D'Alby before finding success under their own names, and a young Karl Lagerfeld designed for the prêt-à-porter label Chloé with great success.

Shape-wise the 1950s continued to be a decade of contrasts. The sheath dress and empire-line dress relied on superb cutting skills to construct a fitted garment that followed the contours of the body with invisible seaming and darts. Completely opposing this refined line, fashion in the decade was also known for volume, and designers played with all manner of billowing shapes, in the form of tulip skirts, balloon-type jackets, huge cocooning capes and generously cut swing coats, sometimes held in place with a half-belt to control the fluidity.

When Christian Dior died suddenly at the age of 52 in 1957, a youthful Yves Saint Laurent was waiting in the wings to take on his mantle. His first collection for Dior in 1958 was a huge success with a refined Trapeze line that fell from narrow shoulders to a wider hemline that just covered the knees, but there was a national outcry at his next collection which introduced a hobble-type skirt, and his time at the house was short-lived. Designers were becoming increasingly in tune with the changes in society and the shift towards a younger client. The image of Bardot, longhaired and barefoot in a cute cotton gingham dress, encapsulated a carefree spirit of the times, which was to dominate the next ten years.

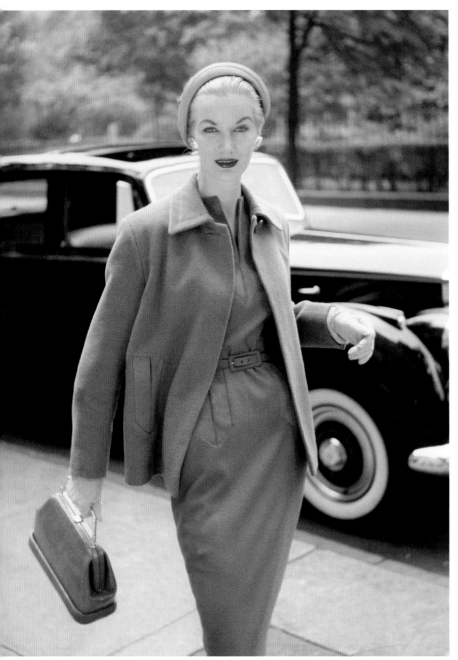

ABOVE: Model wearing Digby Morton's camel's hair-and-wool suit with a felt cloche by Knox, pictured in front of a Rolls-Royce, circa 1953.

on both sides of the Atlantic was Sybil Connolly. Inspired by Givenchy to make clothing that was elegant but comfortable, she worked luxury into poplin, tweed, lace and linen, with designs influenced by Irish country pursuits and arts-and-crafts – riding habits, hooded cloaks and shawls.

Jacques Heim created diffusion lines, Heim Actualité and Heim Jeunes Filles, in 1950, extending into ready-to-wear and specifically catering for America's needs for sportswear. By the end of the decade Jean Louis Henri Bousquet at Cacharel, with Emmanuelle Khanh, created a ready-to-wear company image that was very French, young, and sporty. Libertys of London, meanwhile, was nurturing the talents of Jean Muir.

SIGNATURE 1950S ELEMENTS:

❖ Twinsets and heavily ornate beaded cardigans
❖ Bell-shaped coats
❖ Slim pencil skirts
❖ Boxy collarless jackets
❖ Strapless gowns
❖ Covered buttons
❖ Circular skirts
❖ Half belts
❖ Slacks with foot loops
❖ Oversized collars

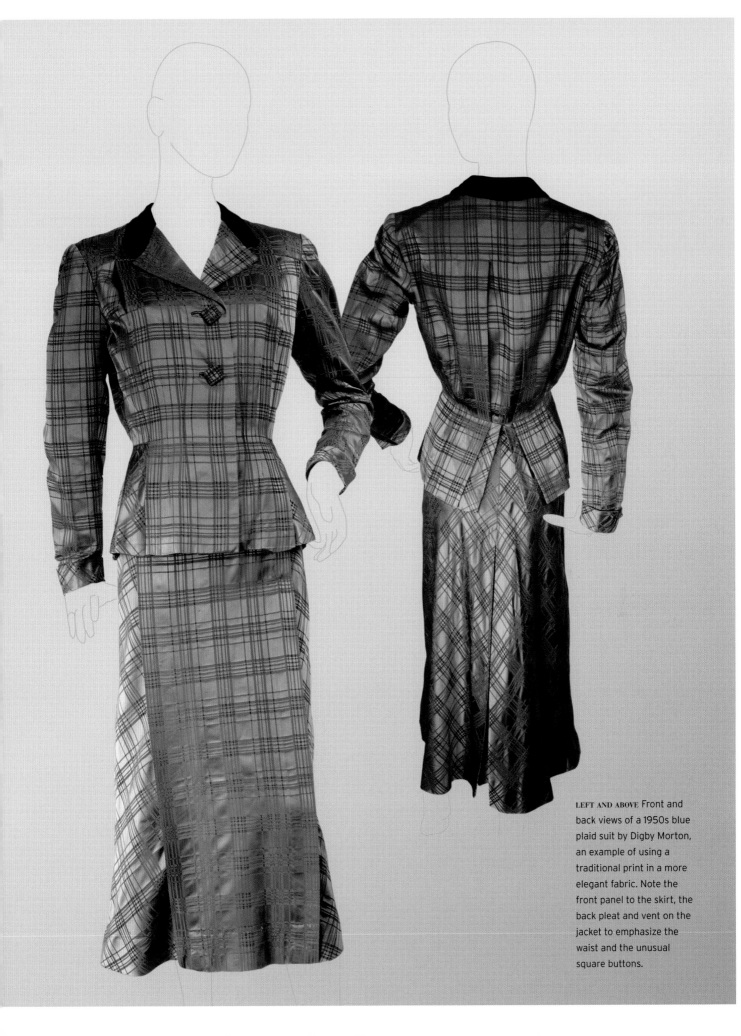

LEFT AND ABOVE Front and back views of a 1950s blue plaid suit by Digby Morton, an example of using a traditional print in a more elegant fabric. Note the front panel to the skirt, the back pleat and vent on the jacket to emphasize the waist and the unusual square buttons.

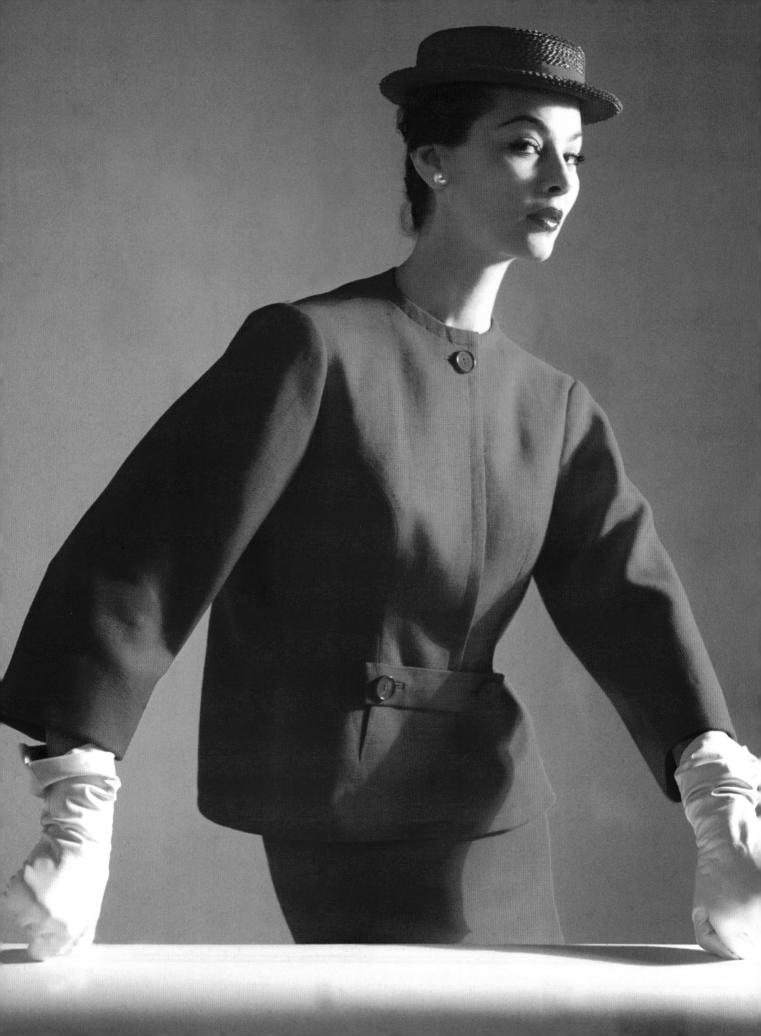

Cristobal Balenciaga and Coco Chanel

Some had criticized Dior's boned bodices as backwards-looking, and by 1952 Spanish-born Cristobal Balenciaga, a master of technical cutting, had started to release the body by eliminating the waistline and broadening the shoulders, cutting a looser, less structured jacket to a new 'midi' length that fell across the hipbones. Without huge fanfare he created clothes suitable for modern living, endlessly refining to make them efficient and elegant. He perfected the semi-fitted suit, called the H- or I-line, that became synonymous with the decade: a long straight jacket, worn over a slim pencil-line skirt, very chic and modern-looking when compared with previous shapes, and cut to just below the knee. Regarded as a sculptor among designers, Balenciaga created collarless blouses as well as balloon tunic sack and chemise dresses. His expertise lay in the detail of his cut, collars and sleeves, which always looked perfectly form-fitting in every situation. Known as one of the foremost designers of the decade, Balenciaga also introduced 'semi-fit' dresses with soft round shoulders.

Coco Chanel, too, had vocally criticized Dior's restrictive shape as stifling for women, and at the age of 70, after 14 years in retirement, she relaunched in 1954 with a collection of boxy collarless jackets, with slightly flared skirts made from soft jersey fabrics. The style was perfect to copy for mass production, providing thousands of 'ordinary' British women with a Parisian original at an affordable ready to wear price tag, courtesy of the high street retailer Wallis. Chanel was scathing about Dior's 'upholstered' clothing and offered an alternative silhouette that was clearly feminine but much less restrictive, and absolutely veered away from the boned nipped-in look. Her classic iconic suits consisted of a cardigan-style collarless and almost boxy-shaped jacket that fell open to the waist, worn over a slim skirt and decorated with trademark gilt buttons, girlish bows and contrast braiding. It was a style that was easy to wear and was made in luxury nubbly tweeds with a contrast silk lining; it became immensely desirable for women of all ages and remains so through to the present day.

OPPOSITE A poppy red linen Balenciaga suit with a fitted front and a loose back line, accessorized with a matching hat and white gloves, 1952.

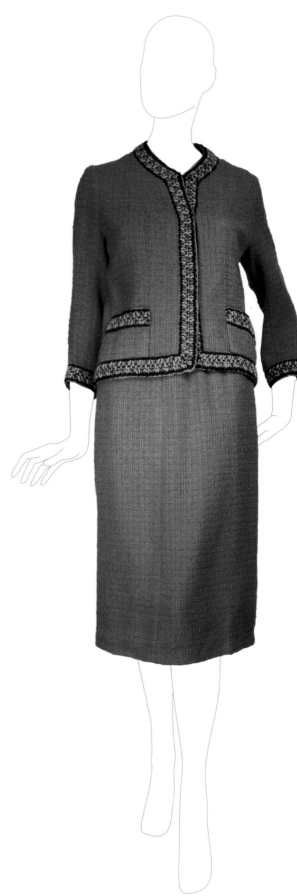

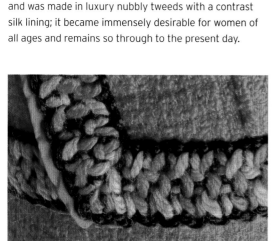

RIGHT Red tweed Chanel suit 1954/5. Cut loose and boxy with the classic front patch pockets, the suit was made for movement.

LEFT Chanel's classic braided trim around the cardigan-style jacket became a trademark of her tailored suits.

Coats and Jackets

The 1950s saw great diversity in the styles of jackets and coats on offer. Dior, Fath, Balenciaga and other couturiers all experimented with less formal styles and a move away from fur. There were practical considerations, too; as so many of the decade's dresses and blouses were sleeveless, there was a greater need for cardigans, jackets and coats to keep the arms warm when the temperature dropped and to coordinate the look.

A shape that was popular from the start of the decade was a wide triangular coat commonly called a tent or duster coat. Based loosely on Jacques Fath's swing coat of the previous decade, it was single-breasted, with wide square armholes. It sat easily over a voluminous silhouette and was worn over cocktail sheath dresses and full-skirted eveningwear for much of the decade. Design details like oversized Peter Pan collars, or buttonless versions with extravagant shawl collars, which became

BELOW AND RIGHT A 1950s jacket and inside collar label by Maria-Louise Bruyère, a French designer popular in the 1940s and 1950s. The jacket may have been originally part of a suit, or worn with a contrasting skirt.

RIGHT AND BELOW RIGHT The bow motif around the rounded collar is repeated on the buttons, creating a very feminine styled jacket.

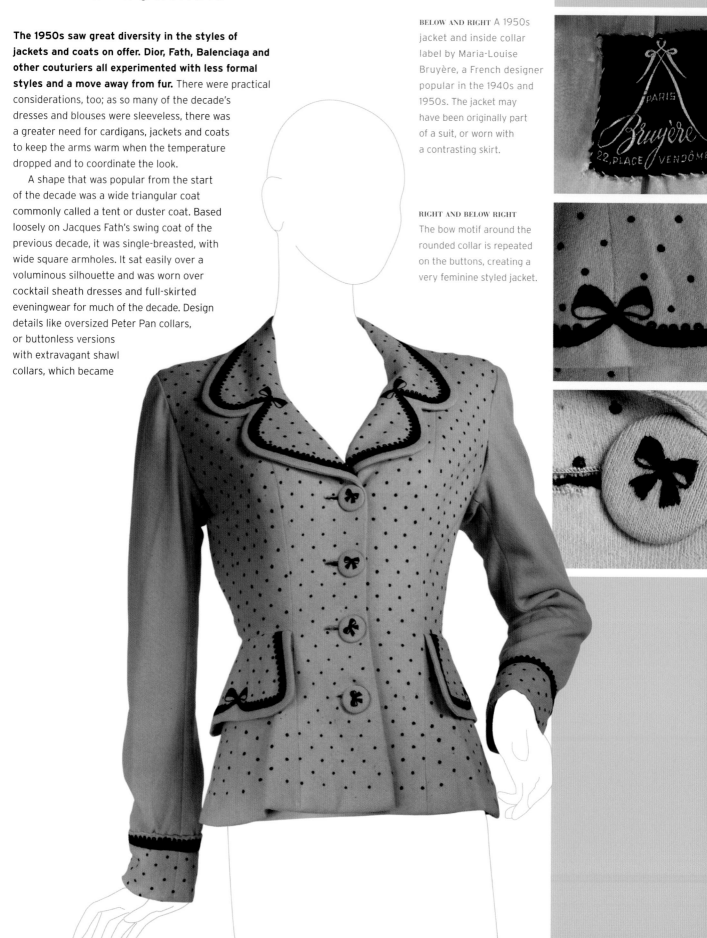

known as clutch coats (because they had to be held together by hand), were all variations on the same theme. Coats often had contrast lining. Popular fabrics included camel, wool velour, Melton cloth, tweed and velvets. Fur was reduced to trims, and beaver, lamb, astrakhan and mink were used.

In Paris there was a definite trend towards tunic coats and flared three-quarter coats. The designer Nina Ricci, who became established in the 1930s but was still a prestigious couturier until the mid-1950s, excelled in making garments that flattered the wearer. Her hip-length boxy jackets are a perfect example of clever cutting that allows maximum freedom and ease, while her coats provided the popular bell-shaped line that sat easily over full skirts. The soft fluid cut was her trademark and an example of Ricci's underlying design philosophy to make women ultra-feminine and beautiful. The very loose topcoat that covered all shapes of clothing was also popular until the end of the decade when shapes started to change dramatically, and billowing shapes gave way to minimalist geometric pieces.

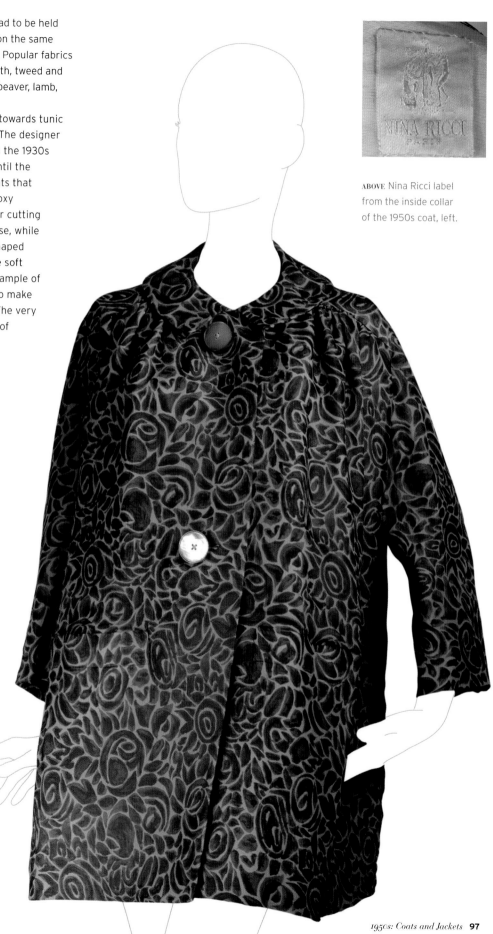

ABOVE Nina Ricci label from the inside collar of the 1950s coat, left.

BELOW One or two buttons were all that was required over clutch coats. Here a mother-of-pearl button is typical of the oversized details of the time.

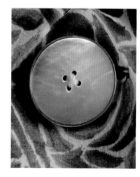

RIGHT Rose-print 1950s coat by Nina Ricci. The Peter Pan collar and soft gathers falling from the shoulderline into a voluminous bell shape were perfect over full-skirted dresses.

Christian Dior and the Corolle Line

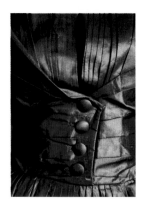

ABOVE AND RIGHT Sapphire silk taffeta dress, with buttoned pleated bodice, by Dior, 1952. Dior, who wanted to be an architect but became a fashion designer, said, 'I created flower women with gentle shoulders and generous bosoms, with tiny waists like stems and skirts belling out like petals.' His 1947 New Look hourglass silhouette harked back to the ultra-feminine belle époque ideal with voluminous long skirt and tiny cinched-in waist, and set the prevailing shape for the 1950s.

OPPOSITE Models posing in one of the last Christian Dior collections, 1957. Note the variety of Dior lines on show, and the move from the hourglass to less restricted forms.

In February 1947 a shy and balding designer from the provinces presented his first collection under his own name; few could have foreseen that a single show, heavily focused on one unfamiliar silhouette, would have such an impact around the world. Like all great designers, Christian Dior had the ability to capture the mood of the time; he recognized women's yearning for a return to femininity after the Second World War, and presented a show where the models looked quite unlike anything that had gone before. He called the collection *Ligne Corolle*, the 'Corolle line', and it was his ambition to make women look like flowers. Charming and ladylike in expensive and glamorous fabrics, his feminine ideal had rounded shoulders, a fully formed bosom and a tiny waist, sitting on top of an enormous full skirt that fell to about 30 cm (12 in) from the floor with sheer stockings and high-heeled pointy shoes. This was an astonishing innovation after 13 years of women wearing square-shouldered Schiaparelli-style suits, and Carmel Snow, the editor of American *Vogue*, dubbed the elegant shape the 'New Look'. In a single collection Dior's reputation as one of the most important couturiers in the world was assured. The look was at once an international success and inspired every fashion house to produce a similar line.

Having trained originally with Robert Piguet in 1938 (where he worked alongside Pierre Balmain) and then at the much larger house of Lucien Lelong until 1946, Dior was acknowledged as an expert cutter who employed complicated dressmaking skills to achieve his finished look. From 1950 new ideas came thick and fast and it was not only the haute couture collections that established Dior's name on a global scale. He was the first designer to license a whole range of products that introduced his label to a new type of consumer. Dior was imaginative and enjoyed playing with proportions, although his clothes were always elegant and in the very best fabrics; each couture presentation had a new theme. In 1953 he presented the Tulip collection, which featured an abundance of floral patterns and colours to stunning effect; 1955 had the A-line, a triangle shape that widened from the shoulders to a dropped waistline and then a voluminous skirt that stuck out, pleated and stiffened. Later that year came the H-line, a long slim jacket that fell to the knee, worn over an even slimmer skirt cut a few inches longer.

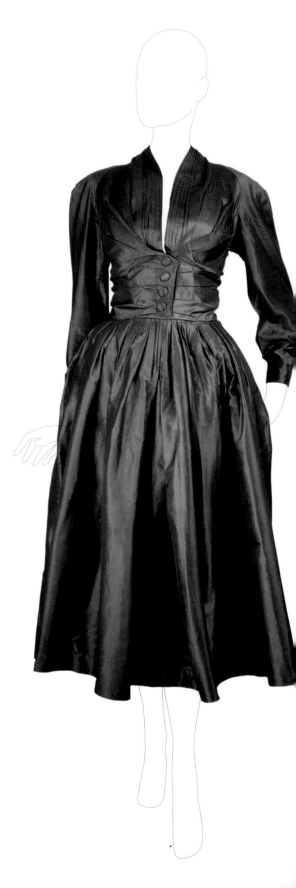

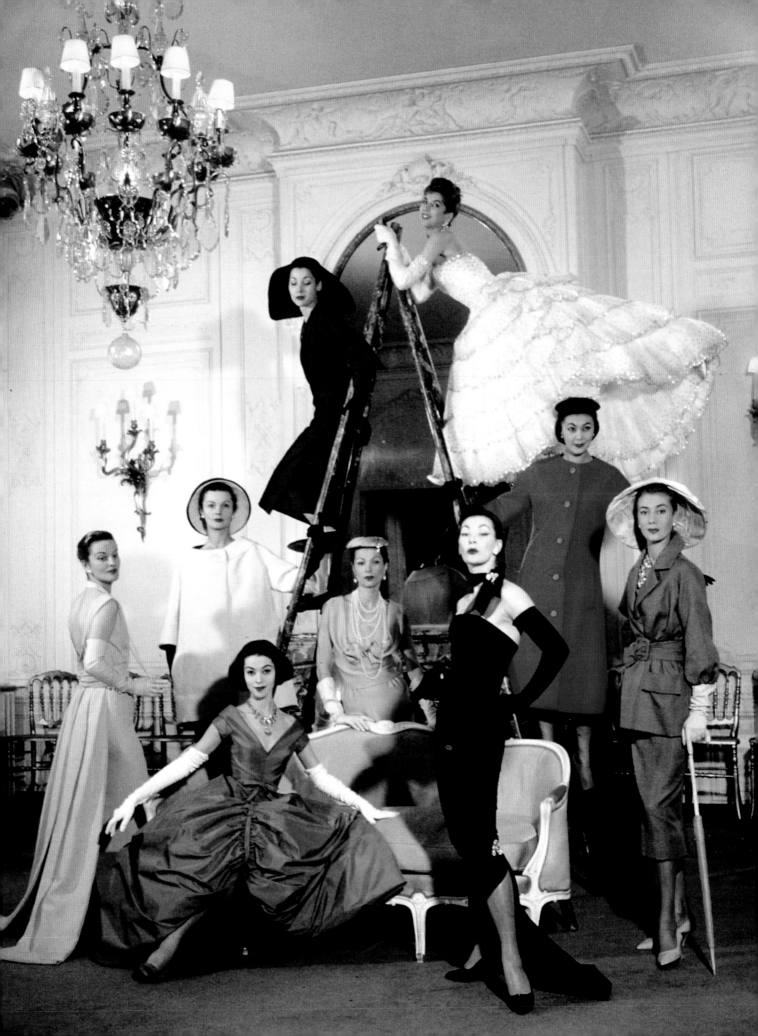

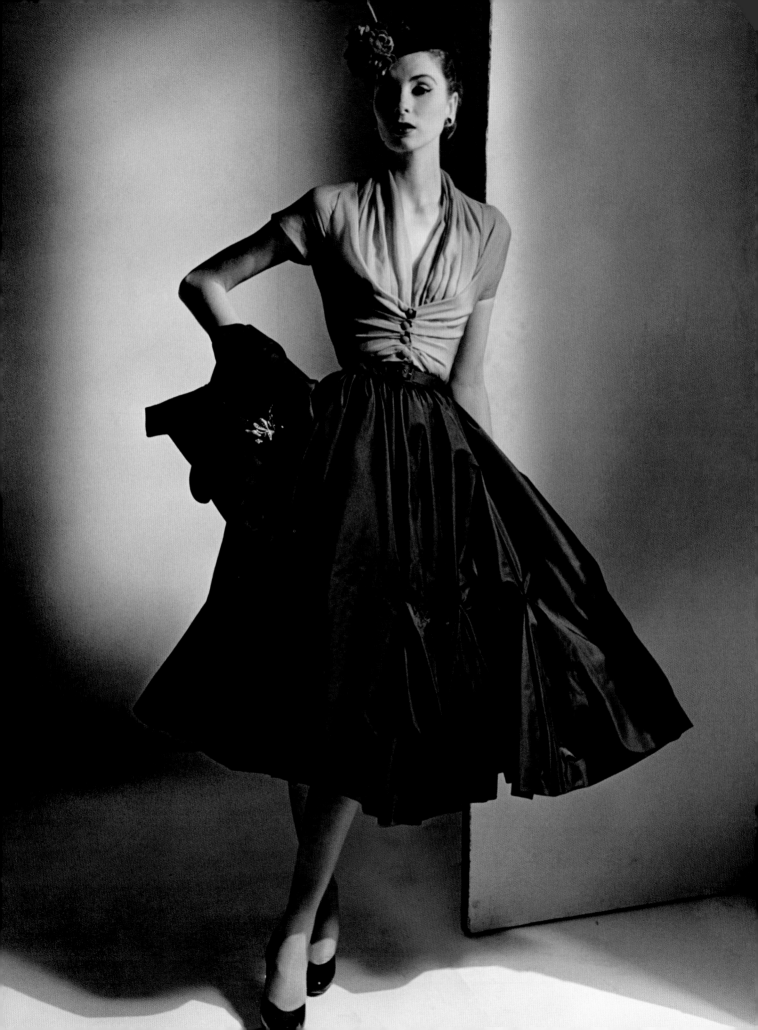

Dior favoured fine-quality men's suiting fabrics in graphic black-and-white check and pinstripe for most of his tailored pieces, and expensive velvet, satin and taffeta for eveningwear. The Y silhouette was created from an oversized V-shaped collar, cut out over the shoulders, or a large stole that was draped around the shoulderline, over a very slim sheath-type body.

From 1947 to 1957 Christian Dior presented his own version of elegance, but his clothes were ruthlessly demanding and women were expected to suffer in pursuit of old-fashioned glamour. For his final collection in 1957 the designer had at last moved attention away from the waist, and his new line appeared to be favouring a more relaxed unstructured shape, based around a simple chemise (a refinement of Givenchy's Sack dress, see page 90) with a stand-up collar and patch pockets.

His death cut short a dazzling career that had single-handedly reestablished Paris as the undisputed fashion capital of the world, and seen him dress the most prestigious women of the time, including Queen Elizabeth II and Princess Margaret, Marlene Dietrich and Princess Grace of Monaco. When he died there were Christian Dior boutiques in 24 different countries, and his company employed more than a thousand people. Today, 50 years after his death, John Galliano is head of design at Christian Dior, and the label, which is still considered to be one of the most prestigious, has gone from strength to strength. It is even now synonymous with elegance, luxury and innovation. Original Christian Dior pieces are hard to come by except in specialist vintage shops, where they often sell for many times the amount they would have in the 1950s. As Dior's clothes were made in the highest-quality fabrics and by superb technicians, they can still be found in good condition.

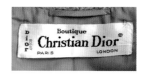

LEFT A green satin two-piece by Christian Dior, circa 1953. The off-the-shoulder bodice with bow detail has complex internal corsetry to accentuate the waist. Many of Dior's dresses had the trademark narrow belt, as shown opposite.

SIGNATURE DIOR ELEMENTS:
- Fitted jackets with peplum at the waist
- Coolie hats
- Very full skirts
- A-line coats, flared out to below the hip
- Pleated A-line skirts, stiffened to hold their own shape
- Trapeze coats with a collarless boat neck
- Deep-cut V-neck, with very wide shoulders
- Hobble skirts cut very long and narrow with a back split
- Strapless self-supporting evening gowns with a fitted bodice and full skirt

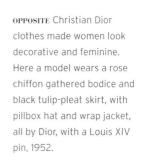

OPPOSITE Christian Dior clothes made women look decorative and feminine. Here a model wears a rose chiffon gathered bodice and black tulip-pleat skirt, with pillbox hat and wrap jacket, all by Dior, with a Louis XIV pin, 1952.

American Style

Before the war, America had bowed to Parisian superiority on the fashion front, but the war proved to be an enormous catalyst to its own fashion industry, which was not prepared to put its own manufacturing businesses on hold for five years. America was forced to look to its own designers – Norman Norell, Hattie Carnegie and Mainbocher (an American living in Paris) – who went on to become leading names at the top end of the business, as well as designers like Claire McCardell who led a thriving ready-to-wear trade.

There were other changes, too, that were responsible for the breakdown of Parisian-led couture. Technological advancements in the textile industry and manufacturing processes had increased during the war, and throughout the 1950s people started to embrace change and look for new ideas in every area of life. Better living accommodation, improved communication, and the expansion of commercial air travel all helped to further these aims, and were a reflection of the social changes taking place across the world.

The early 1950s saw the birth of the modern fashion industry as we now know it. Manufacturers realized that there was a huge demand from 'ordinary' women to follow the diktats of Parisian designers but without the restrictive costs. In Manhattan's Seventh Avenue a deal was arranged with the couture houses in Europe to buy the rights for original designer clothes, and to copy them precisely stitch for stitch. Women were now able to buy good-quality, design-led garments from department stores, and this opened the floodgates for other entrepreneurs to step in and break the stranglehold that Paris held over the fashion world. It was becoming possible for women to choose clothes from a growing ready-to-wear market that were influenced by Paris but related more to their own real lives, for which they required clothes that were based on practicality and ease.

Edith Head and the motion-picture influence

Although Edith Head had no formal design education, her career as Hollywood's most famous costume designer, working under contract for all the major studios and dressing the biggest film stars of the day, spanned more than 60 years, with some of her best work achieved during the 1950s.

Starting out as an assistant at Paramount Pictures in 1927, she was made head of design in 1938 and was responsible for dressing the really glamorous stars of the day, such as Mae West, Ginger Rogers, Grace Kelly and Elizabeth Taylor. Although Head did not consider herself a couturier, she became a great American 'taste maker', known for designing beautiful and flattering clothes that the movie-going public wanted to copy. In *Sunset Boulevard* (1950) her clothes for the ageing silent film star Norma Desmond (Gloria Swanson)

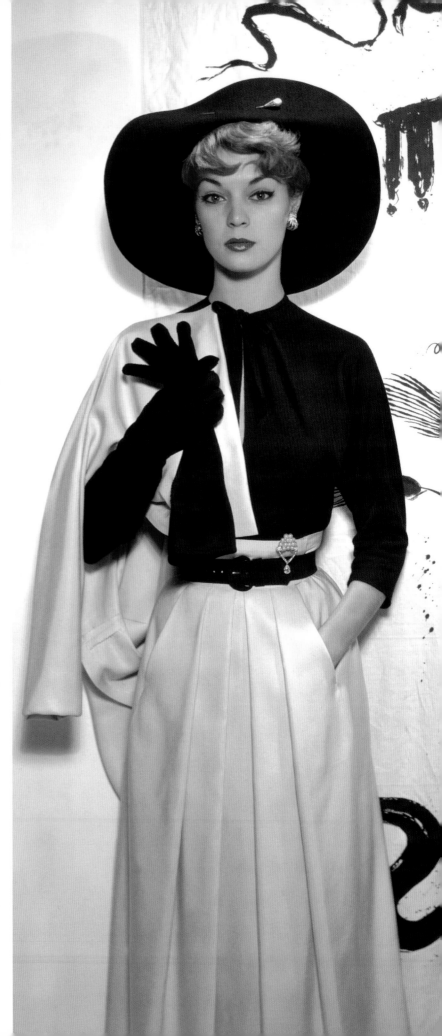

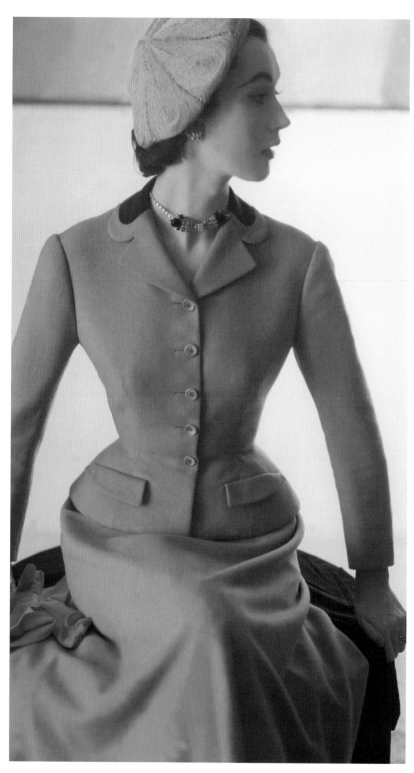

brilliantly captured a bygone era. Although she dressed Audrey Hepburn in some beautifully tailored pieces for *Roman Holiday* (1953), it was Hubert de Givenchy who designed most of Hepburn's wardrobe for *Sabrina* (1954), even though Head collected the Academy Award that year for Best Costume Design for the film. As Head's reputation grew outside Hollywood, the studio publicity department ensured that the name Edith Head became synonymous with home-grown American fashion. As a designer she was extremely versatile but tended towards clean simplistic lines in a subdued palette with minimum details.

Youth trends and casual clothes

Throughout all this the American ready-to-wear market kept quietly expanding, with the emphasis on leisurewear, and clothes that combined functionality with good design. The ever-growing teen market was demanding clothes that related to young lives, not their mothers, and America was the first country to recognize the business potential of a new consumer group who were very different from adults. Designers began to take notice. In the 1940s the teenager as a separate entity simply did not exist; young people copied adult taste, and wore scaled-down versions of their parent's clothes. But in the 1950s companies in America started to see the financial advantages of creating a separate youth market, and adolescents were targeted with their own products made especially for them. This was the beginning of the young woman being seen as a potent commercial force, whereas previously fashion had always been aimed at a mature woman (between 30 and 40 years of age) of comfortable means.

The most notable young fashions of the time were simple and easily adopted by a broad cross-section of people. Marlon Brando, James Dean and Elvis Presley were influencing teenagers who increasingly wanted their own style of fashion and music. Rock 'n' roll had arrived, and with it a teenage look of straight black jeans and leather jacket for boys (as exemplified by Marlon Brando in *The Wild One*, 1953) and for girls a 'poodle' skirt (a long full skirt that often had an overstitched poodle on it), bobby socks and saddle shoes, and a tight sweater. The sporty American look of girls in tight slacks, flat ballet-style pumps and a short-sleeved sweater had a parallel existence at the end of the decade as the Parisian beatniks adopted it as their chic black uniform worn by the existentialist crowd in smoky jazz clubs and cafés.

OPPOSITE Valentina Sanina operated as Valentina. Here is her 1950 oyster-white silk grosgrain skirt and jacket, with black hat, belt, gloves and jersey blouse.

ABOVE Suit by Hattie Carnegie in aquamarine blue wool with a velvet collar, and beret, 1952. Carnegie specialized in creating an entire look.

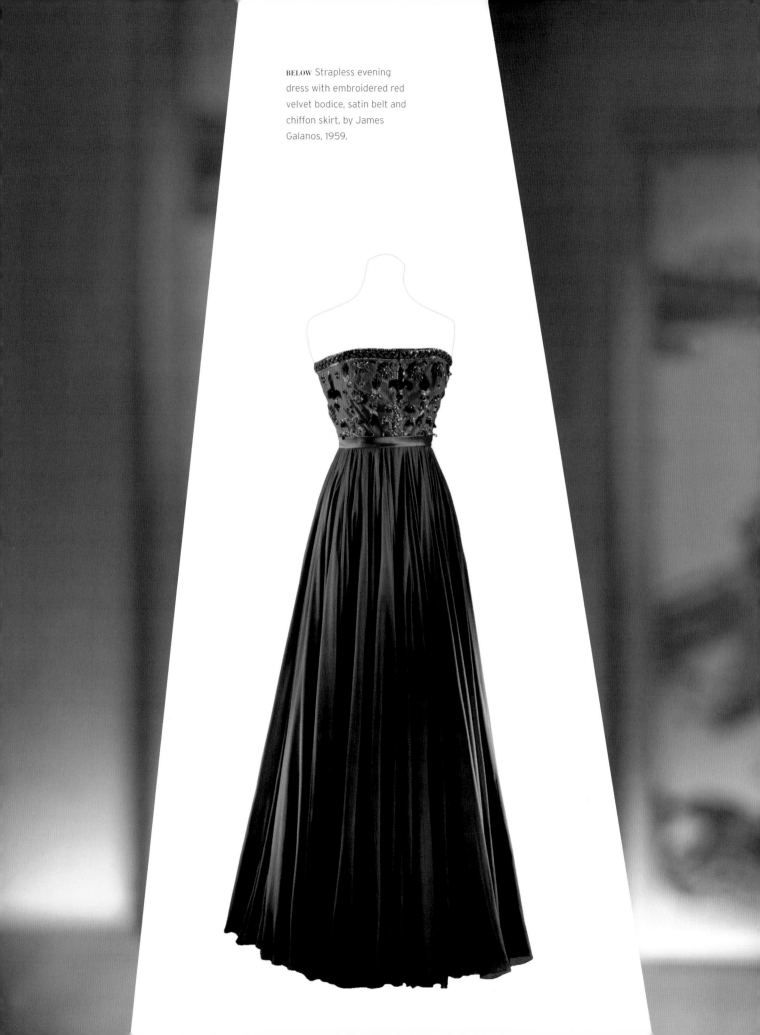

BELOW Strapless evening dress with embroidered red velvet bodice, satin belt and chiffon skirt, by James Galanos, 1959.

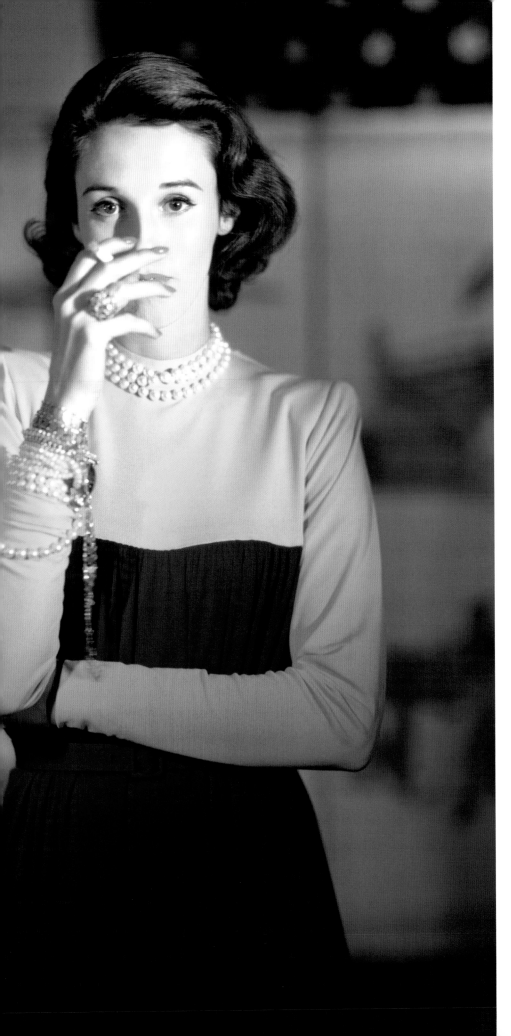

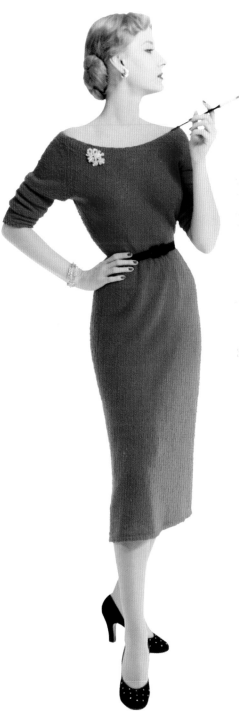

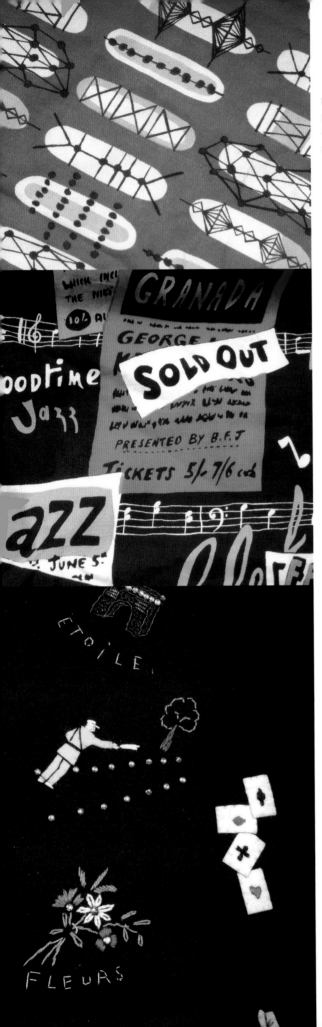

Prints and Fabrics

The 1950s were a decade awash with imaginative prints and surfaces adorned with embroidery and beading – popular for both daywear and glamorous eveningwear. After the drab 1940s, decorative fabrics with highly stylized graphic prints and detailed beading and appliqué stood out as something new and modern. America was the instigator of the explosion in leisure wear, and in the popular way print was used for dresses, circle skirts and shirtdresses.

New developments in fibres and production resulted in fashion knits, which were adopted by the teen market to wear casually over ski pant-style slacks and dirndl skirts. Chunky knits with open-neck collars in soft pastel shades of baby blue and canary yellow were staples of weekend leisurewear, and could even be washed by machine. Fine-gauge knits were commonly embellished with complex glass beading, either in a decorative flower pattern along both sides of a cardigan opening or in paisley-style patterns that adorned the cuffs and neckline. Sequins were used in the same way on cardigans and short-sleeved turtleneck sweaters.

Decorative surface detailing was common for day in the form of ricrac braiding and hand embroidery, but for evening sequins and beads were an essential ingredient of grown-up glamour. Norman Norell created a range of shimmery, sequined dresses that were sheath-like in style with a low neck and cut just above the knee. Strapless prom-style dresses were commonly decorated with sequins or beads around the whole of the bodice area.

Another 1950s staple that people immediately associate with the decade was very loud prints. Used for skirts, slacks and men's shirts, they ranged from florals to small repeat patterns. The popular shirtwaisted dress and gathered skirts that were fitted tight around the waist and gently flared out to below the knee, all came in small all-over prints, many intricate in design. Circles joined up with triangles and elongated trapeziums all interconnected in different colours on a plain background. Bright floral prints of tulips, roses and marigolds were common prints for housecoats and circular skirts, especially in hues of bold turquoise, red and pink.

Leisurewear took off in a big way and in America the wholesome girl-next-door, as typified by Doris Day, often wore a 'poodle' skirt that had very stylized graphic prints of cowboy and western paraphernalia, futuristic atomic prints, or small poodle-dog prints. Some of these skirts had handpainted patterns, or dog cutouts made of felt with a collar and pretend chain embroidered on to the fabric. Gaudy prints and colours were also part of the male wardrobe in the form of short-sleeved Hawaiian shirts, which became standard leisurewear in America, along with boxer-style swimming trunks.

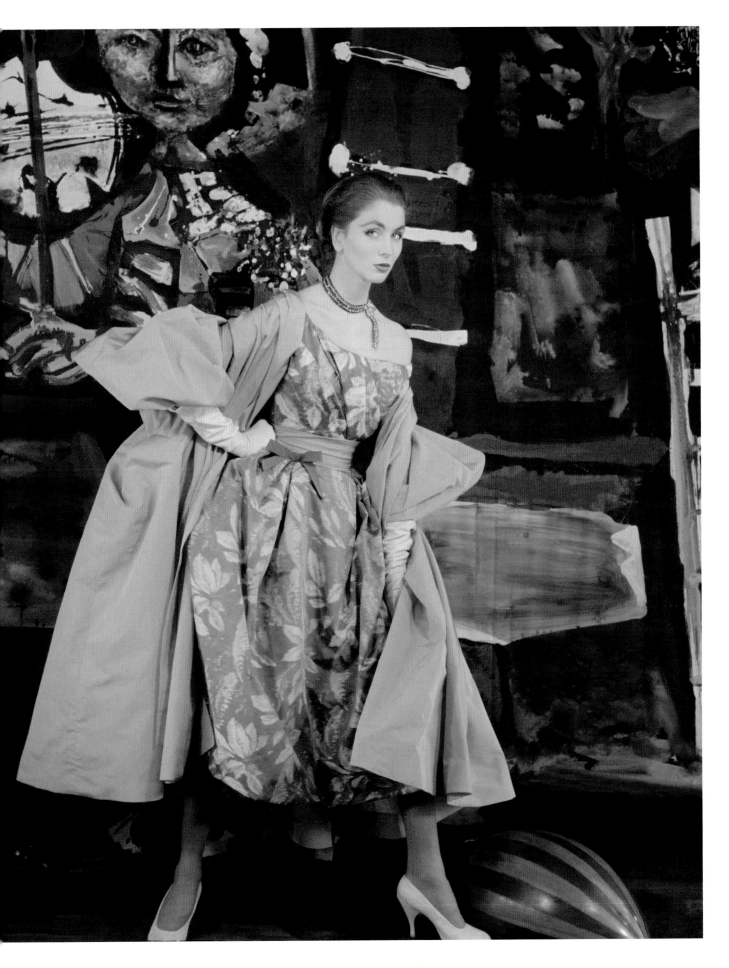

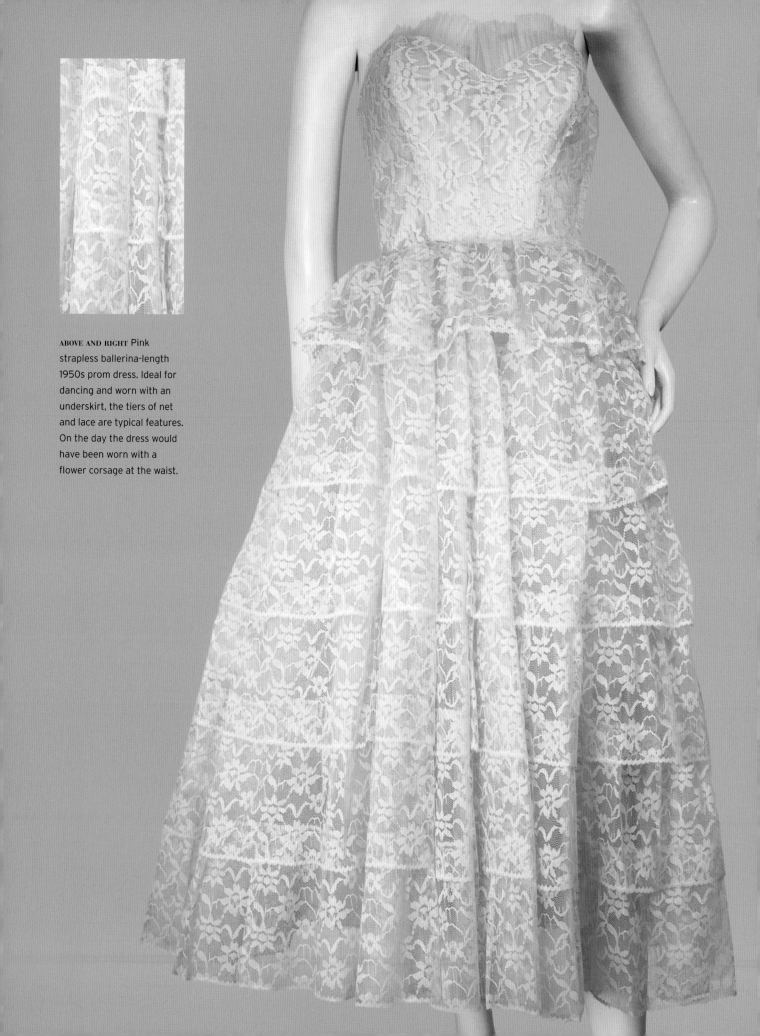

ABOVE AND RIGHT Pink strapless ballerina-length 1950s prom dress. Ideal for dancing and worn with an underskirt, the tiers of net and lace are typical features. On the day the dress would have been worn with a flower corsage at the waist.

Fabrics and synthetics

Mass manufacturing really took off in the 1950s, resulting in the greatest changes for women's clothing in history. The Second World War saw advancements in manufacturing processes and standards of production, all of which were put to good use in the fashion industry when the war was over. For the first part of the century designers were restricted to using basic wool, cotton and silk for their creations, but after the war the developments in manmade fabrics were rapid, and the textile industry provided them with endless new fabric variations to work with.

There are two distinct and defining fabrics that belong to the era. The first is fine English worsted suiting and Irish tweed cloth as favoured by English designers such as Norman Hartnell and Hardy Amies – which were grandly associated with the aristocracy and royalty. These weaves were hugely popular with Parisian designers, too, because of their finesse and quality, and they were used for the formal suits and coats of the early 1950s. Plaid, houndstooth and dogstooth check were perfect for the slim, straight ladylike skirts, and Christian Dior was particularly fond of black-and-white Prince of Wales check for his tailored pieces (see also the Worth suit, page 90).

The ongoing production of synthetics was also influential in the development of 1950s fashions. Nylon, which had been used to make parachutes during the war, was continually refined until it became gossamer-thin. It became integral to the look, used to make layers of stiffened petticoats, which supported the circular skirt. Nylon was also fundamental in the development of foundation garments that were becoming increasingly important to the fashion industry. The self-supporting strapless dresses of the time were all kept in place by an elaborate substructure of nylon corseting, and the invention of 12-denier stockings, which were almost invisible, reinforced the stereotypical ladylike image of the period. Today manmade fibres are considered fine for sportswear, but distinctly tawdry for designer clothes; back then new synthetics like rayon were seen as miracle fabrics because of their silk-like properties to touch, and also because they could hold a shape.

Thick pullovers in baby blue and primrose yellow Courtelle became wardrobe staples worn with a scarf tied at the neck, especially over black stretch pants. Sheer fabrics were very popular for eveningwear, frequently used for decorum on shoulders or arms, and as top layers over a solid fabric for dresses and skirts. This stream of new fabrics – acrylic, polyester, acetate and Spandex – changed women's lives, as they were able to indulge in clean clothes every day. Manufacturers enthusiastically produced and promoted Crimplene blouses in white and pale pastel colours, promising that they could be easily washed and left to drip-dry in minutes.

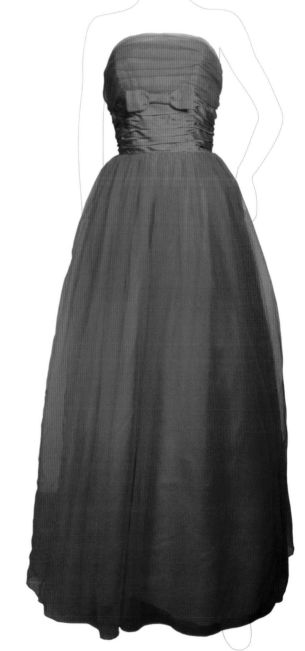

RIGHT Strapless 1950s red nylon ballgown from Harrod's own label, England, with pleated bodice and bow detail. Nylon, a new synthetic, was considered a high-end product and perfectly acceptable in designer fashions.

FEATURES OF 1950S PROM DRESSES:

❖ Fitted strapless bodice
❖ Full skirt to below the knee
❖ Tiers of lace and tulle
❖ Synthetic fabrics, such as acrylic and polyester
❖ Coloured net petticoats
❖ Fabric or paper corsage worn on the bodice or at the waist
❖ Plain bright colours
❖ Worn with matching long gloves and loud costume jewellery in the form of brooches or strings of pearls

Gloves

Women wore short kid leather gloves for formal daywear, and in the evening long satin gloves were worn to complement their strapless cocktail dresses and evening gowns. The fashionable look was to wear them pushed down with big glitzy bracelets over the top.

Slacks

Old-fashioned, ski-pant-style trousers were made from synthetic stretch fabric in plain fabrics or multicoloured plaid. Tailored to fit the body, they had a flat front waistband and side zip opening; they epitomized the casual look in America's growing leisurewear market.

▶Ballet shoes

Simple flat black pumps based on a classic ballet shoe became popular in 1950s America and Europe. They were mass produced and worn with ankle socks and full skirts, or with bare feet and cut-off capri pants.

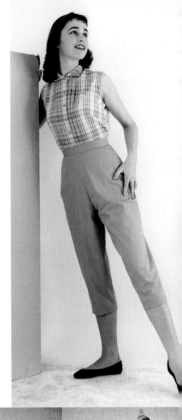

▼Net petticoats

Layers of petticoats were worn under full skirts to give lift and movement; they were stiffened with starch or a sugar solution to keep their form. Tiered petticoats made from nylon tulle gave a softer look that was less ballroom-dancing in style. They gave form and volume to many styles of 1950s ballgowns.

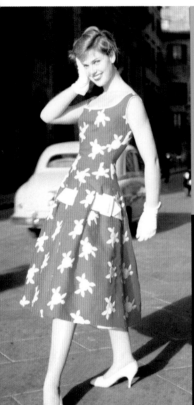

Key looks of the decade

1950s

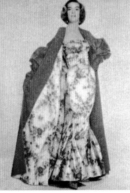
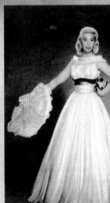
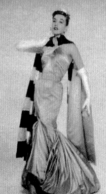

Hats

Pull-down bucket hats, small lampshade-style hats, coolie hats and wide-brimmed flat picture hats made from coloured straw were all popular shapes. Black and white were used to graphic effect and for grand occasions, and women often wore a formal black net veil.

Pencil skirts

A narrow, slim straight skirt called the 'hobble', and first pioneered by Poiret, restricted women's walking. It fell from a narrow waistband with little excess fabric, no gathers or pleats and usually a small back split that allowed for movement.

Empire lines

The Little Black Dress that Givenchy designed for Audrey Hepburn in Breakfast at Tiffany's (1961) is a much-copied classic of the era. The straight empire-line shift dress, cut to the knee with narrow shoulders and a high boat neckline, was given iconic status when she wore it with big black sunglasses and pearls.

Fur stoles

The most popular style of eveningwear was strapless, and the addition of a large fur stole wrapped around bare shoulders, sometimes fastened with a large brooch, became the most fashionable way to keep covered in the evening.

Oversized detailing

The decade's tailoring embraced oversized details in the form of large shawl collars, giant buttons and big turn-back cuffs on wide square-cut sleeves with very deep armholes, known as dolman sleeves.

Trapeze coats

The loose swing coat, that was sometimes called a 'tent' and resembled a triangle in shape, was made to accommodate the wide skirts of the time, and the post-war pregnancy boom. Many were given a diverging set of buttons designed to emphasize the triangle shape of the cut.

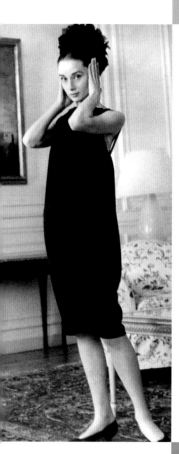

◀ Sack dress

The waistless Givenchy Sack dress, as modelled here by Audrey Hepburn in 1958, finally freed the figure from the restrictive hourglass.

Sheath dress

The fitted sheath clung to a woman's body shape. In satin or silk, it was usually strapless and required considerable corseting.

Wide belts

A small waist was emphasized for almost every fashionable look throughout the decade. Either with a full dirndl skirt or a straight pencil skirt, or with sporty slacks or capri pants, a big wide belt was a must-have fashion accessory.

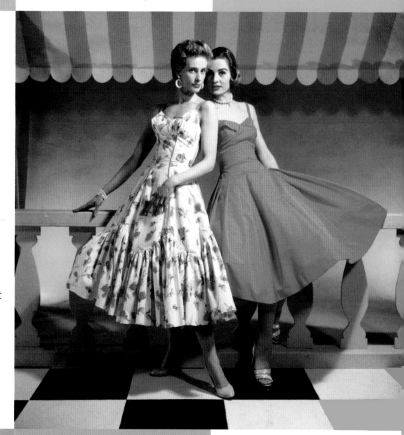

Pedal pushers and capris

Half-length trousers, either cuffed or flounced at the hem or cut narrow, were prominant from high street to high fashion. Capris were slimline pant and most had a small V at the hem to enable greater mobility. Here Natalie Wood models a strapless top and pedal pushers in the 1950s.

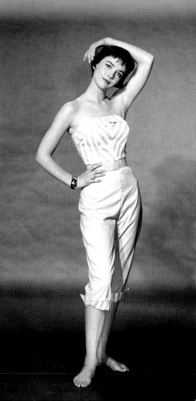

▲ Full skirts

Wide circular skirts were worn for daywear in simple fabrics like gingham and printed cottons. They sometimes had a big bold design, like a poodle or American cowboy motifs, printed on them. For eveningwear full skirts were made from layers of frothy chiffon or rayon in the most vibrant of colours – canary yellow, baby blue and lime green.

Sweater dressing

The short-sleeved turtleneck worn tight and fitted, and the big bulky pastel-coloured sweater were favourites for teenagers and movie stars alike. The invention of the twinset, with its sleeveless crew-necked vest and matching cardigan with neat pearl buttons and decorative beading, became a 1950s staple.

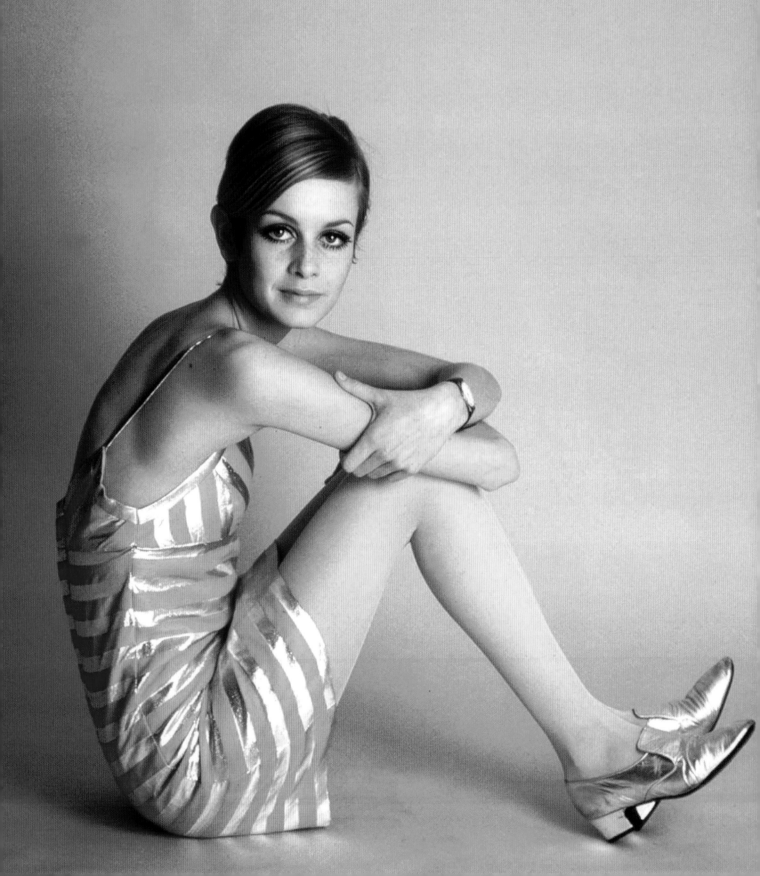

1960s

The Swinging '60s, as they became known, heralded an extraordinary decade of change after the austerity and reconstruction of the 1950s. The fashion zeitgeist was changing direction and whereas in previous generations it was always Paris that had led the way, now the whole world looked to London. When in 1960 a 24-year-old Yves Saint Laurent showed what was to be his final collection for Christian Dior, and sent out a cool Beat collection of black leather suits and knitted caps to an astonished and slightly bewildered audience, he effectively sounded the death knell of French haute couture. With the rumblings of a revolution well under way in a party atmosphere in London, this was a defining moment when fashion turned a corner. Labels such as 'formal' and 'casual' dressing, which existed in the previous decade, ceased to have any meaning at all. As new styles arrived in small London boutiques on a weekly basis, the savvy shopper quickly learnt that fresh stock was delivered in the evenings and they hung around to make sure they were first to grab the latest looks. It was in the 1960s that fashion became absolutely central to a young person's identity. For the first time ever there was a generation of young people with money to spend, looking for ways to express their newfound sense of freedom through fashion, music and lifestyle. The generational power balance had shifted: young people were making things happen for themselves and taking great pleasure in doing so, while simultaneously thumbing their noses at the old-guard Establishment.

The British Explosion

Britain, and London in particular, was where everyone wanted to be, and the 'Youthquake' explosion that affected every area of popular culture gathered pace as the decade wore on. It was a time when young talented people, regardless of class or background, were determined to make revolutionary changes and demand recognition for what they did. Image was everything; fresh-faced photographers such as David Bailey, Terence Donovan and Brian Duffy changed the style of photography from formal studio-based portraiture to energetic street-style 'reality'. The models they worked with – Twiggy, Jean Shrimpton ('the Shrimp') and Verushka – became icons of their time for their playful poses and quirky looks.

The Beatles and the Rolling Stones changed the look and sound of music, and on the streets there were new and exciting boutiques springing up in Carnaby Street and the King's Road. Typically small, dark and deafeningly loud with the current pop music of the day, they flourished overnight and in many cases simply disappeared just as quickly. Owned and run by ambitious individuals, they were united by the weirdest of names: Granny Takes A Trip, Mr Freedom, Hung On You and I Was Lord Kitchener's Valet. Fashion was no longer dictated by middle-aged Parisian designers, and the demand by London's young 'dolly birds' to wear whatever they wanted, whenever and wherever they felt like it, was being met by a host of up-and-coming British design stars who were spilling out from art schools. The Royal College of Art Fashion Department was run by Professor Jayney Ironside, who became a legendary figure for her ability to spot and nurture a generation of young talents, many of whom went on to become internationally famous. Zandra Rhodes, Bill Gibb, Ossie Clark, Marion Foale and Sally Tuffin were all students under her tutorage. These and many others – including Gina Fratini, Anthony Price, Yuki and Thea Porter – were part of a mushrooming band of designers who were responsible for turning London into a leading fashion capital. Not all the bright young things who were helping to build Britain's fashionable reputation had a fashion degree; some had simply arrived at the same place by a different route.

Mary Quant, undoubtedly an early trailblazer of the Youthquake movement, had studied illustration at Goldsmiths, before setting up a tiny shop in 1955 with her then boyfriend and business partner Alexander Plunkett-Green. Barbara Hulanicki, the owner and designer behind the hugely influential Biba boutiques, started out as a fashion illustrator before deciding to try designing something she liked instead of illustrating other people's clothes. Jean Muir, who went on to become one of the leading British names for understated classics, started out as a sketcher for Jaeger.

PAGE 112 Model, muse and icon Twiggy in a gold-and-orange striped minidress in the 1960s.

OPPOSITE A 1960s advertisement for Mary Quant dresses in the new synthetic Courtelle. The classic minidress featured a zip down the front with a circular pull-ring.

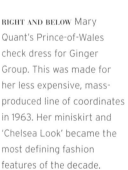

RIGHT AND BELOW Mary Quant's Prince-of-Wales check dress for Ginger Group. This was made for her less expensive, mass-produced line of coordinates in 1963. Her miniskirt and 'Chelsea Look' became the most defining fashion features of the decade.

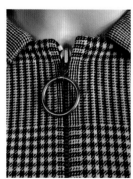

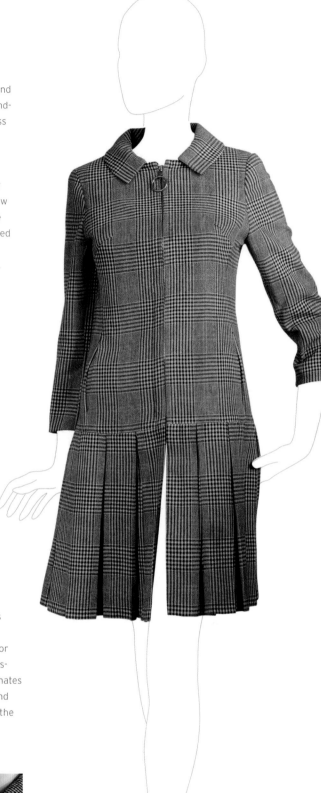

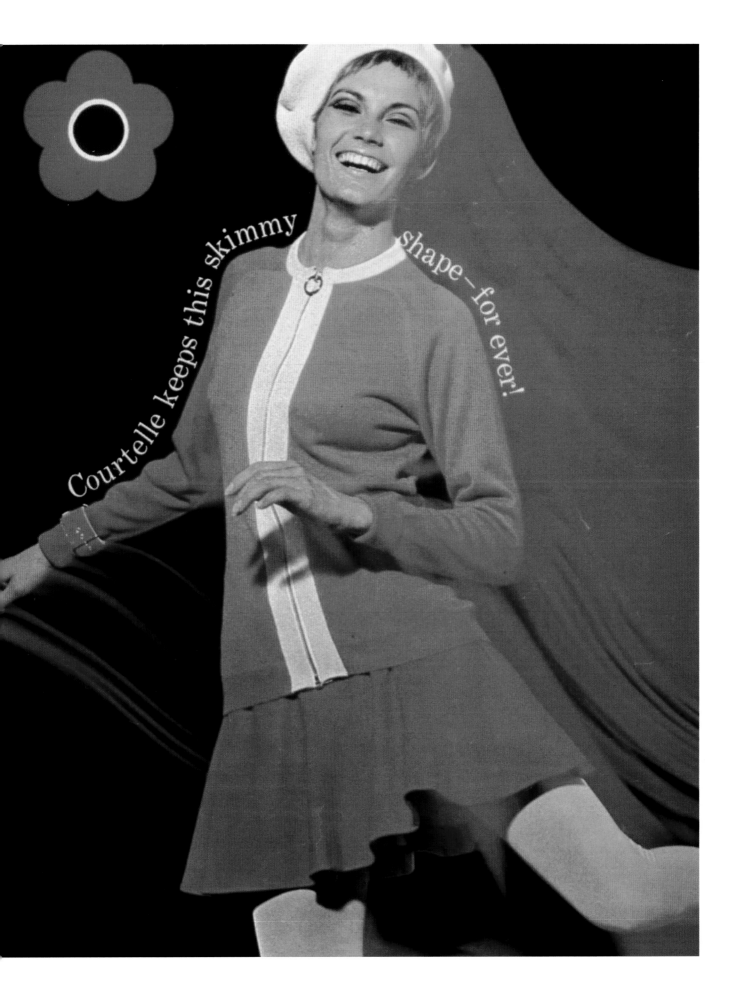

Courtelle keeps this skimmy shape—for ever!

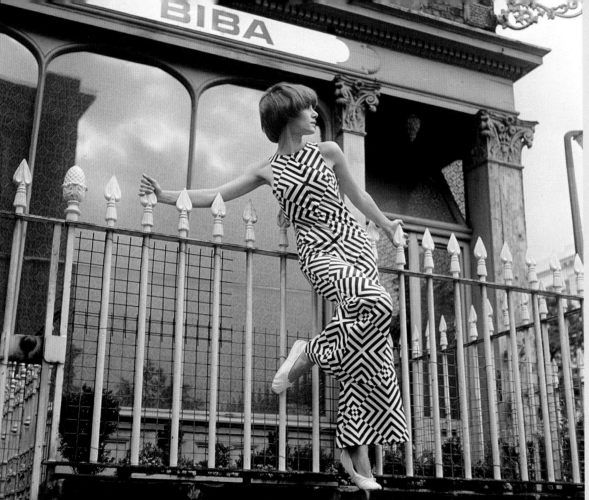

SIGNATURE BIBA ELEMENTS:

- Droopy low-cut necklines with ties
- Button detailing, as long rows of covered buttons on cuffs or at the neck
- Leg-of-mutton sleeves
- All-over small prints
- Funnel collars with buttons
- Bias cutting on long dresses
- Coloured fake-fur shrugs and tippets
- Maxi-length double-breasted trench coats

LEFT Model wearing a Biba Op Art jumpsuit outside the Abingdon Road shop in London, 1967.

Biba

The Biba label was a huge success from the time Barbara Hulanicki opened her first little shop in Abingdon Road, Kensington, in 1964 through to the eventual demise of the Biba lifestyle store in Kensington High Street in 1975. Hulanicki broke all the rules for dressing, and created whole outfits including a matching make-up range, which meant that people could dress entirely in Biba. From head to toe, hats, scarves, underwear, tights and shoes could all be bought in the same soft muted colours to create an entire look – something no other designer had considered at the time.

From her initial mail-order catalogue called Biba's Postal Boutique, which she and her business manager husband Stephen Fitz Simon started in 1963, the Biba style offered a unique look for young women. The clothes were cheap, which made them even more desirable for the young working-class customer who wanted to dress fashionably. For the same price as a Mary Quant dress, a girl could walk out of Biba with a new coat, dress, shoes and hat. The Biba look was also overtly soft and feminine (not the short, sharp, angular tailoring of other 1960s designers), with droopy collars, gathered-in sleeves, flared skirts and long-line waistcoats. Daywear fabrics often had an all-over small print, either mini floral sprays reminiscent of 1940s teadresses or zig-zag geometric designs. Fabrics for

daywear tended to be soft wool jersey or crepe – fabrics that allowed movement and gathering. Trademark design elements were big leg-of-mutton sleeves, falling tight into long cuffs with rows of covered buttons, long rounded collars and waistcoats with flared panels, cut to the same length as the miniskirt. For evening Hulanicki's obsession with the glamorous 1920s and '30s resulted in her 1960s mixture of Art Nouveau and Art Deco. She favoured dark smudgy colours, from the black and gold of the Biba logo to chocolate brown, all shades of grape and smudgy petrol blue. Fabrics were shiny satins and panne velvet, topped off with a matching feather boa. By the early 1970s leopardskin was big, worn with wide fake-fur collars and shrugs.

When Biba closed its doors in 1975, few people would have imagined that the designs would become collectors' items. At the time they were seen as the fashion equivalent of the rock 'n' roll epitaph 'Live Fast, Die Young', clothes that were fantastically appropriate for their immediacy but with little ongoing mileage. They were, of course, incredibly cheap and notoriously badly made, which suited the customer of the time. Twenty years ago, Biba pieces could be found at jumble sales and secondhand market stalls. Now they are seen as covetable pieces of history.

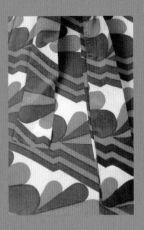

ABOVE AND OPPOSITE LEFT Art Deco print rayon late 1960s Biba dress, with a pussy-bow tie neckline. Past eras, such as Art Deco and Edwardian periods, were evident in Barbara Hulanicki's designs, which eventually included homewares and interiors as well as clothes.

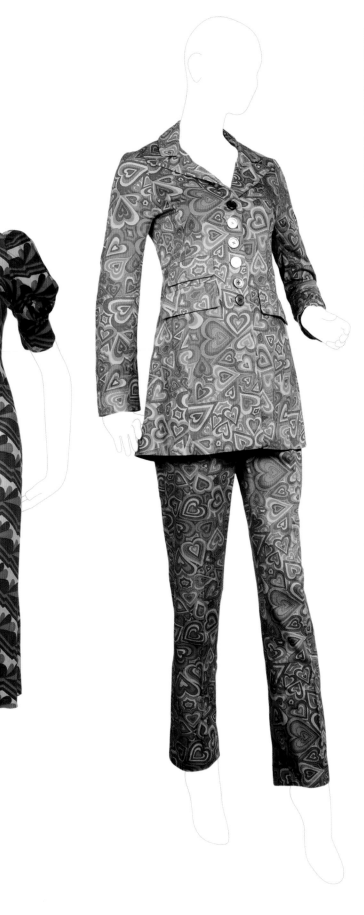

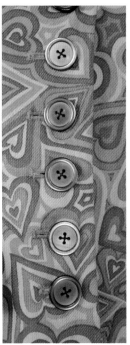

ABOVE AND LEFT Psychedelic-print heart-motif 1967/8 Biba suit from the Abingdon Road shop, featuring a neat line of buttons. Loud and clashing coloured prints were snapped up by the decade's hip young things.

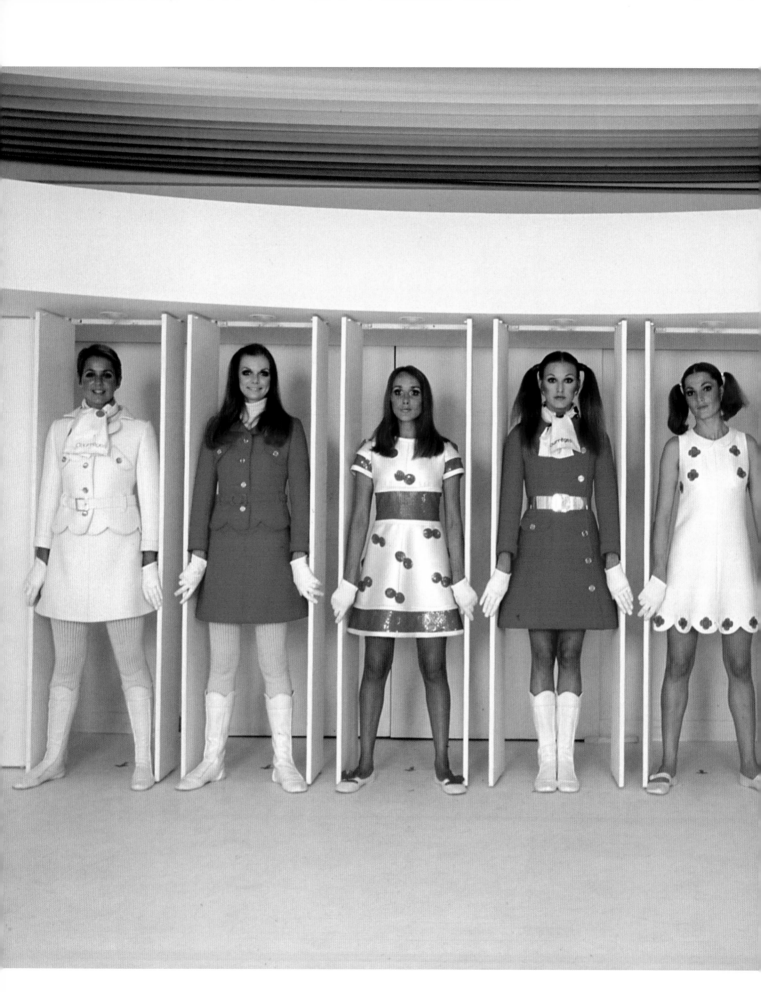

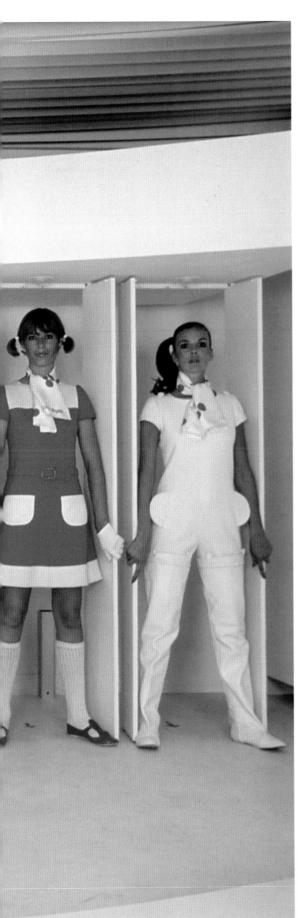

Space Age Design

Where London led, Paris followed, and soon the prêt-à-porter collections of young Parisian designers were generating new headlines around the fashion world. Inspired by the Yuri Gagarin space race in 1961, such designers as André Courrèges and Pierre Cardin produced futuristic collections using a limited colour palette of shimmering white and silver. These 'space age' clothes, based on a fantasy vision of life in the year 2000, were modernistic, minimal and designed around straight shapes and clean-cut lines. Superfluous decoration was discarded in favour of A-line tunics, short straight skirts and flat kid-leather boots.

When French designer André Courrèges showed his Moon Girl collection in 1964, it was a show that was defined by straight lines and boxy shapes without a frill in sight. Simplicity was the key, and he offered lean trouser suits with straight-legged pants that had a slit up the front seam to fall open over his flat boots; square-cut coats with very little detailing, mostly single-breasted with simple pocket tabs at the hips; and the shortest miniskirts in Paris. Accessories of white

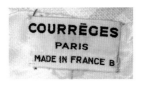

ABOVE AND BELOW Lime-and-white 1960s Courrèges jacket with inside collar label. The jacket exhibits the Bauhaus-influenced designer's streamlined, modernist structuring. By inserting rounded forms into his designs he created a curvilinear shape.

OPPOSITE Red and white ready-to-wear fashions designed by André Courrèges, 1968.

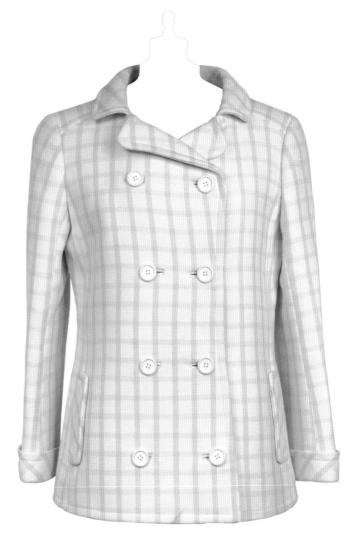

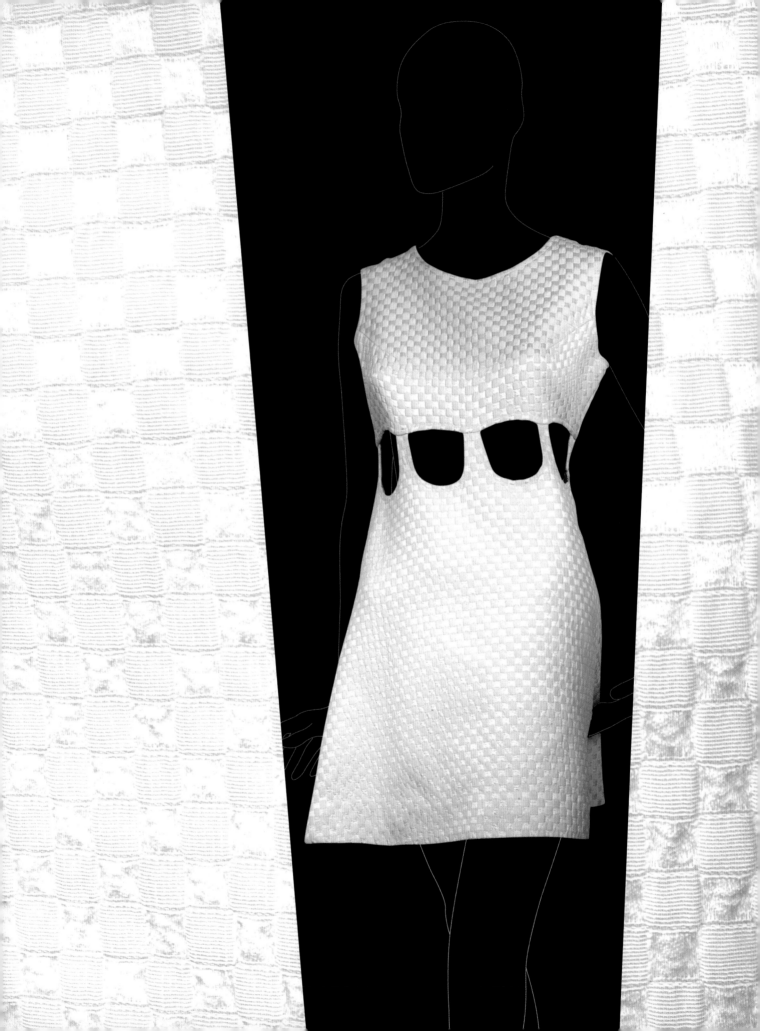

oversized goggle sunglasses and smooth helmet-style hats completed the 'moon girl' look. Freedom of movement was paramount, and his young models, all in white kid booties, strode down the catwalks with a purposeful bounce.

The hard, straight lines of these clothes, together with the angular girls who were wearing them, led inevitably to unisex clothing. Sonny and Cher appeared together in his-and-hers striped hipster pants that were cut low across the hips and worn with a big belt, fringed leather waistcoats and simple T-shirts. It was a must-have look for young couples who wanted to appear identical and share everything.

The hugely talented Yves Saint Laurent was one of the few designers able to make the leap from the sumptuous postwar Paris of the 1950s to the youthful vigour and freedom required by fashion in the 1960s. Having started in haute couture for the house of Dior, he quickly embraced the breakdown of the old society and invented Rive Gauche, his ready-to-wear label, in 1962. As a designer who found inspiration from a world in transition, he exerted a considerable influence throughout the decade. From an early collection based on Mondrian's geometric blocks of colour and graphic black lines used on a white jersey tunic dress, through to his motif moon, heart and face Pop Art dresses, and later his vivid gipsy collection, Saint Laurent's collections captured the mood of the street in a stylized way. Many of his designs, such as safari jackets and transparent dresses, became staples that transcended the decade. Most importantly, his 1966 classic tuxedo suit for women, 'Le Smoking', paved the way to androgynous fashion and 1980s power suits.

'SPACE AGE' STYLES:
- Mini pinafore dresses
- Graphic black-and-white designs and prints
- White and silver plastic
- Plastic detailing
- Metal chain dresses, tops and tunics
- Metal jewellery incorporated into dresses, especially at the neckline
- Cutouts in dresses and trousers
- Oversized patch pockets
- Asymmetric cutting
- See-through mesh
- PVC coats, trousers and dresses

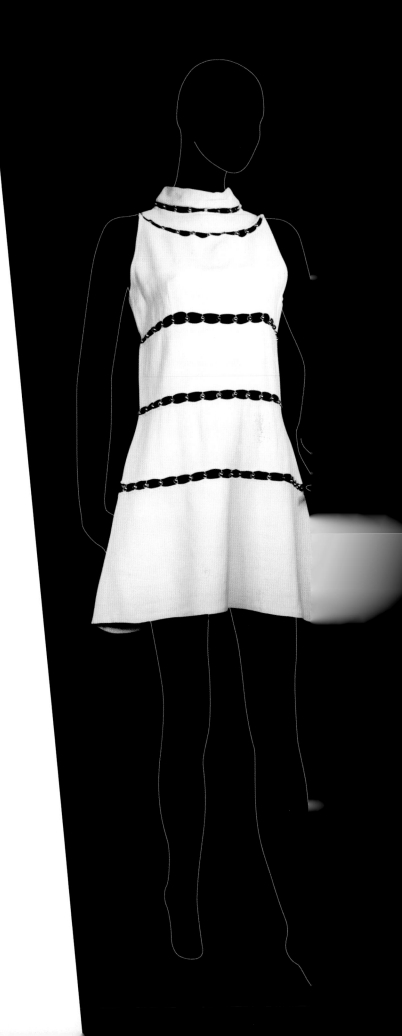

OPPOSITE White Louis Féraud minidress with cut-outs, late 1960s. After his 1960 catwalk collection, Féraud was contracted to Oleg Cassini, which made him available to North America and Britain.

RIGHT Louis Féraud white minidress with silver bead cutouts, late 1960s. White and silver combinations were used to create a futuristic look and denote youth and newness.

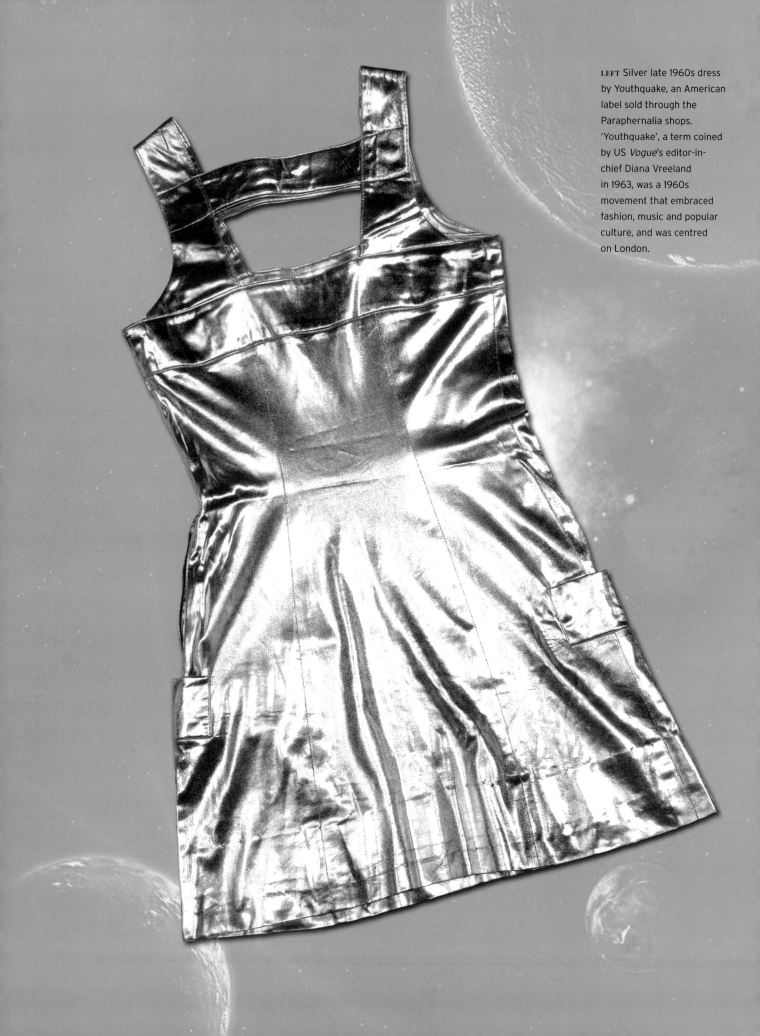

LEFT Silver late 1960s dress by Youthquake, an American label sold through the Paraphernalia shops. 'Youthquake', a term coined by US *Vogue*'s editor-in-chief Diana Vreeland in 1963, was a 1960s movement that embraced fashion, music and popular culture, and was centred on London.

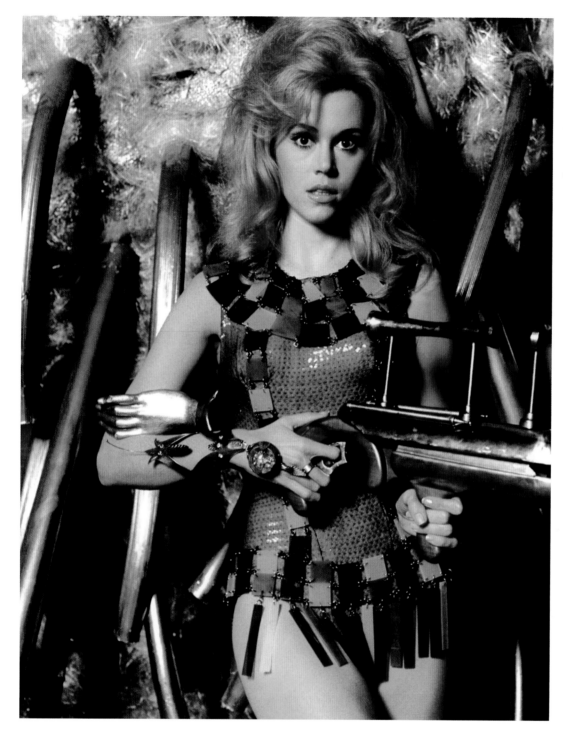

LEFT Jane Fonda wearing a costume by Paco Rabanne in *Barbarella*, 1968. Coco Chanel called Rabanne the 'metallurgist' and he not only experimented with chainmetal, leather and plastic but also with paper, Plexiglas and elastic bandages.

Paco Rabanne took the New Age idea even further by creating clothes from materials not normally associated with fashion. Plastic discs, pieces of scrap metal and chainmail were all crafted into angular shapes that were thought of as half sculpture, half fashion.

His unusual approach to fashion came about ostensibly because he had trained to be an architect not a fashion designer, although during his student years he had sold fashion accessory sketches to Courrèges, Cardin and Balenciaga, who had all encouraged his creativity. In 1966 Rabanne produced a resolutely modern collection of 12 experimental and slightly unwearable dresses, that were shown barefooted models who danced down the catwalk to loud music. Using a rigid plastic called Rhodoid, metal, pliers and a blowtorch, he eliminated sewing and created clothing by lying a woman on his work table and shaping metal parts on to her body. His experimental creations were very much in keeping with what young modern women wanted to be seen in, and Rabanne continued to innovate with paper dresses in 1967 and later seamless dresses made by spraying vinyl chloride on to pre-shaped moulds. He will be remembered for his 1969 gold-metal sculptured dress, and for his costumes for Jane Fonda in the sci-fi movie *Barbarella*.

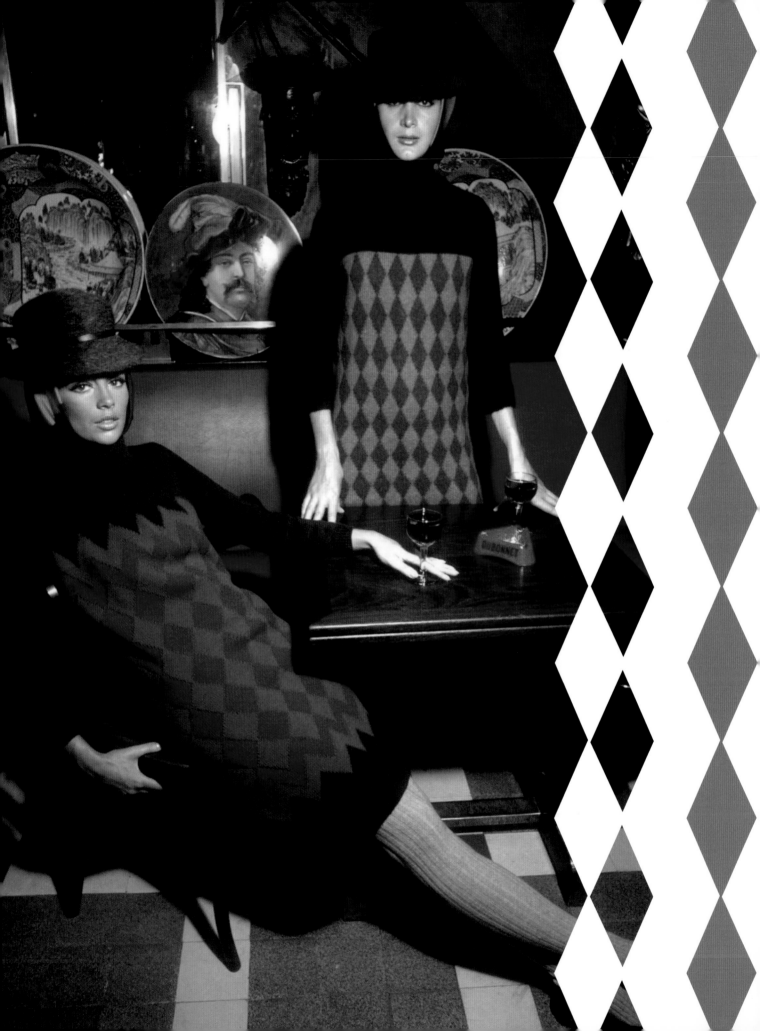

Simple Shapes and Cuts

The endless stream of exciting designers who burst into production at the start of the 1960s were determined that young people should have their own voice when it came to fashion, and that they should be allowed to express themselves visually in a way that reflected the changes in society. For the first time in history – with the exception of Coco Chanel's unrestricted jersey collections in the 1930s – women's clothing was to become comfortable and easy to wear. For most of the decade designers had a very simple mantra, and that was to worship the God of Simplicity. The 'mods' of the early 1960s were ardent devotees of this creed, deeply concerned with their immaculate appearance. They were almost fanatical about their 'uniform' of pointy shoes and narrow straight-legged trousers, worn with a buttondown shirt and a very simple jacket that had three buttons at the front and two vents at the back.

Shift dresses and tunics

Mary Quant's early output was based on very straight simple shift dresses, which bypassed the waist (such a focus of attention in the previous decade) and simply hung to above the knee. These were clothes that were easy to pull on and dash to catch a bus in. Hemlines quickly rose to mid-thigh, but shapes remained very simple, with neat A-line coats, jersey sweater dresses that clung to the body, and endless sleeveless tunics with high-cut armholes and narrow shoulders.

Rudi Gernreich and Pierre Cardin were just two of many designers who produced countless variations on a straight tunic shape – big cutaway armholes, outsized circular pockets and contrast edging were all devices that added visual impact to what was essentially a straightforward sleeveless dress. It helped, of course, that girls all aspired to look like Twiggy – flat-chested, legs like a gazelle and hardly any bottom. The 'no body' body was perfect for hanging unstructured clothes on, as they only needed to fit where they touched, and the fragile 1960s waif was also the ideal shape to wear skinny-rib sweaters, immensely popular at the time.

The miniskirt

From the daring tunic dress that fell to the knee, the straight square-cut miniskirt was not far away. Hemlines continued to rise from just above the knee in 1963 to 15 cm (6 in) above the knee by the end of 1965. By the end of the decade the mini was barely more than a large hipster belt that became know as the micro-mini. The only way to go from here was down. By 1969 it was common to see girls with long ankle-length maxi coats worn over tiny hotpants and micro-minis with patterned tights and clunky square-heeled patent shoes.

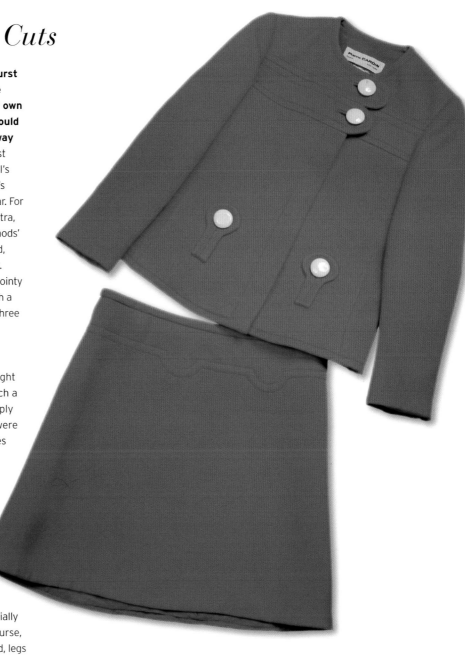

OPPOSITE Yves Saint Laurent handknitted smock dresses with diamond-patterned bodice and sleeves, hem and yoke all in one colour, 1966. The dress on the far left has a polo neck and the other a round neck. Saint Laurent's daring colour combinations and interest in geometrics and modern art can be appreciated in this distinctive pattern.

ABOVE Orange Pierre Cardin suit, late 1960s, with circular shaped detailing. Cardin's simple modernist lines were echoed in the work of André Courrèges, and both men had a deep fascination with futuristic ideas – sharp geometric cuts in necklines, hems and pocket details that seemed to owe more to architecture than to dressmaking.

Knitwear and key advances

New developments in the textile industry were exploited for body-conscious clothing, especially nylon and woolly patterned tights, both of which had just been invented and which looked fantastic with the miniskirt, as long as they were worn by girls who were tall and slim.

In Europe a diminutive style-conscious French woman called Sonia Rykiel started designing comfortable but desirable clothes for herself when she became pregnant. Her design status grew very quickly and her speciality became knitwear, making use of modern technology to produce very fine-gauge sweaters in myriad distinctive colours and stripes. By 1964 Rykiel had been nicknamed the 'Queen of Knitwear' in America where she developed an army of fans for her skinny-knit sweater dresses and cardigans.

In Italy the Missoni family, who had started their knitwear business in 1953, were also producing clothes that were grabbing worldwide attention for their fluidity and imaginative use of colour. Throughout the 1960s and '70s Ottavio ('Tai') and Rosita Missoni helped seal Milan's growing reputation as a fashionable epicentre with their artistic collection of knits. Unlike old-fashioned hand knits that were heavy and bulky, Missoni created exceptionally lightweight pieces with patterns that included stripes, zig-zags and even patchwork. They used modern machinery to produce unimaginable artistry in their pieces, which were often compared to works of art. Such was the success of some of the original Missoni pieces, that the house have re-issued modern copies of the early lines.

Trousers and suits

Although controversial, trousers of all shapes and sizes were introduced, and took off like never before. The upper classes perceived them as somehow being 'poor women's clothing' and many London restaurants and clubs refused entry to women wearing them. It was only after a celebrity endorsement – Cathy McGowan wore them to present 'Ready Steady Go' on British television in 1963 – that trousers became acceptable, almost overnight.

It was the decade of the leg – either revealed by the micro-mini or concealed beneath trousers. Tuffin and Foale were among the first designers to create a mix-and-match trouser and miniskirt option that provided the customer with the choice to decide what to wear with the jacket; a revolutionary idea at the time.

Straight-legged skinny pants, loose 1930s pyjama-style trousers, and wide flares were all acceptable shapes during the decade. As the 'waistless' dress evolved into the tunic, so the design of trousers became much lower cut, sitting on the hips instead of the waist – hence the name 'hipsters', which were the popular unisex choice for skinny boys and girls from 1965. As the decade progressed, flares became increasingly voluminous, to the point where they were cut like full-length culottes.

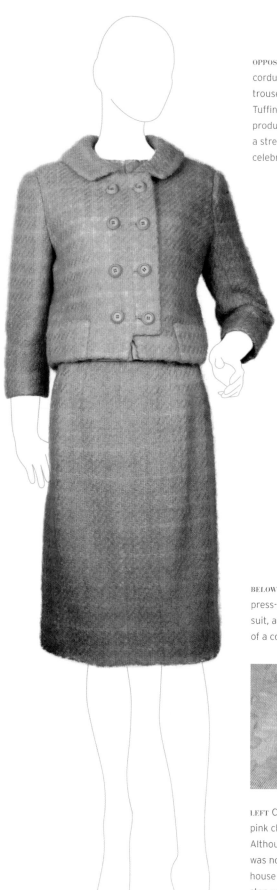

OPPOSITE Narrow-cut corduroy Tuffin and Foale trouser suit from 1964. Sally Tuffin and Marion Foale produced clothes that had a street-style appeal and celebrated youth culture.

BELOW Fabric-covered press-studs on the Dior suit, a distinctive sign of a couture garment.

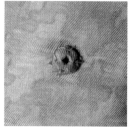

LEFT Christian Dior lime-and-pink checked suit, 1960s. Although the great master was no longer alive, his house continued to keep step with the times, as seen in the fluffy, tactile tweed and modern cut. Note the short half-pockets at the jacket's hem.

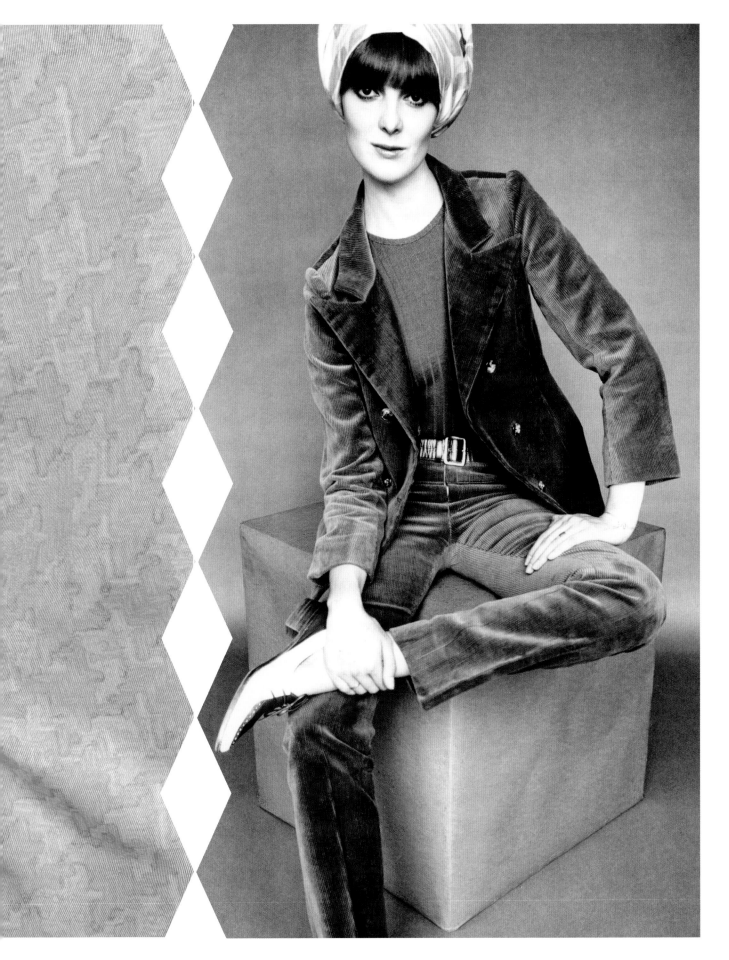

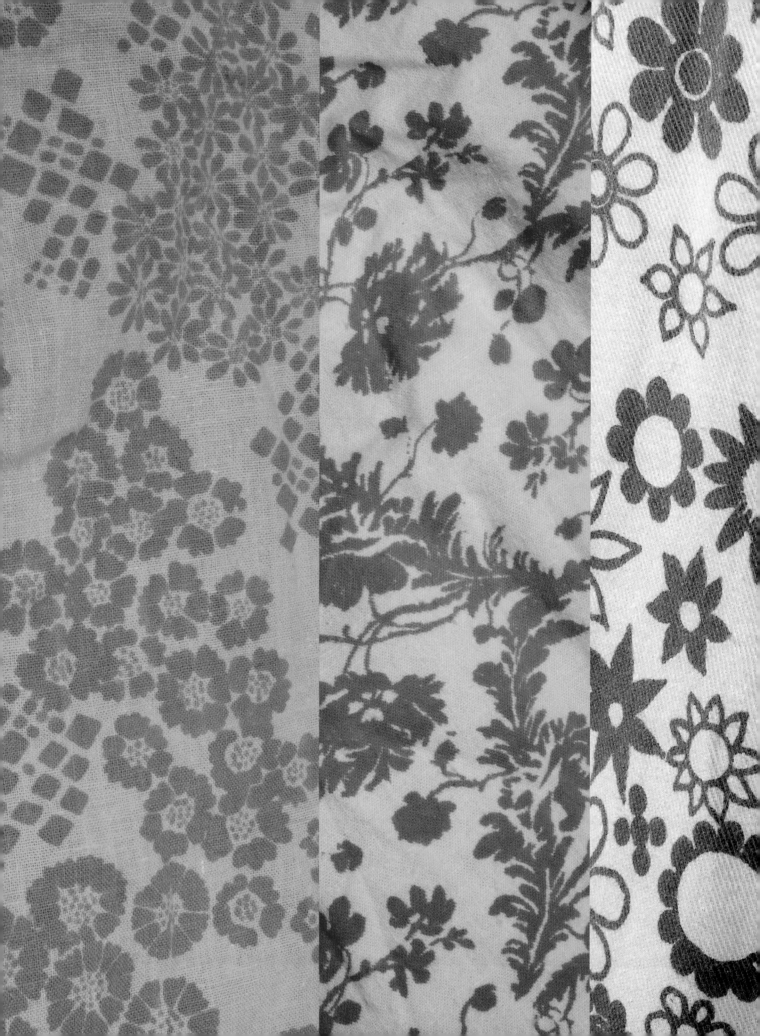

A Feminine Design Ethic

Running parallel to the modern line of André Courrèges and Pierre Cardin were numerous designers who embraced a much more feminine design ethic, and who were producing decidedly girly clothes with frills and gathers and an altogether softer line. Emilio Pucci, the darling of the international jet set with his lurid-print loose-cut kaftan shapes, bell-sleeved tops and pyjama pants, became famous for clothes that relied on a much looser shape and cut. By mid-decade there was also a definite swing to a modern interpretation of old-fashioned Hollywood glamour, and much of Biba's success was built upon Barbara Hulanicki's individual take on 1920s and '30s style. When she started Biba, she was fond of low-cut necklines, wide loose pants, short flared skirts, and women's shirts with exaggerated high collars and full sleeves. As the Biba phenomenon grew, she became known for long bias-cut dresses with feather boas and maxi-length trench coats with big floppy hats.

Influences from the past

Other designers looked to different eras for inspiration. Gina Fratini and Bellville Sassoon were two who became renowned for high romanticism. Their designs contained an element of graceful innocent version of femininity.

Laura Ashley was a British designer who achieved longlasting success with her brand of Old World nostalgia. Integrating ideas from Edwardian and Victorian clothing she produced a range of rustic country girl clothes reminiscent of a Thomas Hardy heroine. Pin-tucked bodices, tiered skirts, full puff-sleeved blouses and long frilled smocks were all trademark pieces that came in Ashley's own prints. Her reinterpretation of original eighteenth- and nineteenth-century patterns, floral springs and paisleys, which were printed on fine lawn cottons in subtle colour combinations, provided her with a look that was instantly recognized and highly coveted on both sides of the Atlantic.

SIGNATURE LAURA ASHLEY ELEMENTS:
- High Edwardian-style necklines
- Full sleeves gathered from the shoulder into a long cuff
- Rows of covered 'ball' buttons on cuffs of sleeves
- Tana lawn cottons
- Pin-tucked bodices
- Lace trims
- Tiered skirts
- Floral sprig prints
- Long smocks
- Frilled aprons

OPPOSITE Laura Ashley prints evoked the natural beauty of the Welsh countryside with florals, paisleys and small romantic prints, which provided a rustic charm and natural simplicity. Her designs reworked influences from past eras, and her florals were usually printed in just two colours, but in many different combinations.

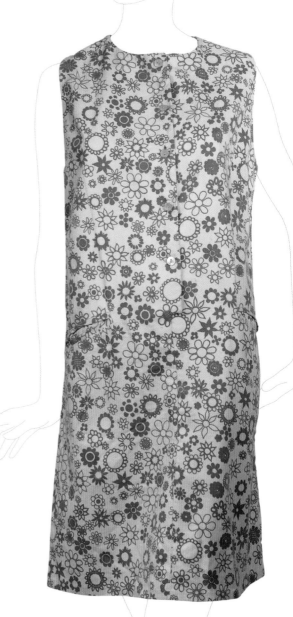

RIGHT An early 1960s Laura Ashley minidress with a button opening at the front. The rigid tunic shape would be replaced by her famous Victorian-style maxi dresses in the late '60s and '70s.

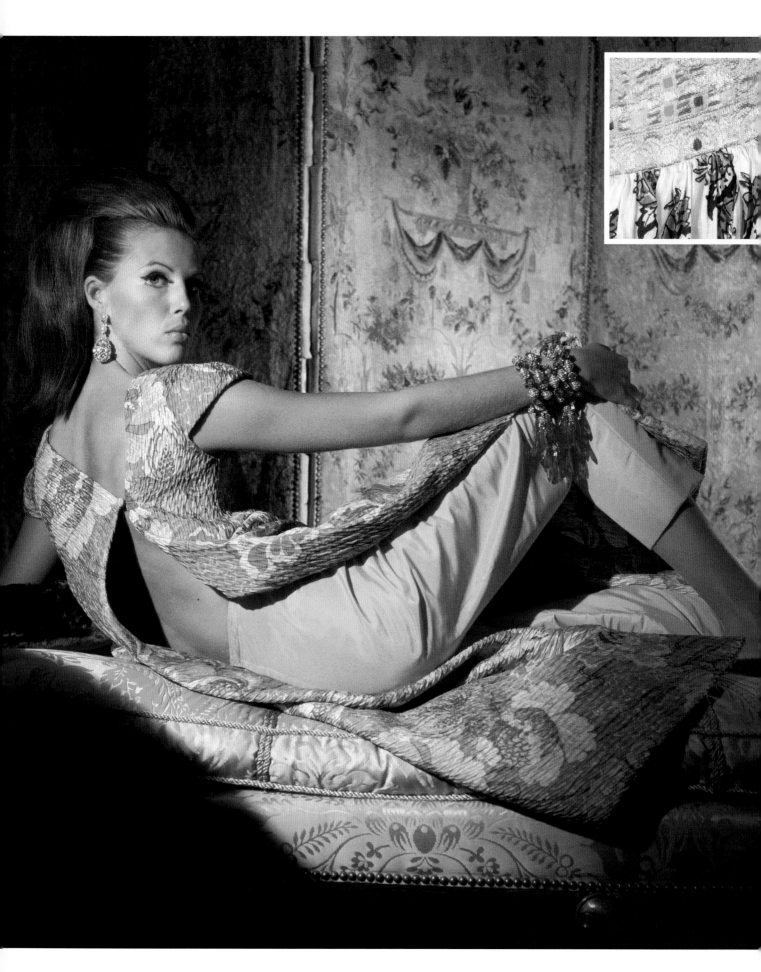

The hippy look and the antifashion movement

The last years of the decade exploded in a riot of colour and confusion as the fashion pendulum swung from the simplified lines of 1960s modern London to the nostalgic secondhand clothes of the hippies, which spanned into the early 1970s.

Pop music had given way to rock and the international hit 'San Francisco (Be Sure to Wear Some Flowers in Your Hair)' was the anthem for a generation of festival-goers who wore painted daisies on their faces, extolled the virtues of free love and invented a street style of utilitarian and ethnic clothes. There was a confusion of gender, with young couples wanting to share everything including their embroidered jeans and to copy each other's look, from long hair to spectacles.

Escapism in the form of secondhand clothes included every sort of imported style: kaftans from India, American worker's jeans, Chairman Mao jackets, Afghan jackets and waistcoats, and ex-army regimental uniform (as worn by the Beatles for the *Sergeant Pepper* album). The hippy look was not a designer's creation, it was about individuality, as everything was picked up from secondhand market stalls and no one could wear an identical outfit. However, this antifashion movement inspired by psychedelic drugs and nostalgia provided a springboard for such British designers as Zandra Rhodes, Thea Porter and Ossie Clark, and also Giorgio di Sant'Angelo and Bill Blass, to launch their own brand of escapism.

Drawing on myriad influences from the past, such as beaded dresses from the 1920s and bias-cut slips with handkerchief hemlines from the 1930s, these designers specialized in beautifully crafted clothes. Their signature pieces were fantasy dresses, embellished with embroidery, quilting and beading. Print was important, as were softer flowing lines, gathered sleeves and fuller shapes that were the antithesis of the short, square-cut lines that had been popular for most of the previous decade.

Other designers who chose to operate outside the system and create their own vision of alternative world clothing were Jean Bouquin, who opened a Bedouin palace-influenced shop in the South of France, crammed with luxurious kaftans, loose baggy pants and exotic African beads.

In London in 1966, Thea Porter opened a small dark shop in Soho's Greek Street, initially full of opulent interior pieces as well as a few ethnic robes that were brought in from her hometown in the Middle East. The shop became a mecca for young student types who wanted to embrace everything Eastern. As the items she imported sold out quickly, Porter decided to design her own dresses to meet demands. Her versions of loose flowing gowns and kaftans that grazed the floor, and were made in a variety of brocades, velvets and lightweight chiffons, often recycled from traditional Eastern textiles, were popular with royalty and the

RIGHT AND OPPOSITE INSET Indian silk, empire-line Thea Porter dress with crimson sleeves trimmed in black velvet, late 1960s. Derived from Middle Eastern and Indian costume, Porter's dresses had easy, flattering shapes and full skirts, which worked several patterns together in one piece.

OPPOSITE Rippled blue silk kaftan printed with large peonies over pink silk taffeta pants, by Bill Blass, 1965. Blass was known for his ability to mix pattern and texture.

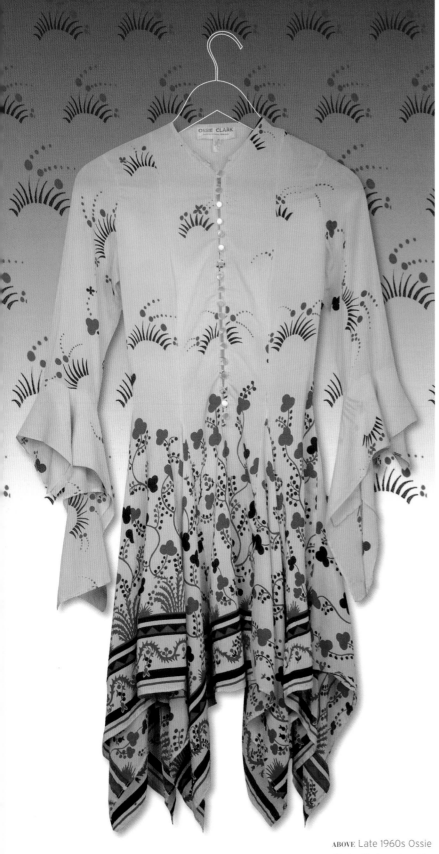

International jet set. Although inspired by the Middle East, Thea Porter's designs were her own romantic interpretation of the exotic, and as fashion moved on rapidly so did she, later producing collections that drew on the last days of the Russian empire, gipsy flounces, and even an exotic knitwear range that was specifically made for the cold English climate.

Ossie Clark, who graduated from the Royal College of Art, London, in 1965, was a master cutter who had an artistic vision and possessed the technical skill to turn it into a reality. He found the miniskirt restrictive and instead concentrated on clothes that were flattering to the female body. His collaboration with his wife, the textile designer Celia Birtwell, produced inspirational fashion and their work together won them instant success. He favoured crepe, jersey and chiffon because of their fluidity and produced clothes that combined intensely complex cutting techniques with a variety of prints, all used on the same garment. At the time this was a revolutionary approach to womenswear and his clothes were coveted by all the superstar glitterati; special commissions were made for Bianca Jagger, Britt Ekland and Verushka. Loose pyjama-style pants in fabulous printed silk, bias-cut chiffon dresses with very full sleeves gathering into a tight cuff, quilted panelling and high-cut oval-shaped waistbands are all Ossie Clark trademarks.

ABOVE Late 1960s Ossie Clark silk dress in a blue-and-red Celia Birtwell print on a cream field. Clark's imaginative cutting marked a shift from hard-edged modernism to feminine romanticism in the 1960s.

RIGHT In the late 1960s Ossie Clark collaborated with the photographer Jim Lee in developing groundbreaking new ways to present his clothes. The 'Airplane' dress, featured above left, is seen here in a 1969 Jim Lee photograph.

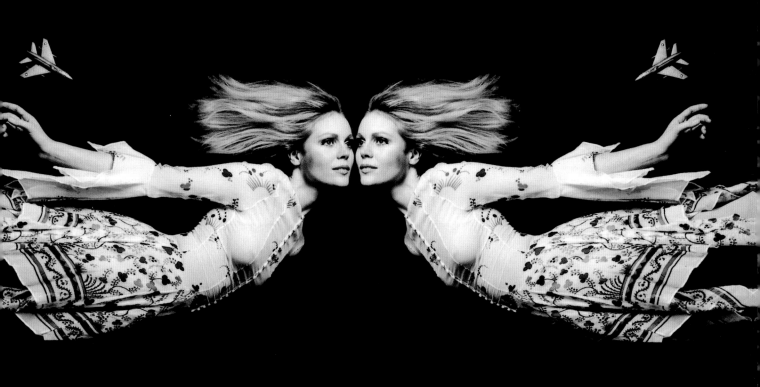

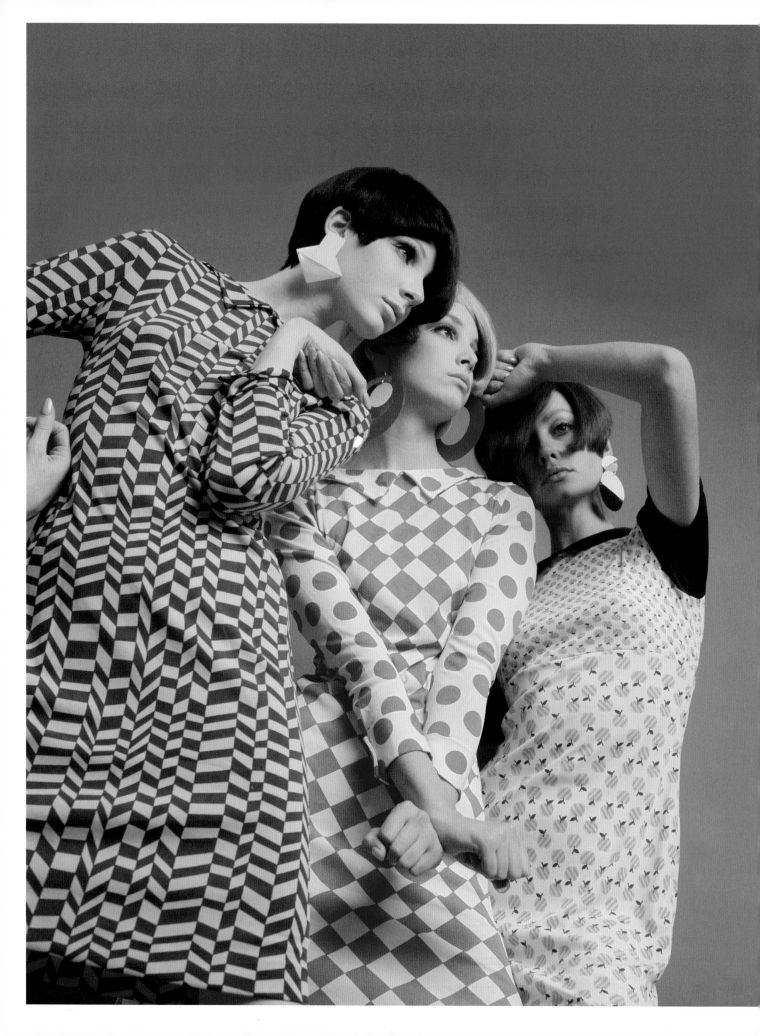

Textiles and Prints

The rapid technological developments in the textile industry in the 1960s led to an unprecedented choice of materials that had never been used before in the fashion industry. Manufacturers had started to develop new easy-care, easy-to-wear fabrics that incorporated polyesters. These brand-new fabrics were comfortable to touch, wrinkle free and required very little time to look after them; in fact, they were a perfect match for the short simple miniskirts and tunic dresses of the era. As the radical change in womenswear continued, designers such as Emanuel Ungaro and Paco Rabanne looked to more unconventional materials like paper, plastics and metal to use instead of soft fabrics. Their choice of material limited their design, but plastic chainmail, with its hard and resolutely 'modern' feel, was a perfect choice for the avant-garde creations of the Parisian haute couture designers.

Mary Quant and Yves Saint Laurent were both fans of another new material that had been borrowed from industrial usage and reinvented as a fashion fabric. PVC (polyvinyl chloride) was a shiny wet-look plastic that was easy to colour and print with flamboyant designs, but also looked exactly right for the times as it was available in plain black or white. It became hugely popular with teenage girls, and required nothing more than a rub down with a damp cloth to keep it looking good. At first it was used for outerwear, double-breasted belted macs, knee-high boots and shiny baker boy caps; then, increasingly, for every style of clothing, from zip-up bomber jackets, bags and belts to tunics and miniskirts.

As the formality of dressing continued to break down, designers abandoned the traditional rules of when and where a particular type of fabric should be worn. Fabrics that had previously been restricted to eveningwear or special occasion dressing were now used extensively for ordinary clothes. Velvets, brocades, satins and lace began to be used for daywear, and it became perfectly acceptable to wear the same outfit to work as later on for an evening out.

Graphic lines and Op Art
The severity of the A-line tunic, and short boxy jackets and coats, provided a perfect canvas for the equally strong dynamic of using just black and white as a colourway. Fashion in the 1960s tended to be very graphic, and John Bates, a British designer who provided all Diana Rigg's costumes for the television

OPPOSITE Dresses by Paco Rabanne featuring spots, chevrons, checks and apple motifs, 1966.

programme *The Avengers* knew how visually powerful this could be. Using only black and white for bold stripes, check and diagonal chevrons, he designed a set of clothes for the character Emma Peel that sparked headlines in nearly every daily paper in the nation. Graphic stripes, spots, checks and zebra print then turned into hypnotic illusions and suddenly the influence of such Op artists as Bridget Riley and Frank Stella filtered through to the fashion industry.

The term 'Op Art' was coined for the dramatic, trick-optic effects of line and contrasting areas of line and colour, and fashion designers picked up these art trends and modified them for use in their clothing designs. André Courrèges, Pierre Cardin, Emanuel Ungaro and Julian Tomchin were all influenced by Op Art and abstract art movements; Yves Saint Laurent, inspired by the paintings of Mondrian, designed geometric patterns in a celebrated line of Mondrian dresses, following with Pop Art dresses in 1966, decorated with comic strips.

BELOW Paper dress with swirly psychedelic design from the 1960s. Although they could be worn only a few times, paper dresses enabled women to try out the latest designs. Now collector's items, they evolved from NASA's experiments with single-use clothing, making them part of the futuristic theme of the decade.

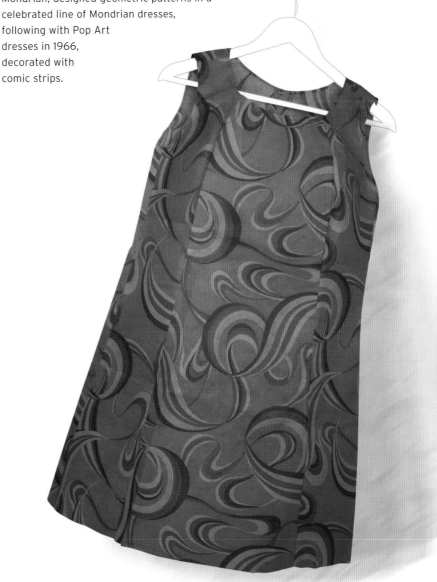

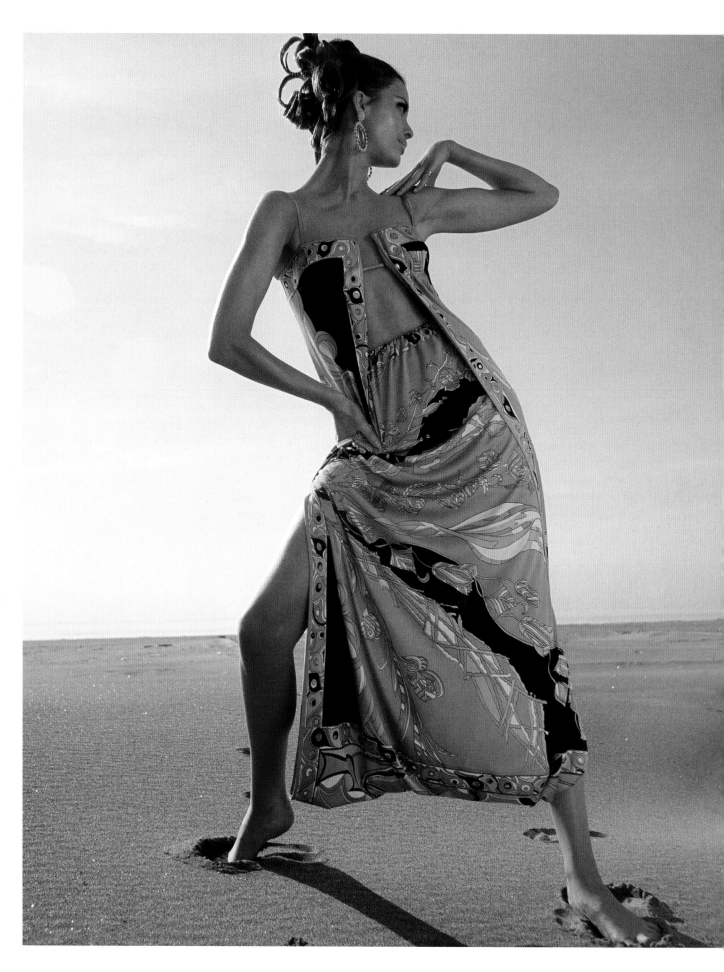

Psychedelia and Emilio Pucci

Every fashionable trend provokes a polar opposite and the backlash against stark monochrome minimalism came in the form of psychedelia. By the mid-1960s designers were drawing inspiration from the Flower Power movement and a cacophony of street styles that combined ethnic pieces with Union Jack prints and as much superfluous decoration as possible. Flowered brocades, embroidery, braiding and fringing were all used to create an extraordinarily flamboyant look that was as popular with men as it was with young girls. Clashing colours and big swirly patterns became the fashionable embodiment of a hallucinogenic LSD trip, and Carnaby Street, London, became a jumble of mismatched prints and styles. In Britain, John Stephen was one of the first to produce completely matching unisex outfits, using wild prints and vibrant colours. Although the young men who wore these clothes had to fight fears of being branded homosexual, ruffled silk shirts, paisley ties and kaftan-style suits made from Eastern prints with mandarin collars were soon being copied for the mass market.

In Europe Italian designer Emilio Pucci was creating a collection that relied on strong swirling patterns on simple elegant clothes. A natural stylist, he began by designing his own ski outfit, which was spotted by a *Harper's Bazaar* editor who asked him to design women's skiwear that she wanted to photograph for a story. The look of ski clothes changed for ever, and a new fashion empire was established. Using gaudy, vibrant colours and luxury fabrics, Pucci's psychedelic clothes defined the 'jet set' age of the 1960s and were favourites with the cognoscenti on both sides of the Atlantic, with Elizabeth Taylor, Twiggy and Joan Collins all proud to be part of Puccimania. The thin silk jersey dresses, palazzo pants and beachwear were wrinkle-resistant and easy to pack, perfect for the international traveller. The designs were heady whirls of colour, often bordered by graphic geometrics, and the unmistakable Pucci print became instantly recognizable for generations to come; it was even featured in the

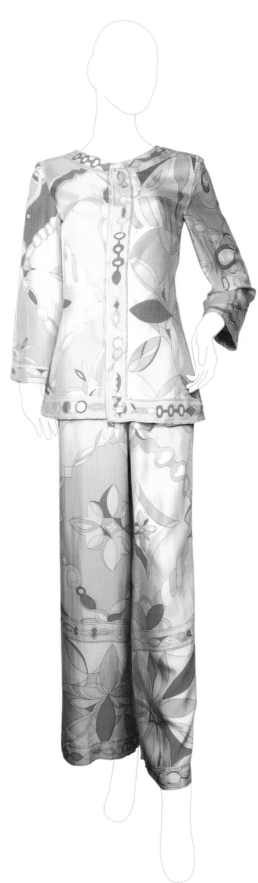

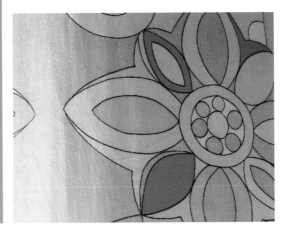

ABOVE, RIGHT AND BELOW RIGHT Yellow and orange silk Pucci psychedelic-print shirt and trousers, late 1960s. These 'palazzo pajamas' would usually have been worn with jewelled sandals. Pucci's swirling patterns and unmistakable colours earned him the title 'Prince of Prints'.

OPPOSITE Model Susan Murray wearing a slit print skirt and thin-strapped top by Emilio Pucci, 1966. In the 1960s Pucci produced capri pants, shorts, resort dresses, silk shirts, trousers and suits, as well as ranges of underwear, sweaters and swimwear for American manufacturers. He pioneered the colour revolution of the decade.

logo of the Apollo 15 space mission and the interior of a Ford Lincoln Continental. Beloved of Americans, Pucci had a long association with New York department store Neiman Marcus, which enabled him to progress from selling his clothing in his boutique on the Isle of Capri (and making all of the clothing in his own home) to major manufacturing. Pucci's designs, styles and fabrics were kept to an incredibly high quality, and he oversaw all his production houses. He was one of the first designers to sign his name in print on the exterior of his clothes, and the Emilio Pucci signature can be seen on original pieces.

The Psychedelic Revolution

By 1966 the clashing colours and gaudy jumble-sale attire that had begun life in London's Carnaby Street had started to lose its way stylistically. For a brief period a new movement appeared, nicknamed the Psychedelic Revolution. Starting in the USA, it revolved around music and the hallucinogenic drug LSD. Swirling colours, kaleidoscopic patterns and a multitude of dizzy-making prints all collided onto unisex shirts, tunics, kaftans and, surprisingly, men's suits. In London the designer Michael Fish, who traded under Mr Fish, had opened a tailor's shop that specialized in making fitted suits for men in the most garish stripes and paisleys. He was also responsible for inventing the oversized kipper tie, often in the same flamboyant fabric to match his shirts and suits.

In America, counterculture guru Timothy Leary's words of advice to 'turn on, tune in and drop out' reflected a general desire to reject Western culture, and seek inspiration from the East. Young people with their

LEFT, RIGHT AND BELOW RIGHT
A late 1960s Neiman Marcus copy of a Christian Dior psychedelic-print silk trouser suit. Note the sleeve slits and ties at the wrist.

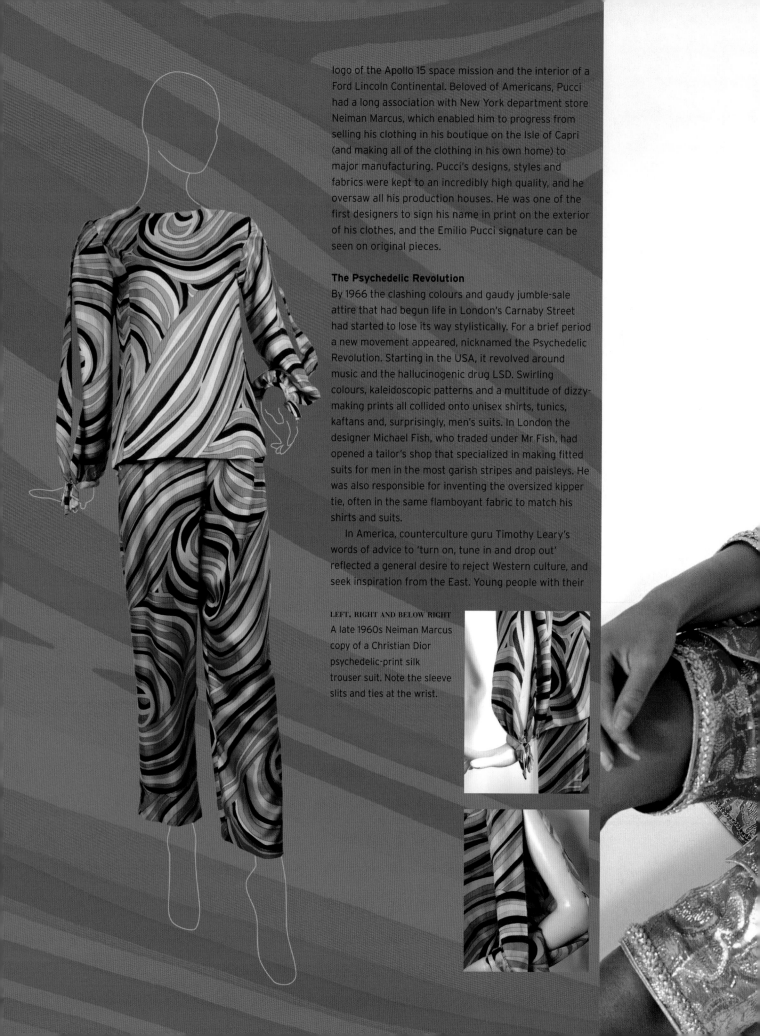

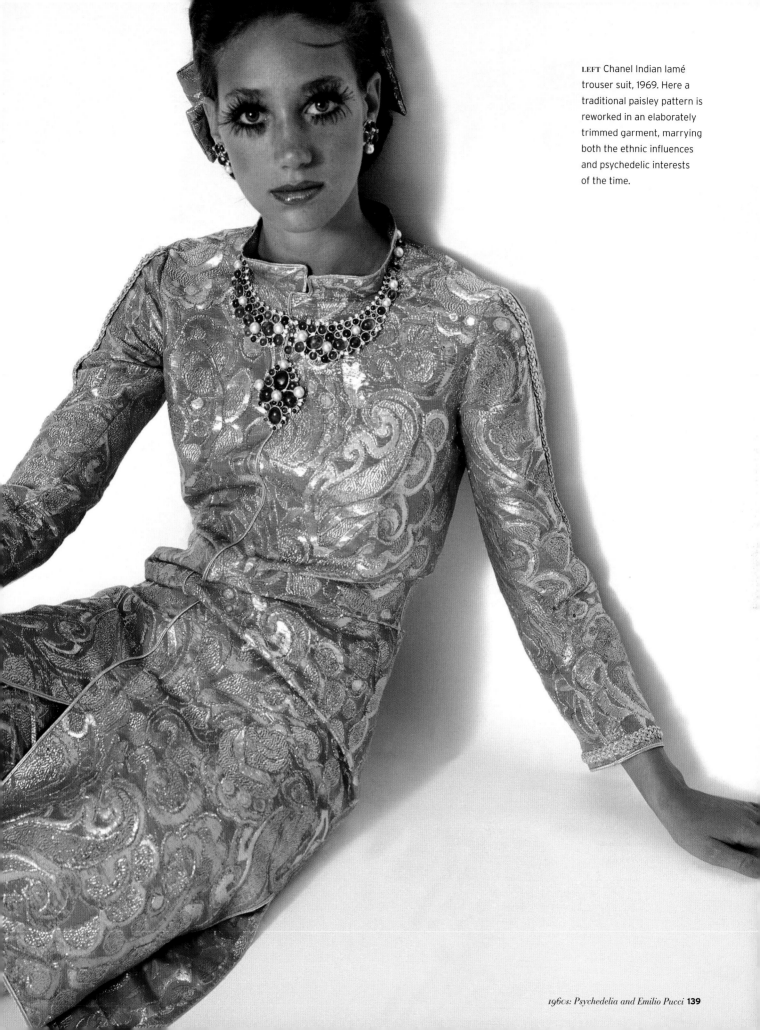

LEFT Chanel Indian lamé trouser suit, 1969. Here a traditional paisley pattern is reworked in an elaborately trimmed garment, marrying both the ethnic influences and psychedelic interests of the time.

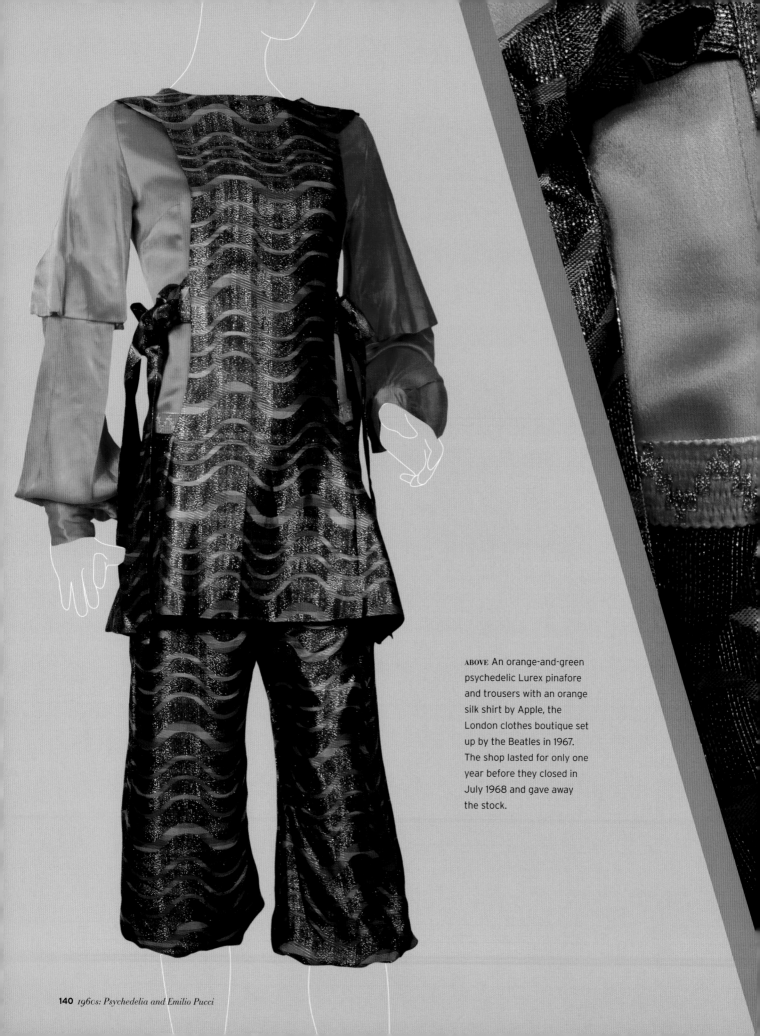

ABOVE An orange-and-green psychedelic Lurex pinafore and trousers with an orange silk shirt by Apple, the London clothes boutique set up by the Beatles in 1967. The shop lasted for only one year before they closed in July 1968 and gave away the stock.

newfound power in society wanted to embrace everything Eastern, from religion to traditional dress, and many European designers were quick to catch on. In 1967 Yves Saint Laurent showed vibrant paisley prints lavished with heavy fringing, Chanel used heavily embellished Indian fabrics for Nehru-styled jackets and Italian designer Count Sarmi produced an opulent evening collection of chiffon harem pants and gold embroidered tunics.

The Psychedelic Revolution quickly turned into the flower power movement, inspired by the folk-rock music of Bob Dylan, Joan Baez and Janis Joplin. With a peace medallion as their symbol, hundreds of young hippies took off to far-flung regions in a hotchpotch of tie-dyed skirts, collarless 'grandad' shirts, paisley headbands and crushed velvet patchwork waistcoats. The bohemian hippy style was commercialized by the such British designers as Ossie Clark and Zandra Rhodes, while Yves Saint Laurent launched his own layered skirt and peasant blouse in 1969, and Giorgio di Sant'Angelo produced a stunning collection of vibrant gipsy skirts that incorporated fringing, beading and multicoloured sashes.

BELOW AND RIGHT Turquoise silk blouse from British boutique, Granny Takes A Trip, 1967/8. Victorian influences can be seen in its leg-of-mutton sleeves and long row of buttons – historical referencing such as this was commonplace in the decade's designs as past prints, textiles and detailing were plundered.

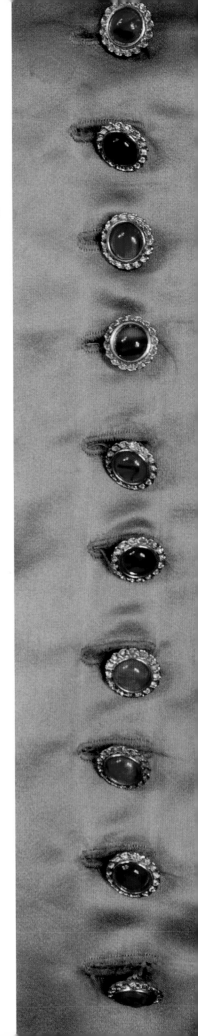

▶Space Age looks

With the moon landing came an avalanche of Space Age clothes, best exemplified by Courrèges with his all-white 'moon girl' collection in 1964. Space-inspired helmets in felted wool or white leather completed the look, as modelled here by Audrey Hepburn, 1965, in Courrèges.

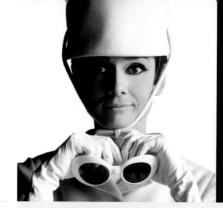

Miniskirts

André Courrèges in Paris and Mary Quant in London can both lay claim to the invention of the mini skirt. Hemlines started creeping higher at the start of the decade, but by 1965 they had risen to mid-thigh and were to become even shorter. Often worn with a big belt hung loosely over the hips, they were adopted by women across the world, not just the young and leggy.

Hosiery

Innovations in the textile industry saw the invention of all-in-one nylon tights, which gave women much more freedom than stockings and suspenders. With the emphasis firmly directed on to the leg, tights quickly became an integral part of the look and were made in strong colours with thick stripes, printed patterns, diamonds and plaid for winter, while white lacy versions were worn under summer dresses.

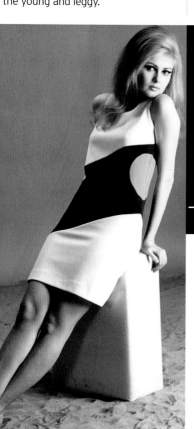

Key looks of the decade

1960s

▼Graphic lines

Mini skirts, shift dresses and short A-line coats were all given the Op Art look as fashion reflected the optical illusions of Bridget Riley's paintings. Thick and thin stripes and geometric checks were used to create strong graphic impact in many of the pared-down simple shapes. Here Natalie Wood models Yves Saint Laurent's Mondrian dress.

▲Synthetics

Polyester, nylon and other manmade fabrics permitted the wearer movement even with slim-cut styles. This 1966 dress by New York designer Gayle Kirkpatrick, modelled by actress Pamela Tiffin, was made in a special stretch nylon developed by Stretchnit.

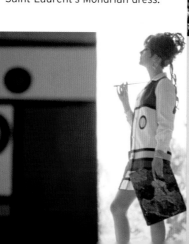

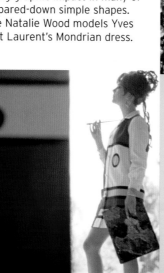

▲Boots

It was a decade of boots in various shapes and styles. Shiny patent boots that came up to and over the knee in black, white and silver were the trendiest footwear to go with the mini. The other strong boot shape, which originated from Paris, was a mid-calf white kidskin boot with a pointy toe and no heel, sometimes with a flat ribbon bow around the top.

Chainmail

[Pa]co Rabanne's resolutely [m]odern designs were made [fro]m a variety of unconventional [m]aterials. Plastic chainmail and [al]uminium appeared in silver, [bl]ack or white. Difficult to work [wi]th, chainmail projected a [fu]turistic image that was very [m]uch in tune with what women [wa]nted. The chainmail and mesh [ca]tsuit below twins chainmail [wi]th the trend for transparency.

Psychedelia

By the middle to late 1960s the emphasis had shifted from London to America, and more specifically to the flower children of San Francisco, with their anti-Vietnam chants, long hair and ragbag of utilitarian and ethnic garments. Brocade jeans, frilly shirts, flower-print tunics, Mao jackets and Indian scarves became a street style emulated by most European designers.

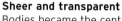

Sheer and transparent

Bodies became the centre of attention with transparent panels of clear plastic or mesh like netting, as in the chaimail catsuit below. Towards the end of the decade see-through clothes became more daring with Yves Saint Laurent's sheer black chiffon blouse and Ossie Clark's gossamer-fine chiffon dresses showing more barely covered flesh than ever before.

▶Plastics

Shiny PVC was used for every item of clothing from over-the-knee boots to mini macs, bags and pinafore dresses. It was easy to colour and to overprint with bold motifs. Connecting circles of hard plastic were popular for belts and earrings. Shown here, Paco Rabanne works vinyl, plastic and steel into a flowery 1967 dress.

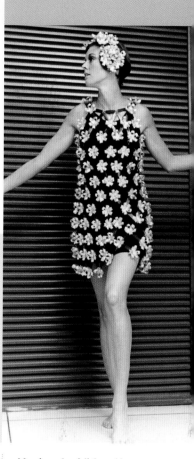

Oversized sunglasses

Huge bug-eyed spectacles in shiny black or white plastic were one of the hottest accessories to match Op Art and Space Age styles. Perfectly round and goggle-like, they were worn more for photographic styling and celebrity 'disguise' than for everyday streetwear.

Maxi and midi lengths

Long coats, skirts and dresses were designed as the antidote to the mini. The maxi fell to the ankle, and the midi was cut to mid-calf. Women were given much more choice to decide what length they felt comfortable in, and they often chose to wear both at the same time: midi knit cardigans were worn over short skirts with boots to show a fleeting glimpse of leg.

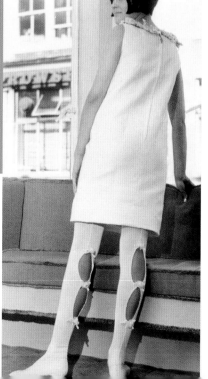

[C]ut-outs

[Sh]apes cut out of dresses [wa]s, especially to reveal the [mi]dsection. Here a 1965 design [by] John Bates teams a simple [shi]ft dress with cut-out stockings [de]corated with roses and bows.

Shift dresses

The most popular shape was an A-line shift that fell in a clean triangular line from shoulder to mid-thigh. Big circular pockets, cutaway armholes and contrast edging around the neck, hem and armholes were defining features. Some were designed to wear over a skinny rib sweater and ribbed tights during the day, or to wear on their own with heels in the evening.

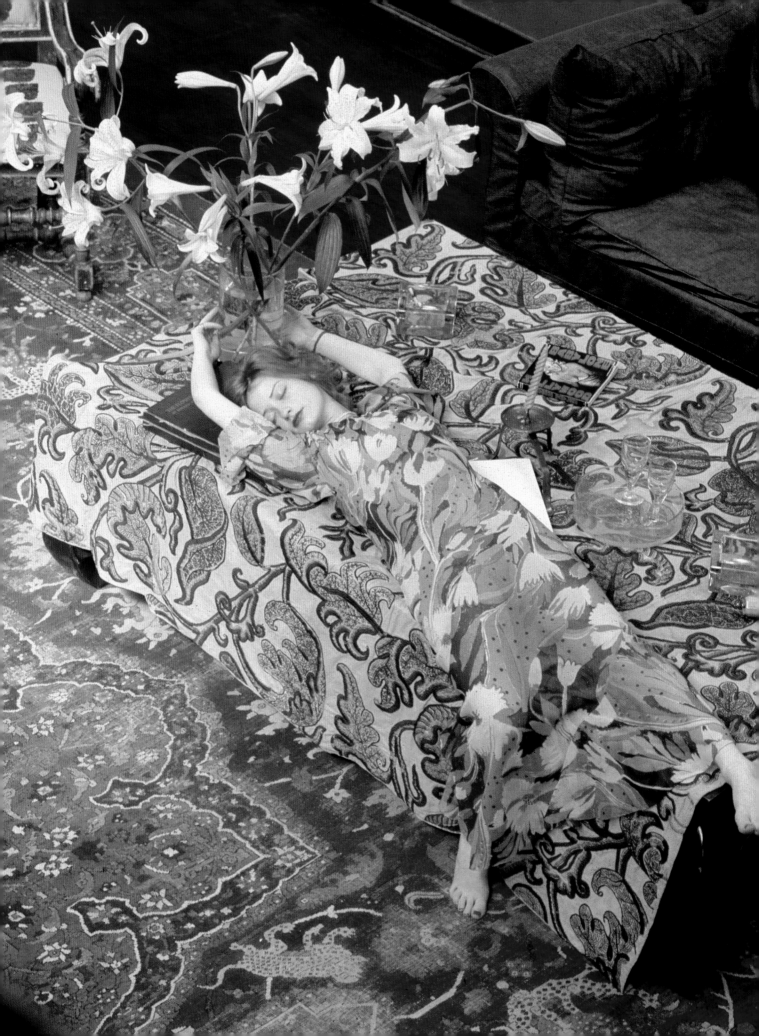

1970s

Clothes with an ethnic, natural and 'rootsy' feel dominated the first few years of the 1970s as people explored New Age thinking and cheaper air travel made it possible to visit far-flung places. The hippy fashions from the previous decade were reworked with a folksy vibe, taking traditional crafts such as knitting, tapestry, weaving and dyeing to the very epicentre of fashion. The Art Deco revival, triggered by the work of Royal College of Art lecturer Bernard Nevill for Liberty, flourished. Barbara Hulanicki's Biba store became a mecca for the vintage look. New inspiration was born through collaborations of fashion and art in the work of designers such as Ossie Clark and Celia Birtwell, and Bill Gibb and Zandra Rhodes. Malcolm McLaren sold 1950s memorabilia at his Let It Rock shop before pulling the plug on the whole retro trend in 1974 and opening a new shop called simply SEX. In 1977 he and partner Vivienne Westwood renamed their shop Seditionaries while simultaneously launching the pop career of the Sex Pistols. Meanwhile, ready-to-wear fashion established a solid base, with Givenchy, Oscar de la Renta, Yves Saint Laurent, Marc Bohan for Dior and Karl Lagerfeld for Chloé wholesaleing around the world. Inspired by the groundbreaking work of British designer Jean Muir and Saint Laurent, Calvin Klein, Geoffrey Beene, Ralph Lauren and others created new, flowing jersey separates and easy-to-wear classics for working women. Diane von Furstenberg's signature wraparound dress was a huge hit and New York's Studio 54 became the most famous discotheque in the world.

Daywear

It's easy to get lost in the drama of 1970s fashion and forget that this was the decade in which ready-to-wear came into its own. Separates were a key component rather than whole outfits in the formal couture sense. Fashion editors showed women how to wear them, pulling together different patterns and fabrics with a couple of key colours. 'Together but apart' was fashion's most wearable message yet.

Ready-to-wear began in the 1960s when a few designers broke away from the rigid, expensive traditions of couture and began producing easy-purchase lines to be sold in their own shops. Oscar de la Renta opened his first ready-to-wear boutique in 1965, with Yves Saint Laurent following in 1966 and Hubert de Givenchy in 1968. By 1970 such shops were forming the cornerstones of the modern fashion industry, making designer clothes accessible to all who could afford them.

Yves Saint Laurent's collections

In the 1970s Saint Laurent's influence became widespread with his partnership with Pierre Bergé, who not only gave him the freedom to design with less financial restraint but also aided him in his expansion from haute couture to ready-to-wear. His 1971 collection, 1940, showed gangster-style trouser suits with double-breasted jackets. Square shoulders, bouffant sleeves and a green fox fur jacket led this 1940s invocation to have a huge effect on daywear, which carried on through to 1973 with black silk two-pieces and dresses of silk crepe de chine featuring simple white floral patterns, short puffed sleeves, nipped-in waists and rounded collars. Similar styles were created by Karl Lagerfeld for Chloé, Cacharel and Ossie Clark.

Saint Laurent had always loved to marry fashion with art and, as the decade continued, he created more adventurous looks harking back to his revolutionary designs of the 1960s influenced by Op Art and Mondrian. In 1979 his 'Homage to Picasso' collection featured strong graphic prints on wool, gabardine and satin. Yet such collections were balanced by his ready-to-wear classics. A strongly wearable nautical collection of sailor-wide linen trousers, knitted matelot tops and bolero jackets in the mid-1970s was followed by his Russian Ballet Opera collection in 1976 and a Mongolian-inspired wool, fur and knitwear collection for autumn/winter 1977.

PAGE **144** Nicky Samuel, 1970s 'It Girl', wearing a Tulip dress by Celia Birtwell, 1971, for a *Vogue* shoot.

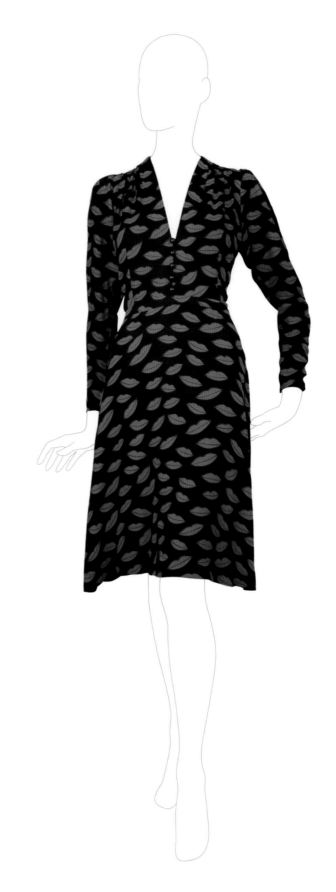

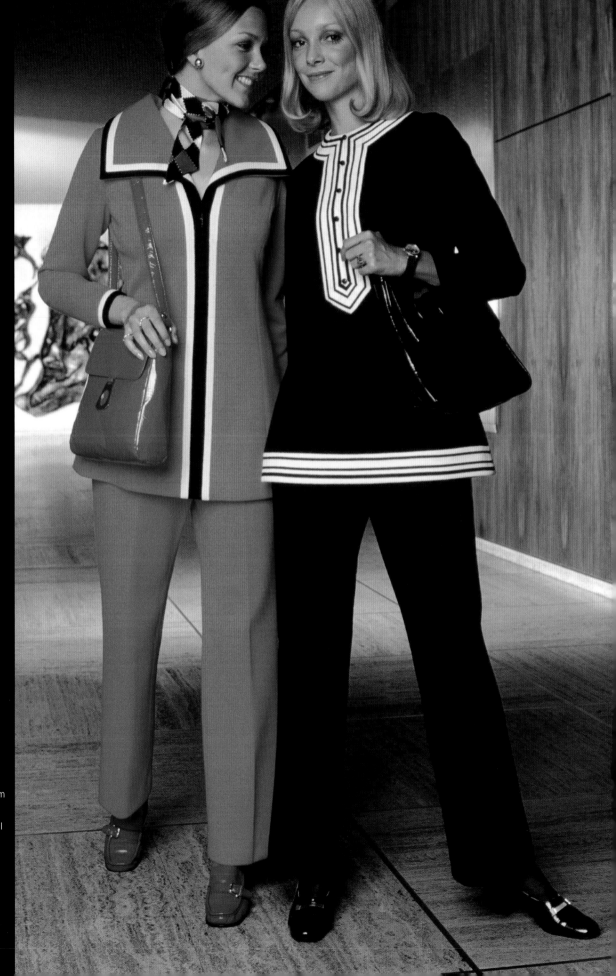

OPPOSITE Early 1970s lips-print dress, by Yves Saint Laurent for his ready-to-wear line, Rive Gauche.

RIGHT Two pantsuits from American label R & K Originals, 1970, are wool knit-polyester blends. The overlong tunic top and wide lapels were typical details of 1970s ready-to-wear.

'Le Smoking', the women's tuxedo introduced by Saint Laurent in the 1960s (see also page 121) and reworked in the 1970s heralded the arrival of the decade's mainstay, the trouser suit, which reflected the trend for all things 'unisex'. Pretty soon, versions were available in wool checks and tweeds, with satin and velvet for evenings, and high street boutiques and chainstores were selling cheaper alternatives in such fabrics as Courtelle and Crimplene to eager customers.

Fluidity and comfort in fashion

While the Parisian fashion houses offered luxurious, even flamboyant daywear shapes in fabrics including cotton drill, felt, heavy wools, crepe and fur, another silhouette took shape. After the shift dresses and hard lines of the 1960s, more feminine clothes reemerged following the shape of the female form with fluidity and movement. Soft, flattering wool jersey fabrics fitted and flared away from the body, creating a new, less restricted silhouette. Jean Muir lowered hemlines after the mini left fashion with nowhere to go, and the midi was reborn. In 1973 *Nova* magazine hailed the arrival of the H-shape, with a low waist and longer hem.

Other Jean Muir designs also caused a stir, keeping them at the cutting edge of style. Jersey culottes and tunics, leather-trimmed pinafores and trademark polo-(turtle-) necks were clothes with a message. Eschewing pretty, sexy and playful, Muir's customers were not afraid to be bold, stylish and vocal. She moved on from her 1960s label Jane & Jane to her own eponymous label in 1966; her muse, British actress Joanna Lumley, had been a 1960s babe, but she chopped off her hair, darkened her lips and reworked her look to match Muir's trademark dark colour palette of black, navy and chocolate brown.

Ease and comfort combined with style were the key elements of these clothes, worn over the latest designs in underwear. Balcony bras, corseted waists and complicated garter/stocking combinations died out with the previous decade, giving way to more comfortable, less structured garments in elasticated fabrics with natural shaping. The aim, said the fashion magazines of the time, was to look as though you were not wearing any underwear at all.

American style

Meanwhile, fledgling New York designers, including Ralph Lauren and Calvin Klein, were establishing their city as a new centre for ready-to-wear. Together with Geoffrey Beene, their classic tailoring with a flourish – including luxurious camel hair coats by Calvin Klein in 1971 – were the building blocks of what was to become the easy, sporty American style, carried through by such fashion models as Lauren Hutton, Patti Hansen and Margaux Hemingway. This was daywear on a far simpler scale than that of the Europeans – in soft, neutral colours with natural accessories.

Ralph Lauren took American history as his theme and moved on from the slick daywear and sportswear of his peers to create 'casual chic'. Preppy slacks, polo shirts and simple sweaters were reminiscent of Princeton in the '20s, then later Western and Native American influences brought a new glamour to casual clothes. Lauren's designs, worn by Robert Redford in the 1974 film *The Great Gatsby,* based on F Scott Fitzgerald's novel, created an era for American style that had not been internationally credited previously. His classic designs for the Polo range said 'no work today', yet denoted the wearer to be a person of means and substance.

Perhaps the most influential look Lauren created was seen on Diane Keaton in Woody Allen's 1977 film *Annie Hall.* Lauren had already begun reworking menswear classics for women but Keaton brought the look to life on screen. Mackintosh coats, men's shirts, jackets and trousers were accessorized with cinched-in belts and hats. Wide belts, ties, kooky sunglasses and fun shoes softened the masculine separates.

Geoffrey Beene and Calvin Klein also created softer versions of masculine styling for the women's market. Both started out by specializing in sportswear, a particular brand of American daywear that never really took off in Europe. Essentially, 'sportswear' was a euphemism for comfortable clothes and off-shoots include the leisure suit or track suit worn every day instead of for sports activities. Soft jerseys, fleece fabrics and easy cotton separates were part of this look and Beene was one of the first designers to use fine synthetic fabrics for his trademark, easy designs. In 1974 the 'Beene Bag' dress was hugely popular, a dress essentially made up of two pieces of fabric with gaps for hands and neck, which draped beautifully in at the knees, fitting anyone who tried it.

Geoffrey Beene pioneered the softly draped jersey dress that appeared in many forms in the 1970s including collections by other great Americans including Roy Halston and Bill Blass. Yet all their versions were overshadowed by the most famous dress of all time, Diane von Furstenberg's wrap dress. In 1972 Belgian-born fashion designer Diane von Furstenberg arrived in New York and, a year later, produced her first line of the wrap dress. It was perfect for the times. Working women were emerging as a force to be reckoned with in the Big Apple and it became possible for a woman to be sexy, attractive and successful all at the same time. American working women loved the professional yet feminine style of the wrap dress. Three years later, this drip-dry cotton jersey garment, cut to flatter and available in a number of natural wood-block prints, had sold five million copies. The DVF brand was born and 'Feel like a woman, wear a dress!' became von Furstenberg's trademark phrase. Re-launched in the 1990s, von Furstenberg's name once again became synonymous with grown-up, feminine chic.

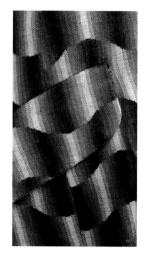

ABOVE AND OPPOSITE LEFT Brown wool early 1970s suit by British boutique label Biba. The trouser suit gained prominence in the 1970s, here with wide trouser legs and turn-ups. The amazing optical effect of the weave can be seen in detail, above.

OPPOSITE RIGHT Jean Muir grey pinafore dress with leather trim, early 1970s, a fine example of her sharp tailoring skills and the immaculate precision of her designs. She was known for her ability to work jersey, leather, wool and cashmere into fluid but perfectly proportioned shapes.

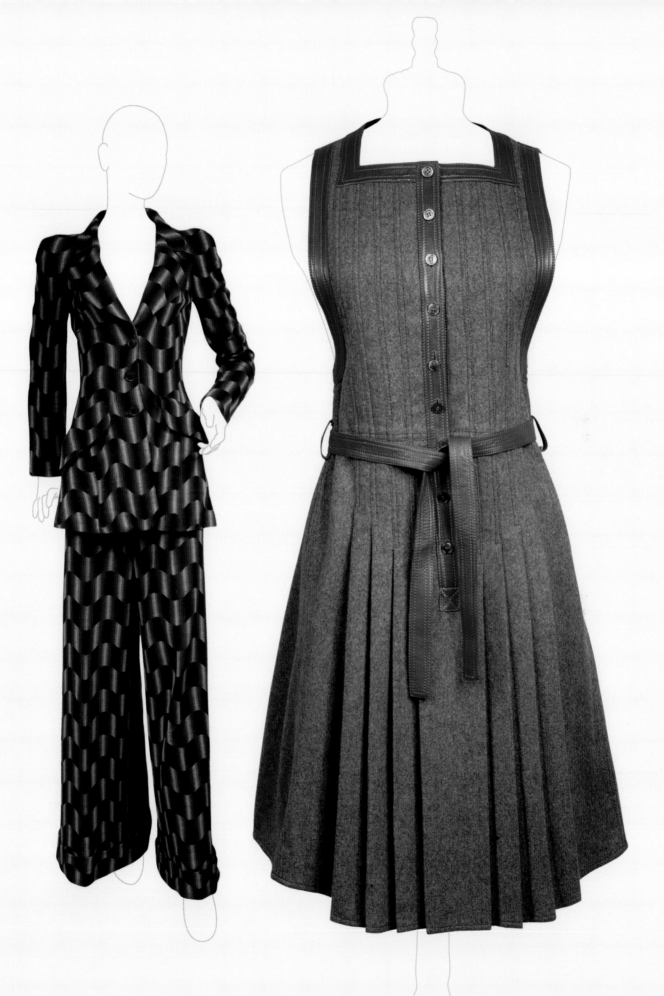

Back-to-Nature Fashions

The rebellious political mood of the 1960s spilled over into fashion. By 1970 nobody wanted to dress like their parents and there was a reaction against the mass production of food and fashion among the politically aware. 'Back to nature' was the slogan of the times along with renewed interest in fantasy, magic and the spirit. The Beatles had been to India, sparking the popularity of yoga and Eastern concepts of spiritual development. Morocco became a holiday destination for rich hippies like Talitha Getty and designers such as Ossie Clark and Yves Saint Laurent.

Wearing the clothes of ethnic cultures that lived closer to nature was equated with freedom from the bonds of Western life – somehow people felt closer to Mother Earth in the naturally dyed, heavy cottons or cheesecloth of India or the colourful, stripey knitwear of Peru. Embellished fabrics from Greece, Turkey and further into Arabia featuring mirrors, beading, bells and intricate embroidery were hot. Styling details including layers, toggle-fastenings, ponchos and shawls as accessories, ricrac edging and embroidered purses on long cord or string worn across the body all added to the look. Eclecticism was the mark of the rich hippy: she still wore furs, but not the traditional, unfashionable Bond Street mink. Instead, she went for floor-length white Afghan lambskin, or patchwork rabbit creations from gipsy dealers and junk markets.

The folk look drifted across the Atlantic from America, where the hippy movement was born in the 1960s. Bob Dylan, the Byrds, the Mamas and Papas and Janis Joplin were all proponents of rock-folk fusion and its fashion off-shoots. In Europe the mood was more political. Hippy-folk vibes were alive and kicking in Amsterdam after John Lennon and Yoko Ono infamously spent their honeymoon in bed in room 902 of the Amsterdam Hilton in 1969. In Paris, Sonia Rykiel produced folkish bag-belts, echoing the 'peasant' feel of the moment. She, along with Dorothee Bis also began creating funky knitwear, aimed at young, feisty Parisians, still sore from the student riots of the 1960s.

British designers

London's Portobello Road market became a magnet for those seeking the ethnic look as stallholders diversified from antiques and junk into ethnic bric-à-brac and clothing. Canny boutique owners also saw a gap in the fashion market. Thea Porter imported Middle Eastern artefacts into her shop in Greek Street, London, and produced a series of one-off garments heavily influenced by her childhood years spent in pre-war Beirut. Like Zandra Rhodes, she produced her own prints in cottons and silks, sewing together different, vivid panels of clashing colours in flamboyant, Eastern-inspired designs. Porter can take the credit for putting

the kaftan on the fashion map, a garment rapidly adopted by such stars as Elizabeth Taylor and Barbra Streisand on the lookout for a touch of Bohemia.

One of the key designers of the decade was Bill Gibb, a farmer's son from Fraserburgh in Scotland, who was named *Vogue* Designer of the Year in 1970. A lover of fantasy, he based his collections around natural themes like the forest floor or mountains and sea. Wild, colourful prints clashed in the same garments, coupled with nostalgic, medieval styling. Long sleeves, tight bodices, scoop necks, lacings, ribbons and overskirts all featured in his designs made up in silks, chiffon and cotton. A typical Gibb evening dress from 1971, in his own hand-printed silk blues and reds, had huge, double-gathered sleeves, a peplum waist, full skirt and asymmetric braid around collar, cuffs, panels and hems, contrasting with two different print patterns on skirt and sleeves.

As the 1970s evolved, elements of traditional Indian, Mexican, Russian and Eastern European dress made it into all the big collections. Zandra Rhodes' early designs were inspired by ethnic cultures as diverse as those of Ukrainian peasants and North American Indians. Her Chevron shawl design drew inspiration from the quilting and stitching of the Russian Steppes, which she found in a picture book. Quilted on calico, Rhodes' circular coat with zig-zag hem summed up her amazing work at this time. Two years later, Rhodes' classic show at the Roundhouse, London, in 1972 – with designs inspired by Native American culture and featuring lightweight,

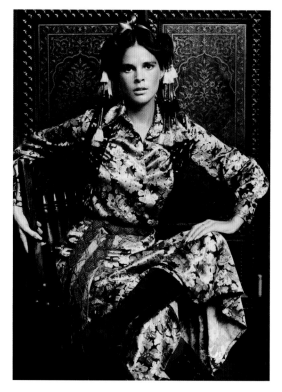

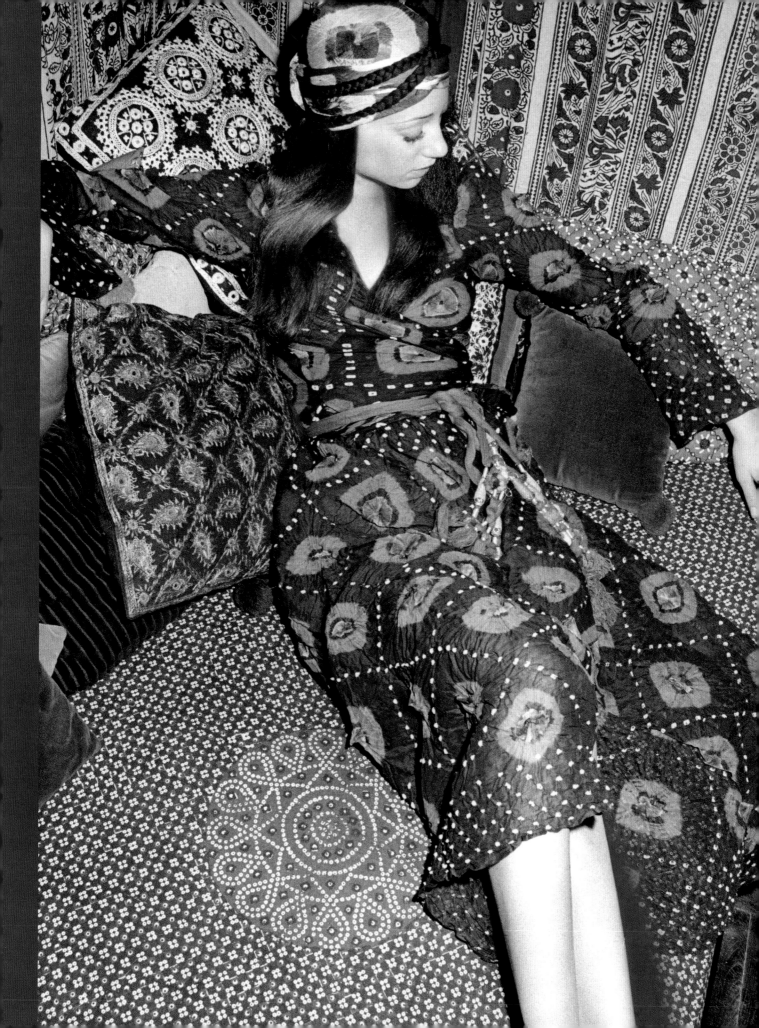

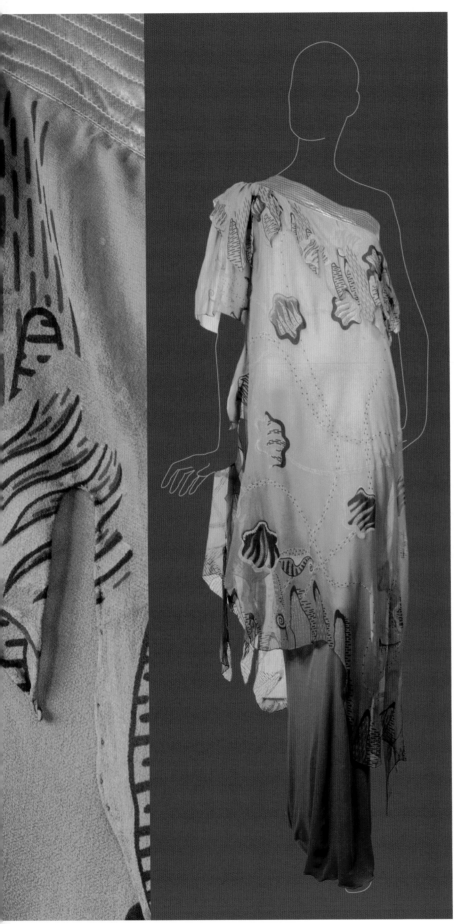

feather prints with string and bead detailing in muted natural blues, rusts, creams and black – put her on the fashion map. Her delightful printed designs, including the famous Butterflies series, cut into flattering silk, slimline ensembles and shifts or billowing chiffon creations remained her mainstays until 1977. However, as punk took hold, she decided that her butterflies felt too fragile for the changing climate and she created her first dresses in plain black or shocking pink silk jersey. In these, ripped and pinned with chains, 'street' and couture crossed paths again, and Rhodes was dubbed the 'Priestess of Punk' (see also pages 172–3).

Ethnic and natural trends also paved the way for innovative print designers who took their inspiration from nature. Celia Birtwell's flower-inspired fabrics became fashionable, their bold, swirling patterns contrasting with the pretty, traditional florals sold by Laura Ashley. Soon a crop of designers would emerge who would take all these elements and bring something new to the picture. Textile print designers Veronica Marsh and Althea McNish created bold, colourful designs for a new generation of buyers in Britain.

International designers

Meanwhile, in America, Patti Cappalli's range for Addenda spread the same vibrant new agenda. Pablo and Delia, two designers who arrived in London from Argentina, created fantasy-based prints for evening gowns and, by 1973, had set themselves up as London's coolest design couple and enjoyed a brief stay at the top of the arts-inspired fashion movement. The pair branched out into daywear, creating pinafores, blouses and wearable separates before their eventual demise as a design partnership in the late 1970s, though Delia Cancela went on to become a respected artist in Argentina. Meanwhile, in Europe, mainstream designers dabbled with looks inspired by the fantasists, but they were still shaking off the hard lines of couture.

SIGNATURE ZANDRA RHODES ELEMENTS:

❖ Asymmetrical hems and necklines
❖ Circular cutting on coats and capes
❖ Cactus, shells and butterfly designs
❖ Feather adornment
❖ 'Handkerchief' and cut-into hemlines
❖ Kaftan shapes
❖ Multi-layered chiffon
❖ 'Conceptual Chic' silk jersey evening dresses with ripped out holes, safety pin and chain detailing
❖ Vibrant colours

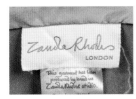

ABOVE AND OPPOSITE Grey and pink chiffon one-shoulder Zandra Rhodes dress over jersey lining with quilted satin band and slashed handrolled edges, 1974, with label detail.

RIGHT Zandra Rhodes's groundbreaking Chevron Shawl print on an unbleached quilted calico coat, 1970.

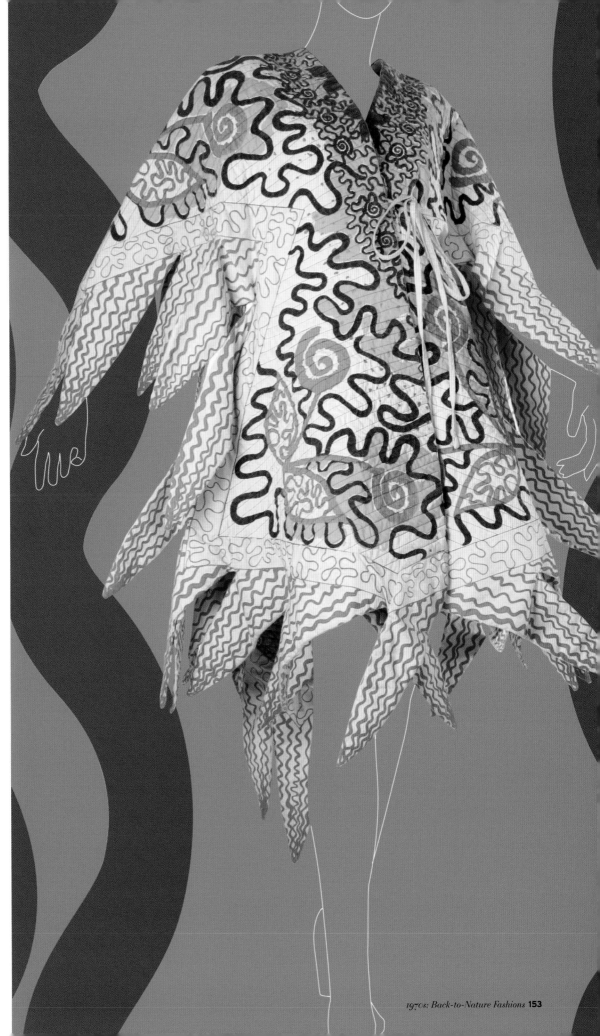

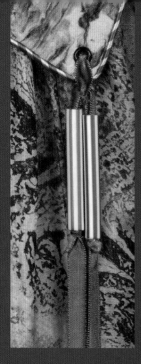

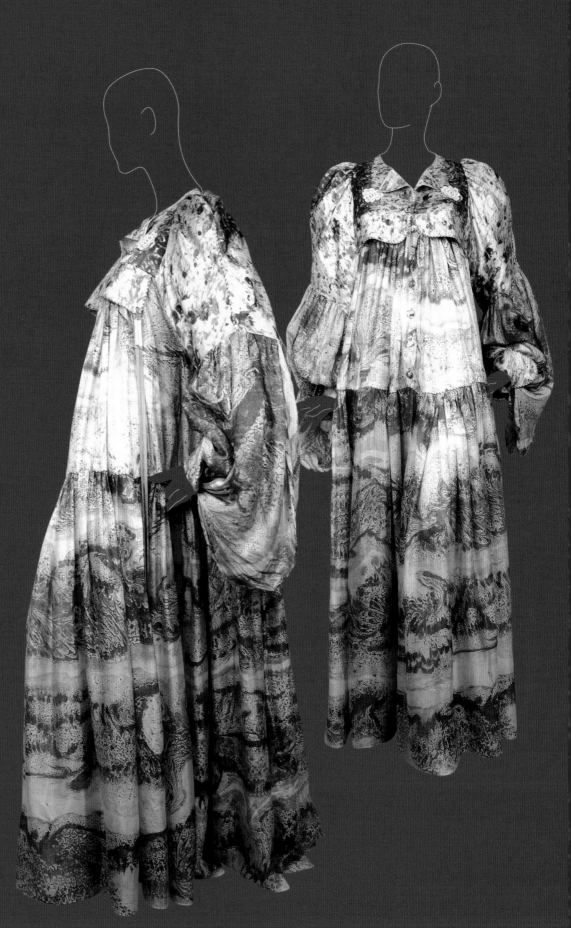

ABOVE AND RIGHT A craftsman costumer, Bill Gibb merged embroidery, slashed sleeves, satin and prints together in his truly imaginative hippy-style dresses. With its incredible decoration and details, worked across a voluminous surface of fabric, the overall print of this 1970 Bill Gibb dress reads like an Italian marbled-paper masterpiece.

OPPOSITE Under deep pleated layers, the sleeve is secured with hidden buttons along an interior panel of fabric in an alternative print.

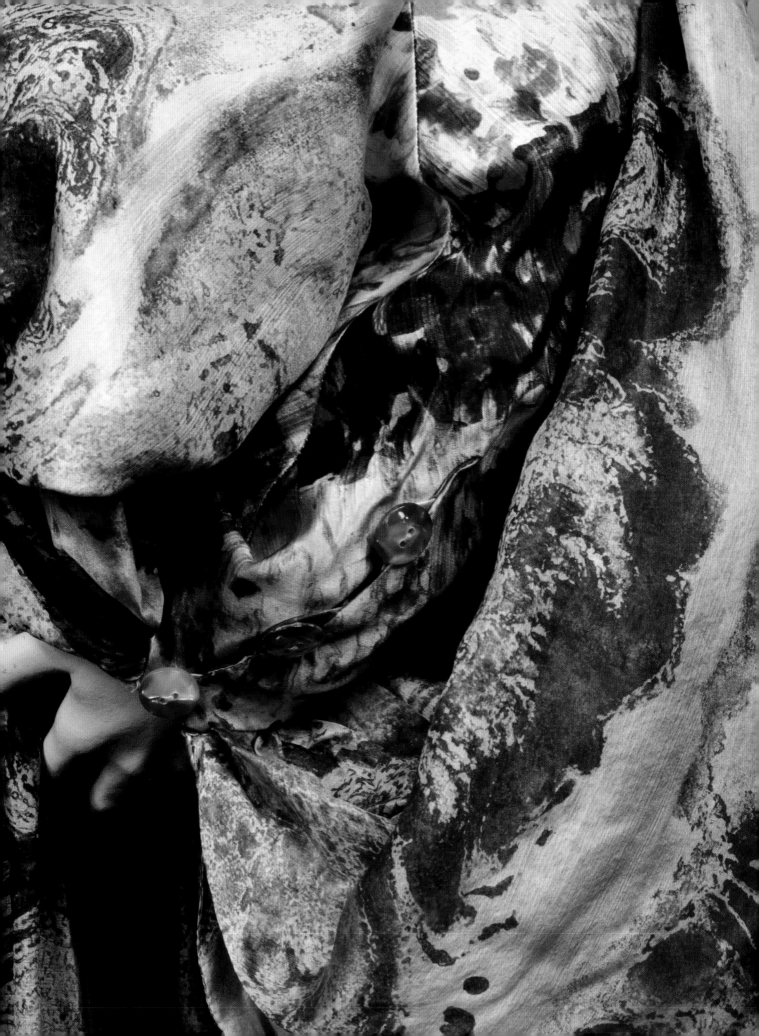

Ossie Clark and Celia Birtwell

The bohemian flavour of the 1970s, in which art and fashion amalgamated beautifully, was nowhere more apparent than in the work of fashion designer Ossie Clark and his wife Celia Birtwell, whom he married in 1969. Born in Liverpool but dubbed 'Ossie' because he had spent time in Oswaldtwhistle in Lancashire as an evacuee toddler during the Second World War, Clark graduated from the Royal College of Art in 1965. He became a cult figure on London's fashion scene: during his peak between 1968 and 1974 each new collection of essentially similar garments was heralded by *Vogue* and the fashion media as 'groundbreaking'.

As his success increased, his circle of friends grew to encompass artists like David Hockney and Patrick Proctor and rock stars such as Bryan Ferry and the Rolling Stones – in 1972–3 Clark designed Mick Jagger's stage catsuits. His early shows, featuring favourite models that included Patti Boyd, Patti D'Arbanville, Gala Mitchell and transsexual Amanda Lear, were true rock 'n' roll events. Parading the catwalk at Chelsea Town Hall in 1970 and the Royal Court Theatre in 1971, the models 'did their own thing', revealing a wild glamour that epitomized Ossie's philosophy of classic with a definite twist.

Clark's skill lay in his ability to cut and shape fabric around the female form with a subtle extravagance that was sexy and chic. He pioneered the midi and maxi lengths in the late 1960s, where other design houses, including Dior, had failed. Until their divorce in 1974, Clark and Birtwell created their designs for Quorum, the Chelsea fashion boutique owned by Alice Pollock, a designer whose mini fashion empire was the hub of swinging London. Birtwell's print designs came to life in her husband's chiffon trouser suits of 1970. Cream, with swirling, Art Deco-inspired plant and flower patterns on

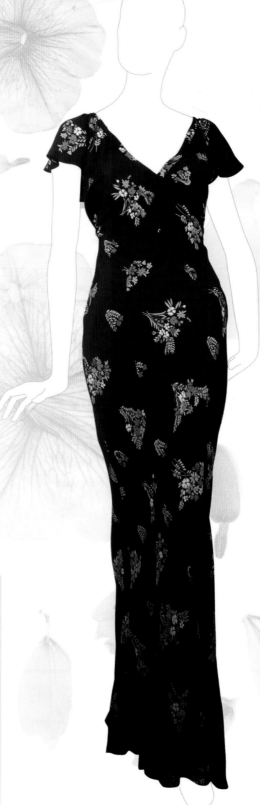

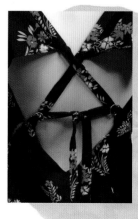

ABOVE AND LEFT Ossie Clark dress with Celia Birtwell floral print, 1972. The bias-cut length hugs the body while the back ties secure the sleeves and neckline.

SIGNATURE OSSIE CLARK ELEMENTS:

❖ Rounded or pointed collars or deep V-necks
❖ Bias cutting
❖ Fitted, peplum jackets
❖ Tulip-shaped skirts
❖ Maxi coats
❖ Ruffles
❖ Puffed-out sleeves between narrow shoulders and narrow cuffs
❖ Chiffon trouser suits
❖ Gently fitted shapes
❖ Layering; e.g. shorter sleeves over long, or minidresses over trousers

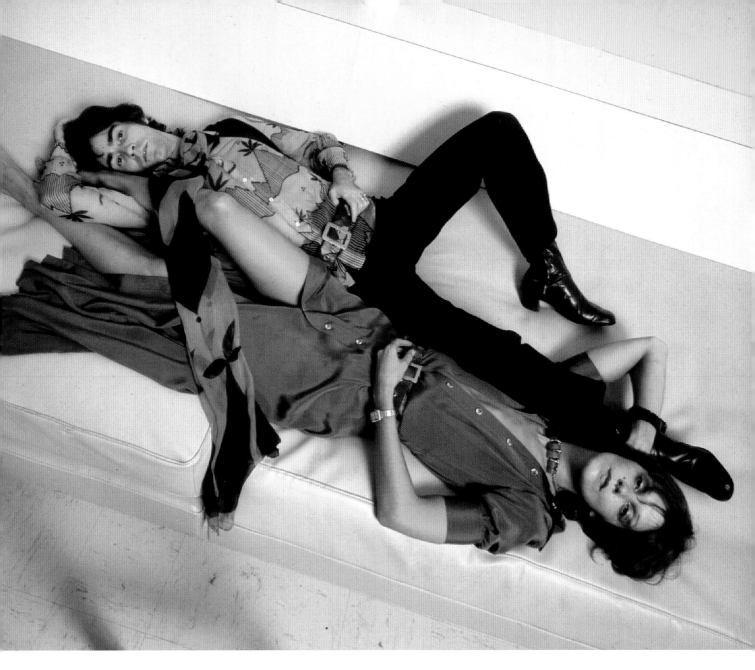

the wide sleeves and the skirt of the mini overdress, and around the hems of flared trousers, this was daywear of the prettiest kind. Clark would incorporate her floral prints in evening dresses, alternating swathes of contrasting prints in a bias-cut, floor-length satin or crepe de chine spiral.

Alongside his coveted frocks, Clark's tailoring was equally desirable. Totally new ideas, like floral-printed wool fashioned into a beautiful fitted winter coat, inspired a whole generation of copies. Among other pieces were three-piece trouser suits in Birtwell-print velvet and zipped bomber jackets in patent pythonskin or similar three-buttoned, closely fitted versions in black, brown, navy or deep red. There are few Ossie Clark originals to be found in the modern vintage market. Most of the garments he made for his London clients (including Nicky Samuel – wife of Nigel Weymouth, owner of 1970s boutique Granny Takes A Trip – and Alfred Radley, whose family business backed

Clark and Quorum financially) have stayed in their family's private collections or they have simply been worn out by their lucky owners. There were copies around, but Clark's style was too perfectionist for many to be able to mimic adequately. He revived the bias-cut dress after picking up 1930s originals in Portobello Market during the 1960s and taking them home to experiment with. The bias became one of his signature shapes – the flexibility and slight stretchiness of bias cuts on fine fabrics like crepe de chine mean that they fit in the most flattering way. Although Clark's designs favoured large-breasted body shapes with narrow hips, his clothes flattered anyone who could fit into them comfortably. After their divorce, the couple went their separate ways and there is no denying the loss to British fashion of this dynamic duo's joint creative powers. Hardworking, dedicated Birtwell continues to design today and deserves state recognition – a damehood at least – for her services to British fashion.

ABOVE Ossie Clark with friend and collaborator Alice Pollock of Quorum in a photograph by Lord Snowdon.

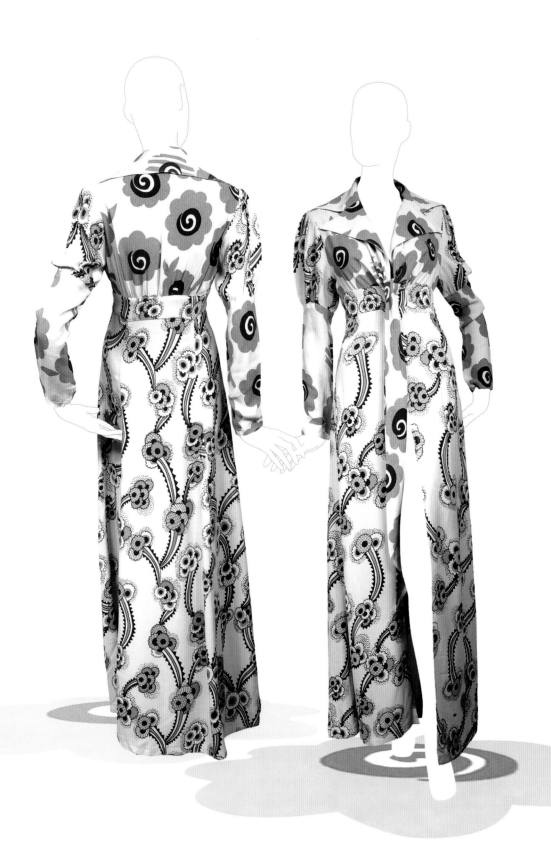

LEFT Front and back views of a 1971 Ossie Clark–Celia Birtwell coat with puffed sleeves, pointed lapel and Birtwell's famous Floating Daisy print. With its tie-front fastening, the coat was made to be worn over a coordinating dress in the same colourway.

OPPOSITE An alternative variation of the Floating Daisy design in another Clark-Birtwell coat, this time featuring the floral print alongside a grid design on the bodice, rounded collar and sleeves. The buttons intersect the grid neatly down the bodice.

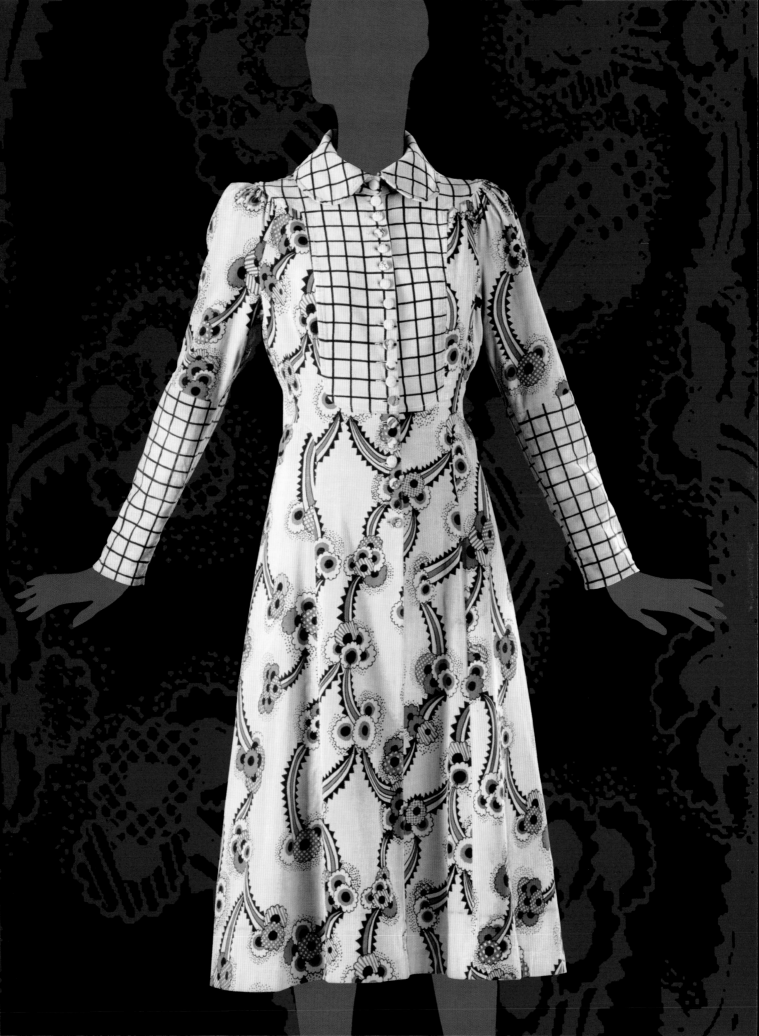

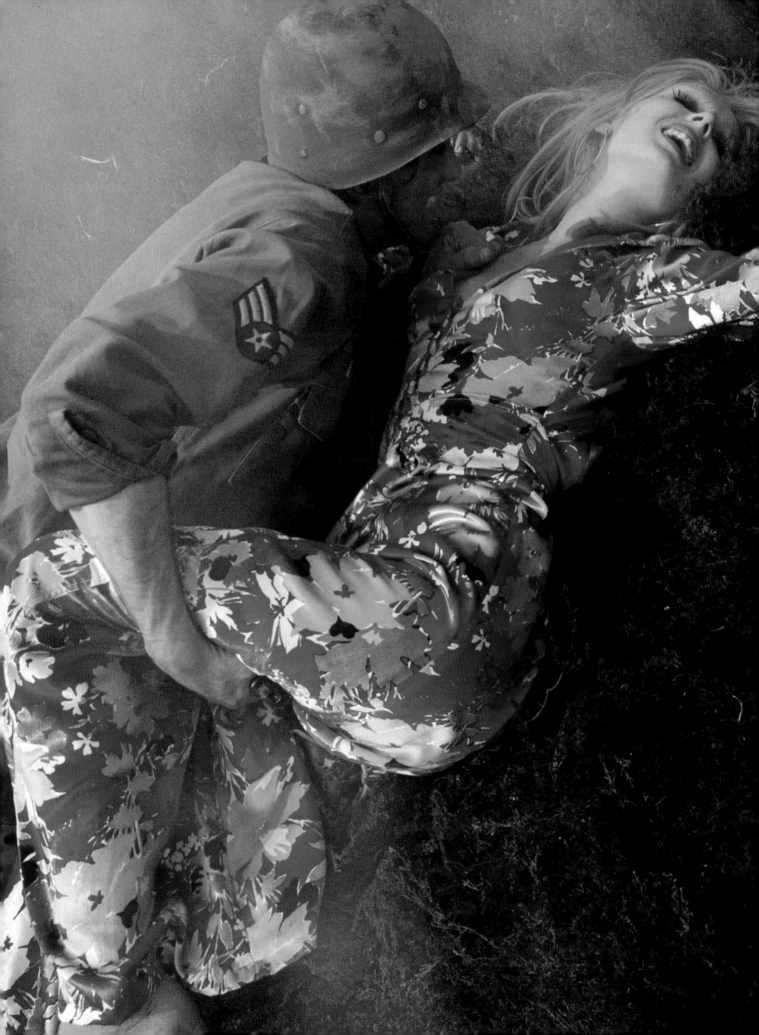

BELOW TOP Celia Birtwell's Floating Daisy pattern. Clusters of dark-eyed flowers are linked by stripey stems in a curving pattern that reflected Ossie Clark's form-fitting bias cut to the dress.

BELOW BOTTOM This floral print mingles poppies with trailing stems. Here the motifs appear in red and blue on a cream ground. Other typical Birtwell motifs included geometrics, leaves, fruit and stars.

BELOW TOP This exotic print is typically exuberantly Birtwell – a mix of graphic and natural motifs – stripes, waves, palm leaves and clover-like trails in blue and black on a lemon yellow field.

BELOW BOTTOM Oversized blue flowers on a long coat make a high-impact statement. Birtwell's textiles were inspired by nature: scattered lilies and tulips, trailing leaves and stems.

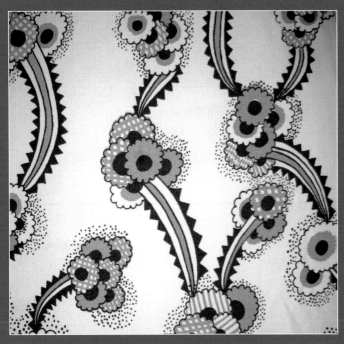

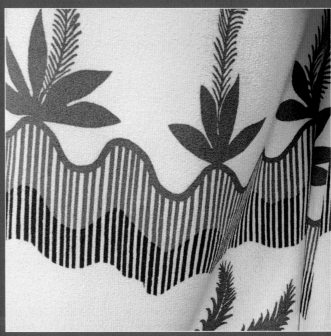

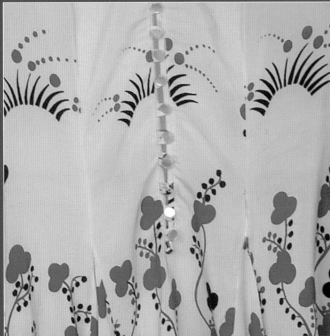

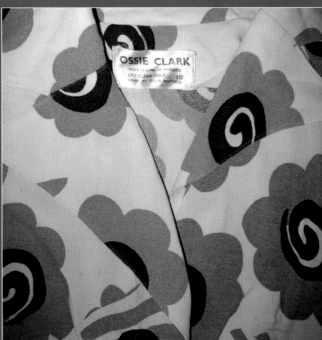

OPPOSITE A 1974 advertisement for an Ossie Clark dress with a Birtwell print, by Jim Lee. The designs are as wearable and covetable today as they were in the 1970s.

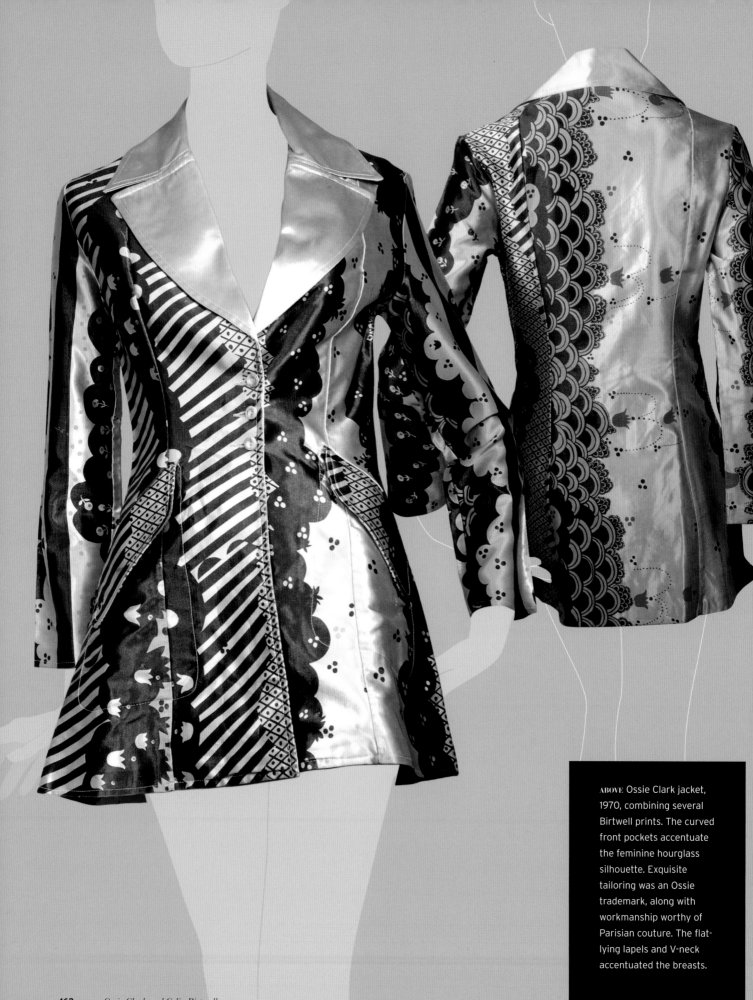

ABOVE: Ossie Clark jacket, 1970, combining several Birtwell prints. The curved front pockets accentuate the feminine hourglass silhouette. Exquisite tailoring was an Ossie trademark, along with workmanship worthy of Parisian couture. The flat-lying lapels and V-neck accentuated the breasts.

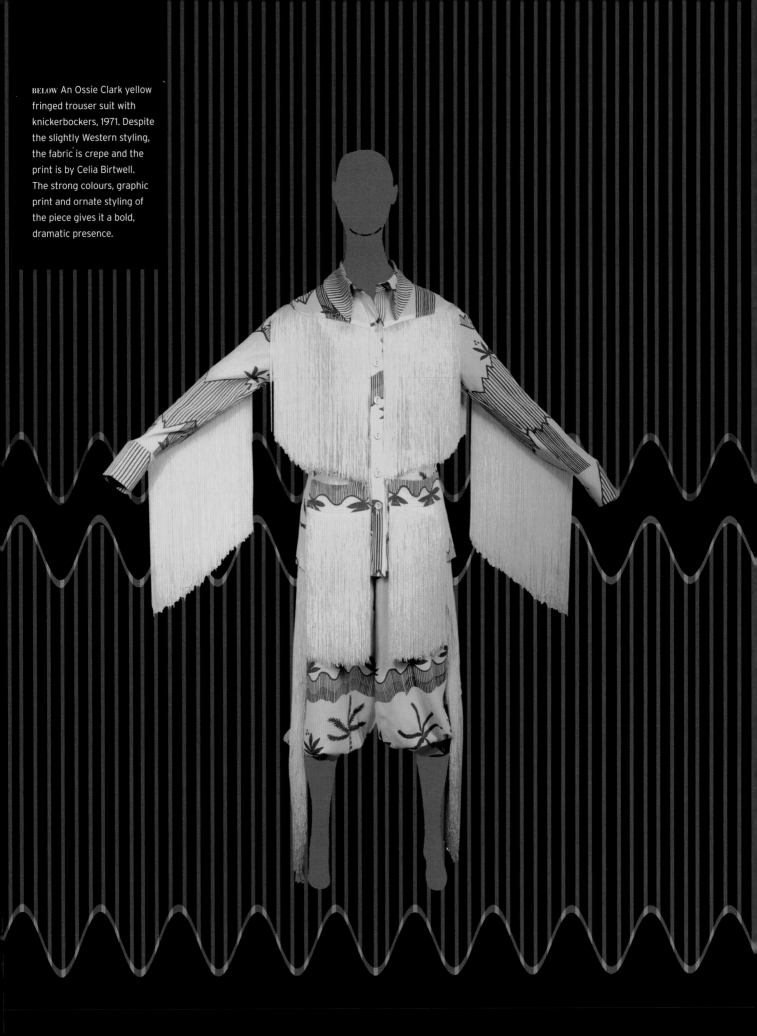

Decorative Arts and Crafts Revivals

Organic farming and self-sufficiency thrived alongside a revival of interest in traditional handcrafts in the 1970s. Night classes in knitting, macramé, embroidery, weaving and pottery began to appear. Detail became a crucial element of fashion, emerging all the way through the decade in different ways, from handcrafted knitted, woven and embroidered fabrics through to patchwork and pleating mid-decade, followed by another appliqué revival at the end of the decade.

Several designers of the 1970s were noted for their interest in reviving traditional craftsmanship. In Britain, Laura Ashley's early designs were inspired by country crafts, and yokes, smocking, embroidery, brocade and lace details set her clothes apart from more mass-produced versions. They helped to supply a growing market for traditional and even Victorian-style clothes.

Bill Gibb used wool, reworking such traditional knits as Fair Isle and Arran into different patterns and weaves with new properties. He put knitted waistcoats over evening dresses and gave the whole concept of knitting a new image. Crochet, knobbly textures, beading and unusually small or large stitches came to characterize his work, as more designers followed his lead and began to work with knitted fabrics. Gibb also liked to take traditional Scottish woven fabrics, including tweed, and give them a new twist. One of his 1970 designs features a heavily patterned pigskin jacket worn over a knife-pleated, checked tweed skirt. Although Gibb teamed up with American knitwear designer Kaffe Fassett on several occasions in joint ventures, he was destined never to capitalize on his creativity owing to constant financial difficulties.

Knitted fabrics were not just craft-inspired, folksy and ethnic-looking. Since the 1960s, designers including Sonia Rykiel and Missoni had been fashioning garments from stretchy knits. By the early 1970s such looks were big fashion news at other major houses, including Krizia. Missoni's trademark zig-zag, finely striped, multicolour knits helped to establish it as Milan's biggest fashion company, planting the northern Italian city firmly on the fashion map. Meanwhile, British names like Jeff Banks and Daniel Hechter entered the market with stylish knitted tank tops and V-necked, deep-ribbed, cuff-sleeved sweaters. The tabard-style overtop – a wide-sleeved, long-lined tunic, often belted at the waist and worn over a turtleneck sweater – was big news in 1976. Further down the fashion chain, knitwear became popular on the high street, with cheaper brands producing sporty hotpants, vests, leggings and legwarmers in cheaper acrylic knits.

LEFT Missoni 1970s top and fringed overshirt. The exceptional colours and textures have made Missoni pieces highly collectible and as popular today as since their inception by sisters Tai and Rosita Missoni in 1953. Worldwide attention started in the late '60s, and the 1970s saw them producing dresses, coats, skirts and trousers as well as sweaters.

OPPOSITE The back view of a 1979 knitted coat by Kaffe Fassett, who was known for his rich many-coloured palette and geometric patterns. The muted colours and full sleeves, which draw on Renaissance and Eastern dress, show his influential creative skills. The colours and shape also recall the work of Missoni and Bill Gibb; indeed, his early collections were commissioned by both.

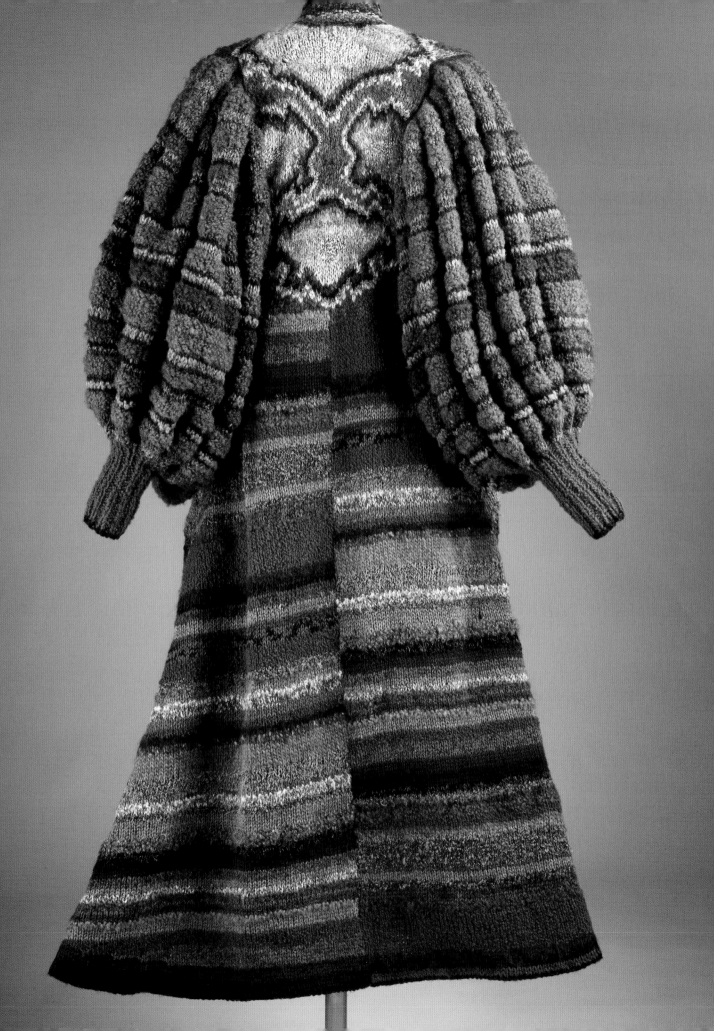

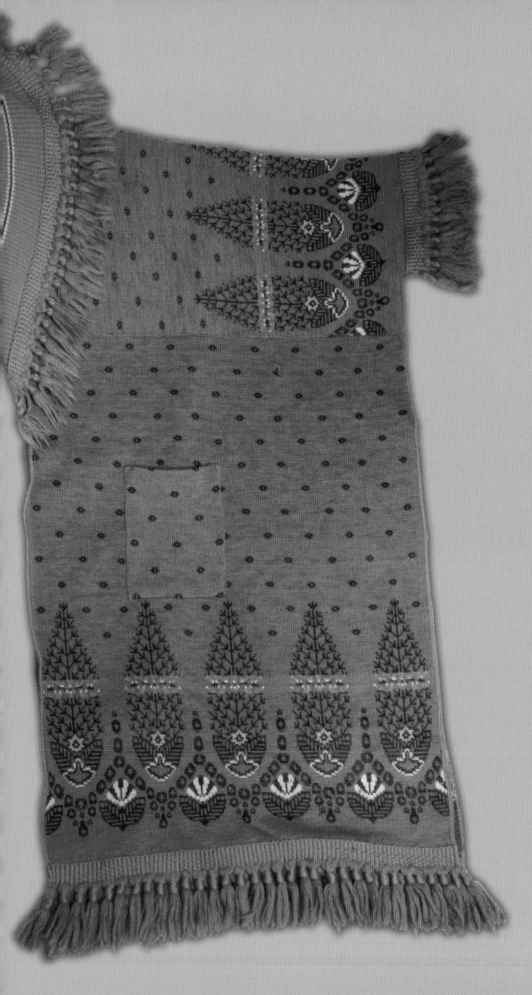

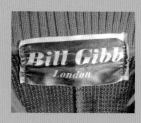

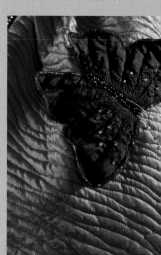

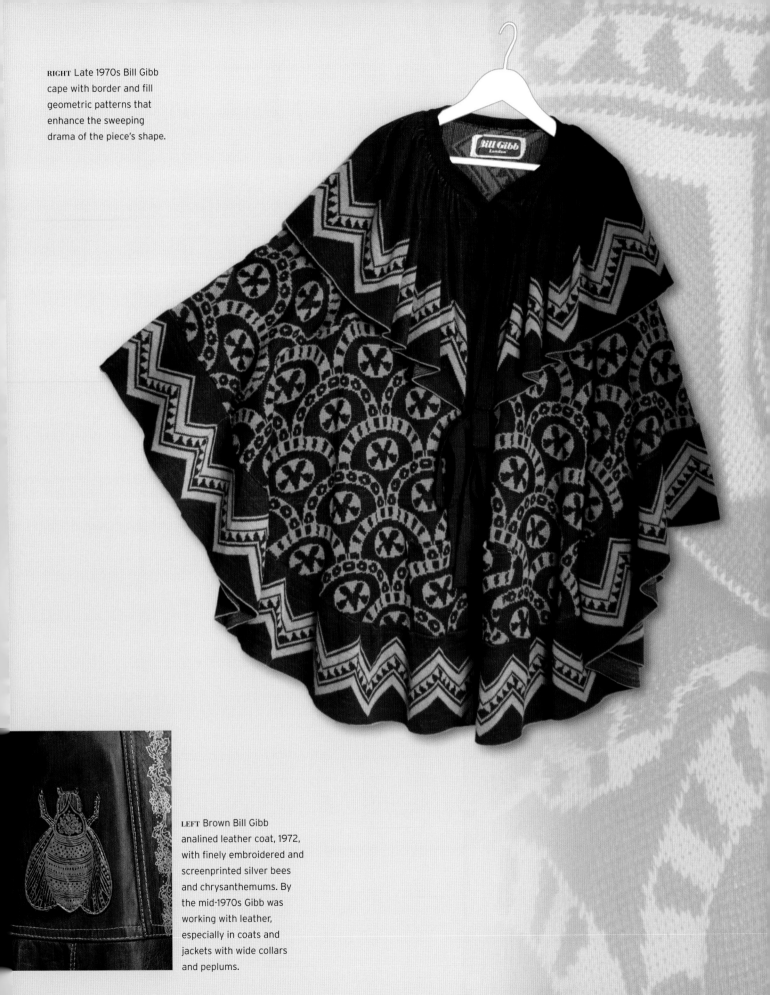

RIGHT Late 1970s Bill Gibb cape with border and fill geometric patterns that enhance the sweeping drama of the piece's shape.

LEFT Brown Bill Gibb analined leather coat, 1972, with finely embroidered and screenprinted silver bees and chrysanthemums. By the mid-1970s Gibb was working with leather, especially in coats and jackets with wide collars and peplums.

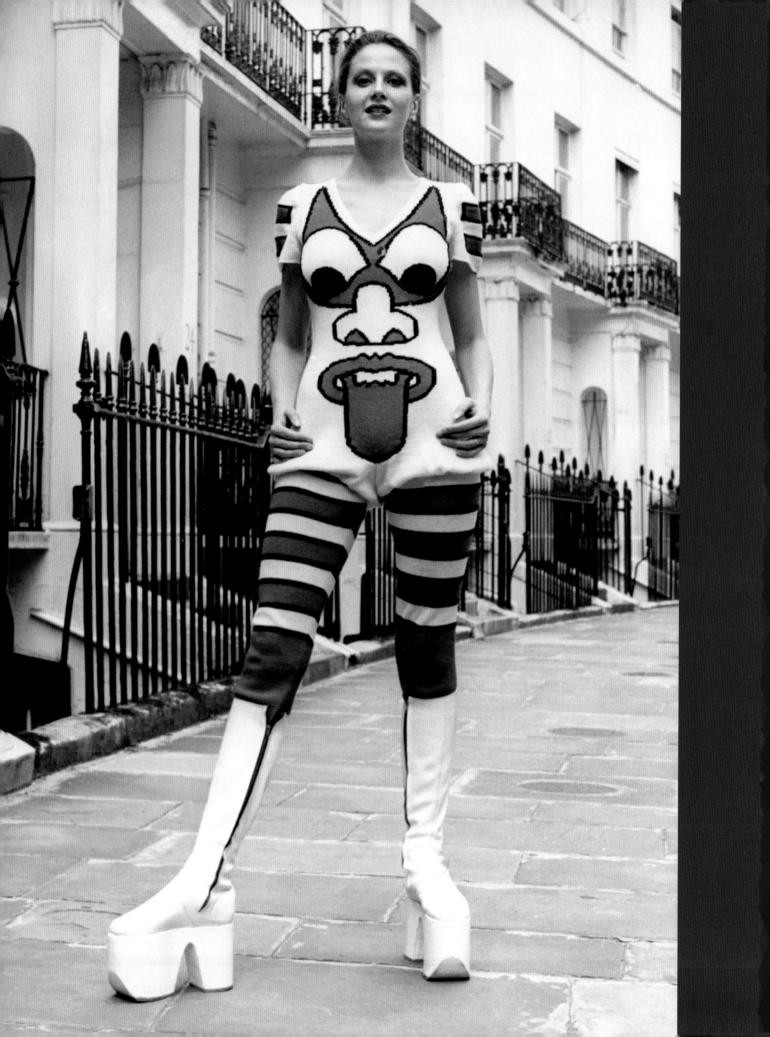

Japanese Visionaries

Although Japanese fashion had been traditional for centuries, the dawn of the techno-revolution sparked design interest in all things cultural and by the early 1970s new design names began to emerge. Fashion was the natural medium for the inspired creativity of Kansai Yamamoto, Issey Miyake and Kenzo Takada, and later Hanae Mori, Yohji Yamamoto and Rei Kawakubo of Comme des Garçons. Described as 'funny' and 'quirky' by fashion journalists, there is no doubt that their work introduced an element of fun as well as some amazing styling.

Issey Miyake's early designs show his genius with fabric, as in his red silkprint evening dress with sash waist and layers of fabric that seemed to show no traditional fastenings at all. The broad spectrum of his inventiveness was demonstrated in one fashion shoot that had models wearing – among other outfits – thigh-high red suede boots with wraparound ties over chequerboard leggings with a matching jacket in red and white, and multicoloured, three-way-striped combinations topped with a matching miniskirt in greens, blues and reds.

Kansai Yamamoto took elements from traditional Kabuki theatre costume, including a giant red mask that he printed on to modern kimonos, T-shirts and knitwear. After his first London design house was opened in 1971, his clothes were quickly snatched up by the fashion cognoscenti, eager for yet another take on the vogue for all things Eastern and ethnic.

A Japanese fashion explosion followed and no one epitomized this look better than model Marie Helvin or Yoko Ono. As the oriental influence on fashion took hold, the designers themselves branched out. Kenzo Takada began his career with a Paris boutique – Jungle Jap, so called after the jungle patterns and prints of which he was so fond. Starting with simple smocks, wide-legged trousers, wraparound skirts and long tops in plain, dark-coloured cottons or padded fabrics, he went on to produce pretty western-style floral prints with Victorian design detailing, including pinned and tucked bodices and billowing petticoat and skirt ensembles that were in keeping with the vintage fashion feel of the early 1970s. Later, as knitwear became a key medium, Kenzo introduced his signature stripey knits. Layering the knits over each other, he created an easy-to-wear trend and was the first to show a bulky sweater over a short miniskirt with a belt at the hips, creating an enduring, youthful fashion shape that has transcended time.

Quilting was also a distinctive element of the work of many of the Japanese designers, including Kansai Yamamoto, whose 1972 spring collection featured a green quilted velvet trouser suit with cropped flares and a silver quilted macintosh with matching hat.

OPPOSITE Artist and political activist Caroline Coon models a red-and-white, handknitted, woollen jumpsuit, by Japanese designer Kansai Yamamoto, 1971, featuring his Kabuki theatre mask.

BELOW Shirtdress in a navy-and-white, Japanese-inspired print, by Hanae Mori, with a twined rope belt by Yves Saint Laurent, and a purple suede watch cap by Mr John, 1970. Mori established her haute couture collection and fashion house in Paris in 1977, becoming known for her restrained elegance and delicacy.

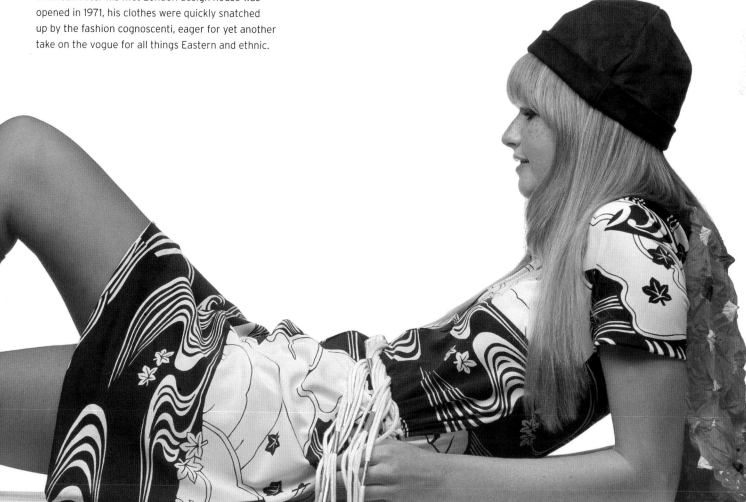

Punk Fashions

Invented by Malcolm McLaren and Vivienne Westwood, punk fashion certainly came as a surprise to everyone. It started out as extreme bondage gear sold in SEX, the King's Road emporium that the pair later relabelled Seditionaries. The overall 'look', as sold by McLaren and Westwood, combined the traditional components of bondage gear, including rubber, leather, studs, straps and buckles, with other elements. Muslin and cotton T-shirts, shirts, narrow trousers and vests were ripped up and then pinned back together again to form loose, layered garments. Skintight leather jeans, mini-kilts, dyed cotton drill trousers with the legs joined together with straps formed the foundation of the punk outfit. The biker jacket, the classic teenage garment of rebellion, was also part of the style, but this time in red patent leather or pink plastic.

Punk separated street fashion from the elitist, higher end of the market for good. The fashion press just did not get it and labelled the punks 'trash'. Punk rock was as much a part of the fashion movement as the clothes, characterized by the same anarchic subversion and anti-Establishment stance, although the music itself soon evolved into New Wave, then fizzled out into a mêlée of different sounds.

Punk fashion revolutionized the way people dressed, kicking off a number of trends with far-reaching influences. Until 1977, trousers had been steadily flaring outwards, reaching anything up to 50 cm (20 in) wide. By autumn of that year, the punks were wearing drainpipe jeans – industrial Wranglers and Levis that they had customized themselves. This in itself was almost as shocking for many as the safety pins, snot and swearing. To balance the new skinny leg shapes brought in by punk, shoulders were padded out and built up. These changes spread into mainstream fashion and by 1978 'straight leg' trousers were everywhere, and padded shoulders and longer-line jackets featured in collections by Marc Bohan at Dior, Adrian Cartmel for Manson, Yves Saint Laurent's Rive Gauche and Genny at Regine.

For a brief moment, street trends and fashion met up on the disco dance floor. Inspired by the safety pins, buckles and badges of punk, Karl Lagerfeld created big, star-shaped pins and brooches for Chloé. Throughout the 1970s, Lagerfeld's designs stayed closest of all the designers' to the 'street' in terms of trends. His youthful touch and intrinsic understanding of the fashion zeitgeist kept him on track and slightly apart from the haughtier couturiers. Marc Bohan at Dior also designed with a youthful 'trendy' touch, clearly influenced by the shapes and colours of punk.

In fact, punk gave couture a new direction. Strong colours including bright pink and red, and checks inspired by tartans appeared in the late 1970s collections of the major houses. When Marc Bohan finally left Dior in 1992, it was felt that a new spirit was needed at the classic fashion house, but during the late 1970s Bohan was truly the master of sexy, funky chic on the international fashion circuit. Back then, Dior developed a slick glamour, reinvented later in the 1990s by John Galliano. A quick flick through the pages of *Vogue* from those later years of the 1970s reveals the divide between mainstream couture fashion and the funkier, punkier, night-time dressing inspired by punk.

Zandra Rhodes' 'Conceptual Chic' look, featuring punk-style evening gowns ripped and torn to shreds, capitalized on the feeling of division that was everywhere in popular culture post-punk. Meanwhile, future design talents were preparing for their own onslaught, which came in the 1980s, when, thanks to government recognition and fashion pioneers such as public relations master Lynne Franks, British fashion came into its own. Betty Jackson worked for Radley (though Ossie Clark, their chief designer at the time reputedly refused to speak to her), Katharine Hamnett was designing jeans for Tuttabankem and Antony Price created looks for chainstore Stirling Cooper. All these names and more would emerge, with their own directional, groundbreaking looks, in the ten years after punk.

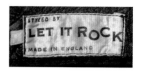

ABOVE AND BELOW Vivienne Westwood dog-collar knit for the Let It Rock label, from the 1971 Let It Rock shop, which was supplanted in name by Too Fast To Live, Too Young To Die in 1972, SEX in 1974, Seditionaries in 1977 and World's End from 1980. In the beginning Let It Rock focused on 1950s revival pieces but, as this piece from the period shows, Westwood's and McLaren's subversive turn towards punk was fast approaching.

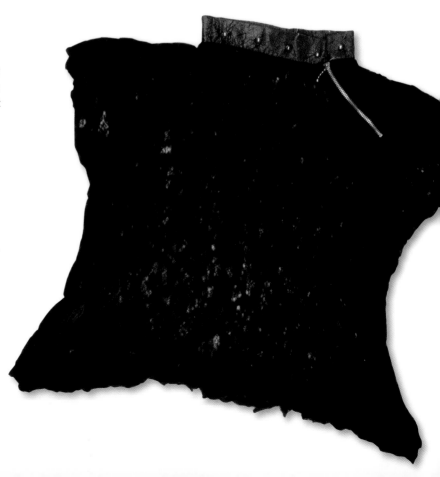

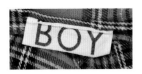

ABOVE AND RIGHT Westwood's clothes born from her 1976 Bondage collection were studded, buckled, strapped, chained and zippered. The BOY bondage trousers, label above and pictured right, are an exact copy of Westwood's Seditionaries' originals. BOY bought the rights to sell a limited range from Westwood and McLaren from 1976 until the early 1980s. The Cambridge Rapist T-shirt is from the SEX label, 1976.

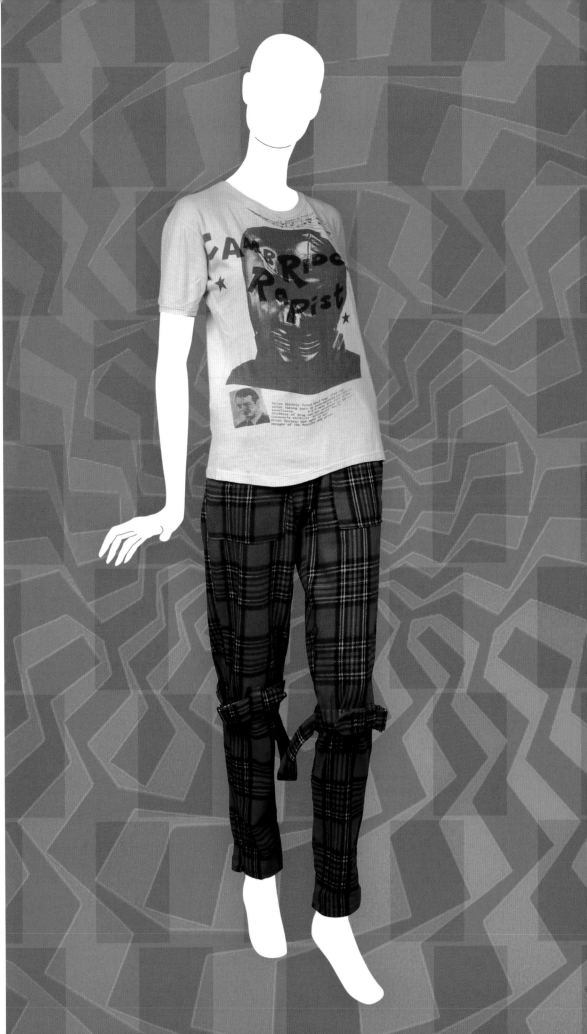

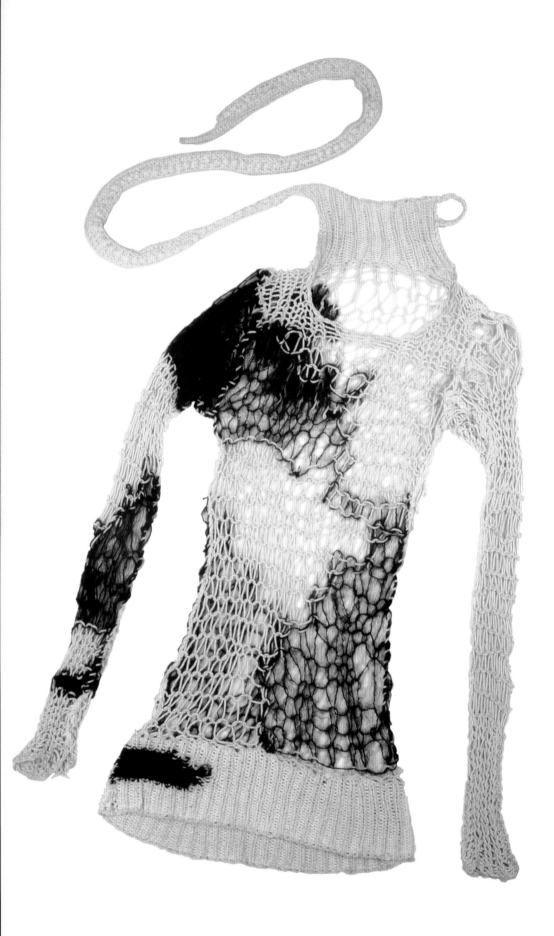

LEFT Black-and-white Hangman jumper by Westwood and McLaren's Seditionaries, 1977. Reminiscent of a straightjacket with the overlong arms, the 'noose' neck fastening loops around to enclose the collar by a tie long enough to hang oneself from. The chaotic, uneven weave of the knit and the noose-tie shape were details that greatly influenced the work of other designers.

OPPOSITE Detail from a Zandra Rhodes Conceptual Chic dress, 1977, in black rayon jersey. Its punk styling is evidenced in the asymmetrical holes, beaded safety pins, ball-link chains and diamanté decoration.

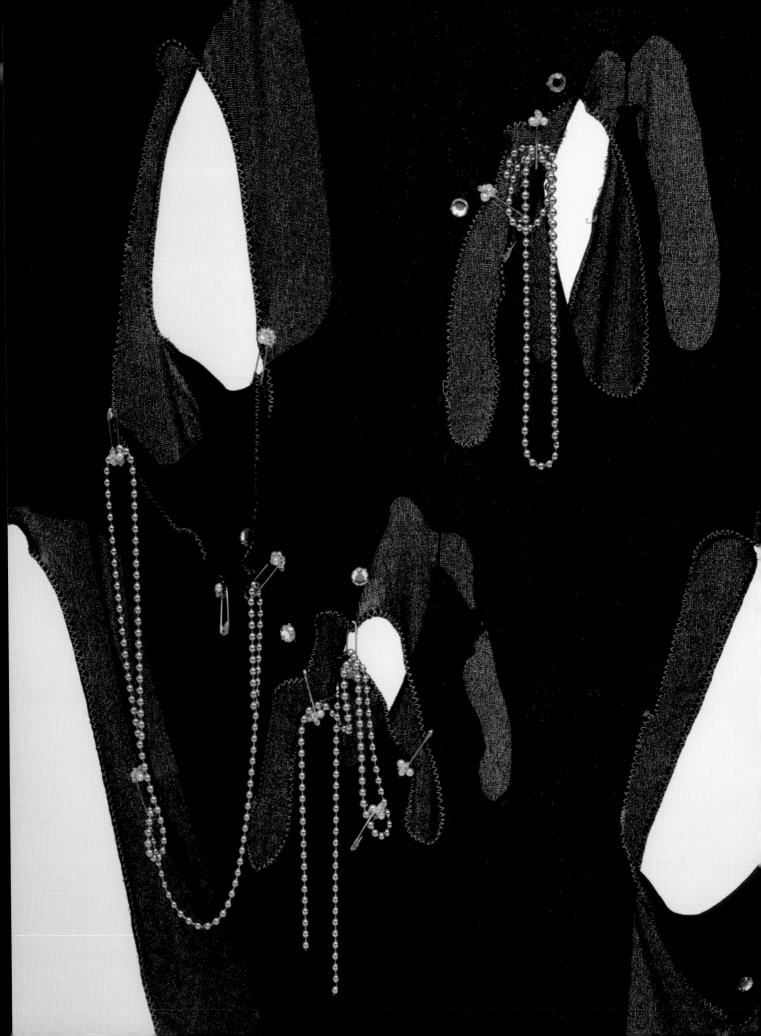

Denim and Leather

'Blue jean baby, LA lady, seamstress for the band,' sang Elton John in his 1971 song 'Tiny Dancer', based on Maxine Taupin, wife of his songwriting partner Bernie. The words epitomized the modern idea of jeans as the sexy, casual uniform of the rock 'n' roll elite. Denim had crept up on fashion in the 1960s, with Yves Saint Laurent creating cool brushed-denim trouser suits. The great designer was later to lament that his one regret on looking back over his career was that he 'did not invent the blue jean'. Naturally, other designers cashed in. Soon there were top-end purveyors including Fiorucci, whose stores in London sold a glamorous, continental denim style as sported on the beaches of San Tropez. Also in London, Katherine Hamnett launched her career designing kooky hotpants and denim mini ensembles for the label Tuttabankem. Until the late 1970s, when denim suddenly went upmarket, patchwork, studded, panelled, bleached and fringed leather and denim styles interwove to create a unisex look that increased in flamboyance.

The Americans, who invented denim jeans during the middle of the nineteenth century courtesy of Levi Strauss, came up with 'designer' jeans aimed specifically at women looking for the perfect fit. First came Gloria Vanderbilt's version in 1978 with its Swan insignia and diamanté sparkle. Vanderbilt jeans were cut like fitted, straight-legged women's trousers and were supposedly of better quality than high street versions. Female shoppers went for the designer jeans concept in droves. Although Vanderbilt jeans did not stay cool for long, their legacy spawned the huge industry that lives on today. In 1979, when 15-year-old starlet Brooke Shields told the world, 'You know what comes between me and my Calvins? Nothing,' the label jean had arrived. The Calvin Klein jeans modelled by Shields were high-waisted and straight-legged, tapering in slightly at the ankle.

In 1970, Roberto Cavalli set up shop selling a small range of sexy leather separates. Soon leather waistcoats, jackets, skirts and trousers became as cool as denim. When denim went 'designer', the leather jacket was quickly snatched up and reworked by Thierry Mugler and Claude Montana. Karl Lagerfeld at Chloé also helped to put leather on the designer map. Mugler's autumn 1978 collection featured a white velvet, diamanté-studded jumpsuit and bronze leather jackets that had studded diagonal fastenings, astronaut padding details and matching skull caps. Meanwhile, Jap (Kenzo Takada's line) delivered pink leather tuxedos. By 1979 soft pigskin and suede were trademark tailoring materials in collections by Maxfield Parrish, Bruce Oldfield and Nicole Fahri for Stephen Marks. Fahri's punched suede blazer in beige with narrow lapels and soft gathered and padded shoulders tapped into the decade's love of suede.

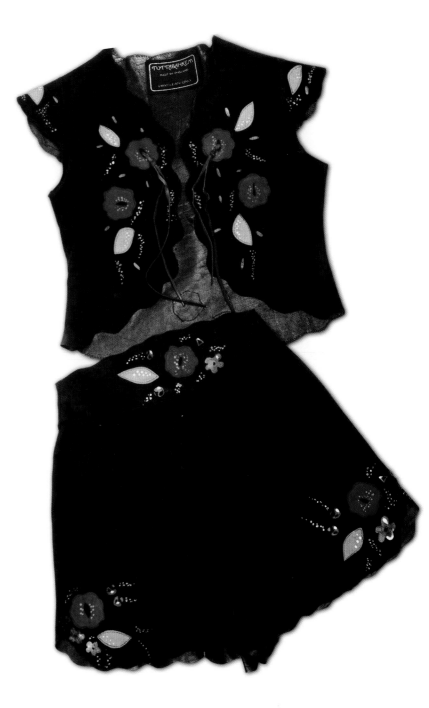

ABOVE Tuttabankem leather appliqué hotpants and waistcoat, 1970/1. Tuttabankem was cofounded in 1970 by Katherine Hamnett and Anne Buck, who sold their pieces to Henri Bendel, Saks, Browns and Alexander's of Rome before Hamnett launched her own label in 1975.

OPPOSITE Russian model, Veruschka in the Borghese Gardens in Rome, wearing a light suede vest and shorts with a dark shirt and leather belts by Gucci, with knee-high black leather boots by Valentino, 1971.

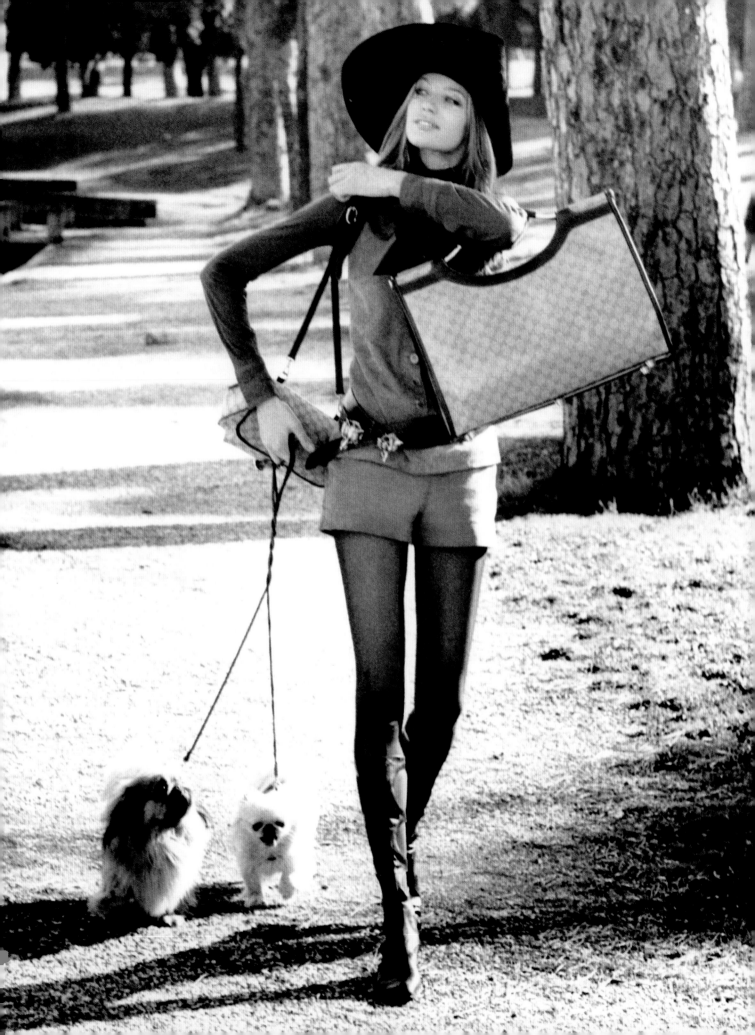

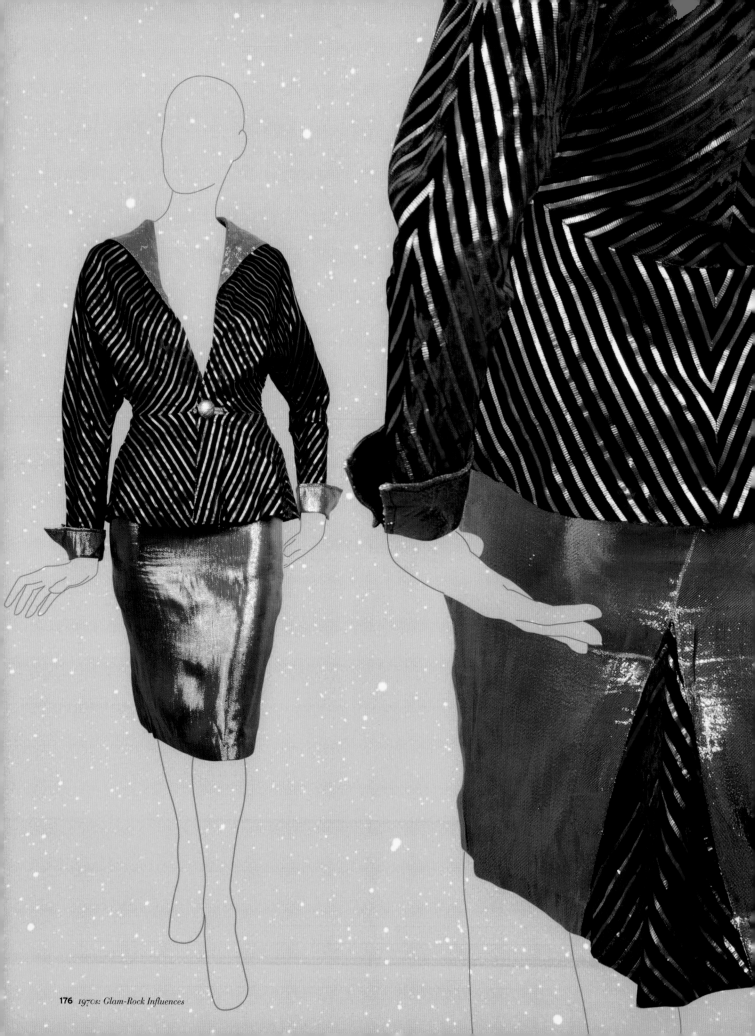

Glam-Rock Influences

Glam, or glitter, rock dominated the music charts from 1973 to 1975, but the sparkly stage costumes went unnoticed until the real trendsetters – David Bowie, Roxy Music and T-Rex in Britain and Alice Cooper, Iggy Pop and New York Dolls in America – came on the scene. Rock revolutionaries in tights, wigs and make-up, they were the musical and visual antidote to the hairy monsters of heavy rock, mixing rock music with art, cross-dressing with heterosexuality, debauchery with elegance. Former art students and, in the case of Roxy Music's Bryan Ferry, a teacher, they soon gathered a fashion following. Elitist and style-obsessed, they ran with a crowd of like-minded souls who by the end of the 1970s were dressing even more outrageously and starting their own clubs, fashion and art movements.

Performing as Ziggy Stardust at London's Hammersmith Palais in 1973, David Bowie epitomized glam-rock style. He wore his legendary jockstrap, stockings, platforms and minidress ensemble. New, super stylish and slightly scary, Bowie sent the old rockers packing, and London fashion divided.

Old schoolers like Ossie Clark stuck with Clapton and the Stones, while new bloods like Anthony Price dressed the glam rockers in fitted suits (boys) and corset-boned dresses (girls) in shiny silks and satins.

Glam rock's fun side showed itself in funky T-shirts emblazoned with iconic images like Minnie Mouse, as sold by boutique Mr Freedom. At Barbara Hulanicki's Biba store, T-Rex and Roxy Music fans could buy their mainstays of feather boas in pinks, purples and black, velvet bell bottoms and Lurex jackets. Glam rockers also loved the iconic fashion shapes of the 1950s, such as high collars, crepe soles and quiffs. The 1920s look of dark make-up, fur collars and slinky retro-style frocks could be found in vintage velvet frock coats, floor-length satin gowns, and diamanté, python, crocodile and patent leather accessories. The glam look reached back across the Channel, influencing the work of design houses including Pierre Balmain and Jean Patou. Fernand Ledoux produced wide-legged, ostrich-trimmed catsuits in 1973 and Ted Lapidus created exquisite, jewelled '30s-style evening gowns in 1975.

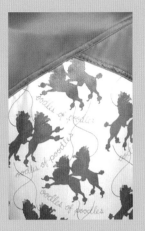

ABOVE AND BELOW FAR LEFT Mr Freedom Oodles of Poodles satin shirt in western style, early 1970s, with yoke detail. British boutiques such as Mr Freedom and Granny Takes A Trip sold glam-rock styles to the masses.

BELOW LEFT Mr Freedom bow-motif yellow satin hotpant dungarees, early 1970s.

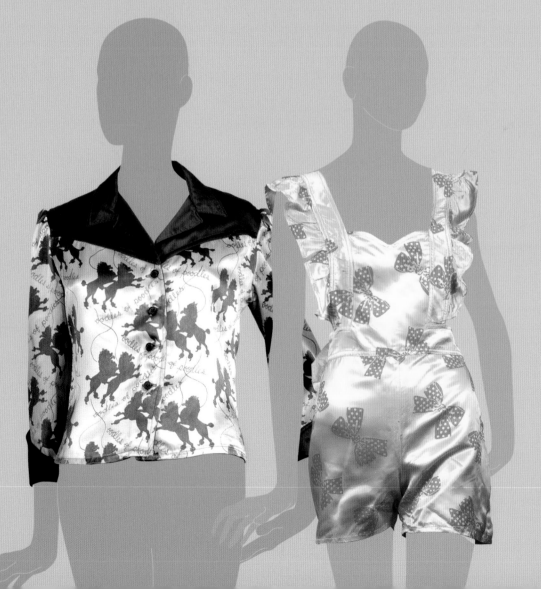

OPPOSITE Glitter-rock-influenced jacket and skirt, early 1970s, from British boutique, Granny Takes A Trip.

Divine Disco

Disco started out in the clubs of New York and was musically characterized by black dance music, electronically enhanced to provide a zooped-up, pounding dance beat or layered, orchestral sound.

In 1976 Steve Rubell's and Ian Schrager's New York club Studio 54 set the scene. On the dance floor, fabrics shimmered and sparkled to get you noticed. This was a dance-based look and nightclubs were packed with women in leotards, footless tights, sparkly leggings, ankle socks with stilettos, silk scarves tied as belts, diamanté hair accessories and glitter make-up. Fuchsia pink, lilac and electric blue were favourite colours, while satin, lamé, polyester, velour and other synthetics were the preferred fabrics.

New York designers including Roy Halston, Bill Blass and Geoffrey Beene had the grown-up version of the disco look taped down. The form-following, softly draped jersey dresses that Beene had been creating were perfect when translated into sheeny fabrics for the dance floor. Halston made his name as the designer of choice for the Studio 54 A-list crowd. His deep V-necked, backless, Grecian-style silk jersey dresses revealed the perfect parts of his star clients, who included Bianca Jagger and Joan Collins. Sadly, Halston's superclients deserted when he signed a high street diffusion-line contract with JC Penney's. Recently regenerated, however, his label is once again becoming synonymous with New York style.

As new silhouettes took over post-punk, designers moved away from snug, fitted shapes towards more fluid outlines. By 1978 silk jersey and crepe de chine suited the new draped shapes, which fell from a neckline or strapless top. Karl Lagerfeld for Chloé created black crepe de chine Grecian-inspired dresses not unlike those of Beene, as well as jackets and skirts that tapered at wrists and ankles. Yves Saint Laurent designed silk pyjamas in satin worn with an oversized satin jacket, pulled in at the waist. Sashes, belts and cummerbunds in gold or coloured leather and stiletto sandals in gold or silver completed the look.

In street style the disco look incorporated drainpipe trousers in shiny satin, sequinned boob tubes and ruched details on skirts and trousers. Shoulders broadened – silk jersey tops featured padded shoulders and front ruching. British chain Miss Selfridge's black satin slit pencil skirt and matching waistcoat was worn over a sequin boob tube, Lurex footless tights and black stilettos. Details like a pillbox hat with a mini veil brought the look to life. Other typical outfits included oversized T-shirts sporting roller-disco motifs and tied at the side, or long, slinky shirts worn open over a shiny swimsuit and leggings and belted with a scarf. Disco was the last great look of the 1970s, encapsulating the glamorous, thrill-seeking side of fashion's most revolutionary decade.

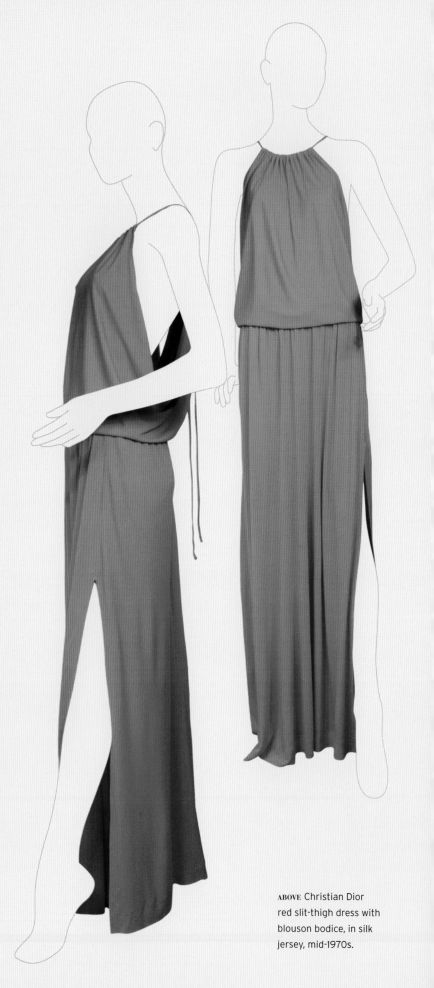

ABOVE Christian Dior red slit-thigh dress with blouson bodice, in silk jersey, mid-1970s.

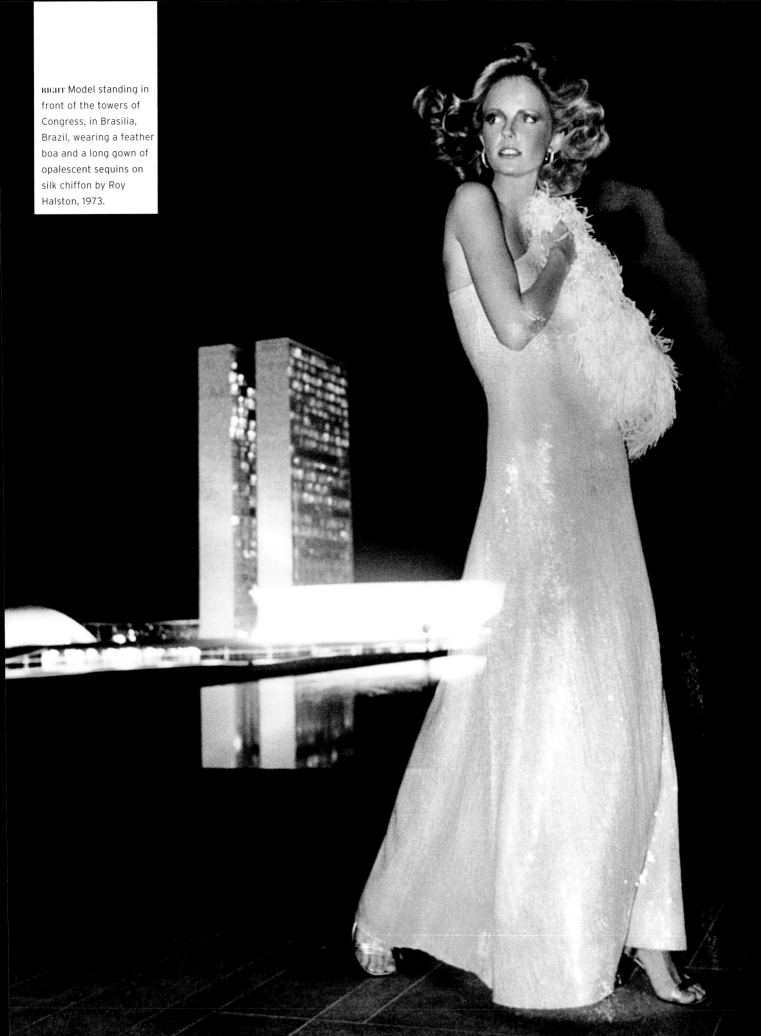

Bodystockings

A one-piece close-fitting garment made of elastic material and enveloping the whole body like a leotard. Originally worn by dancers, it became popular during the disco craze and was part of the slinky look of fluid 1970s fabrics that also harked back to 1930s Hollywood glamour.

Maxi skirts

The ankle- or floor-length skirt was a counter to the 1960s miniskirt (considered politically incorrect by many 1970s feminists). In dress form the maxi was often worn with a choker and crochet shawl and had an A-line skirt with a fitted bodice.

Diana décolleté

An asymmetric neckline with one bare shoulder, first seen in the second half of the nineteenth century and adopted by Elsa Schiaparelli in the 1930s, and Madame Grès in the 1950s, it regained popularity in the late 1970s, especially under the development of Roy Halston.

Wraparound

Diane von Furstenberg's signature wrap dress was a classic that spawned wraparound skirts and tops for the mass market. Her simple knit jersey wrap launched in 1972.

Parkas

A comfortable, lined, long outer garment with large pockets, usually made of tough cotton fabric with a removable lining; initially designed as an all-weather jacket for soldiers. It became very popular with young people in the 1970s.

Key looks of the decade

1970s

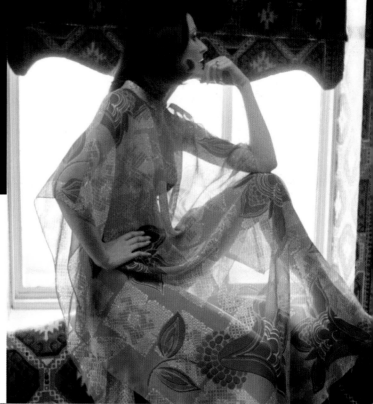

Jumpsuits

One-piece 'Charlie's Angels' pantsuit, usually with short legs made of elastic material, such as jersey. Along with this trend came tube dresses, with a reduced figure-hugging outline in plain colours of white, beige or pastels.

▼Unisex

In the 1970s Rudi Gernreich explored unisex fashion, which he carried to an extreme by using identical clothing on totally hairless male and female models. The androgynous look of Diane Keaton in *Annie Hall,* as below, and musician Patti Smith were part of the trend.

Carmen and gipsy looks

A flamenco style and part of the ethnic fashion of the decade. The look was modelled on Spanish flamenco costume, usually narrow at the hips, thighs and knees and ending in a wide skirt, with lace or frills at the off-the-shoulder neckline. Similarly, the gipsy look was characterized by frilled or unevenly hemmed skirts worn with blouses tied above the waist.

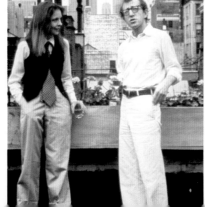

Gauchos, knickerbockers and jodhpurs

Mid-length trousers included the calf-length wide-bottomed gauchos, based on South American cowboys; full breeches gathered below the knee; and traditional riding breeches, very full from hip to knee, narrow on the calves and usually with a leather insert on the inside leg.

▲Kaftans

Along with kimonos, muumuus, djellaba (a Moroccan hooded rol or jalabiya (a loose eastern robe and other styles from India and Africa, kaftans were translated into westernized loungewear. They were especially suited as eveningwear when designed in exotic fabrics and edged in metallic trims, as this one in go thread for Pierre Cardin, 1973.

Folkloric

very type of ethnic image set trend. A peasant fashion for eyelets with lacing, braid trim and false bibbed blouses became universal. The ethnic influence, s seen in this 1970 Zandra Rhodes piece, was so strong hat it revived craft skills from ar-flung places, seen in Tibetan and Chinese quilted jackets, quare armhole waistcoats, atchworking and macramé.

Flares and trousersuits

Trousers and 'pantsuits' were serious fashions in the 1970s. They began gently flared then reached wide bell-bottom proportions by about 1975, after which they slowly reduced to straight and wide until, by the end of the decade, they were finally narrow again. Popular fabrics included heavy crepes, wool jersey knits, Courtelle jersey and woven polyester suiting such as Trevira.

Patterns, prints and colours

An abundance of floral motifs and nature patterns emerged, although geometrics and stripes continued from the 1960s, albeit in prints and patterns (such as in African and Native American textiles) rather than in form and cut. Typified by a sober neutral palette of white, black, beiges and olives, earth tones were the mark of the day, set off by mustard, brick red and dark orange.

Eastern influences

Kenzo, Yuki and Zoran were all 1970s labels that developed from an eastern minimalist point. As epitomized by Rei Kawakubo and Comme des Garçons, along with Issey Miyake and Yohji Yamomoto, the movement produced clothes that were refined, fluid and sculptural. In Kawakubo's case this included ruching and asymmetry.

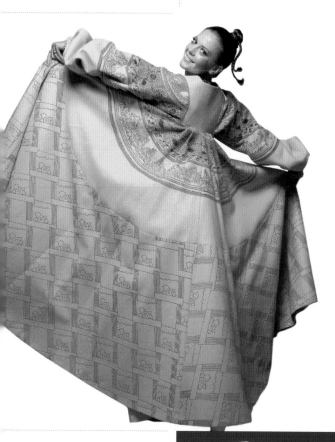

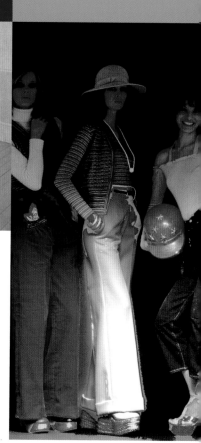

Hotpants

oming into fashion in the early 970s, these were extremely rief shorts that barely covered he bottom, and appeared in elvet or lurex for eveningwear. hey were often worn under a uttoned maxi or midi skirt with he front opened to reveal lots of g. As is typical of synthetics of he period, these items are rarely ound in good condition.

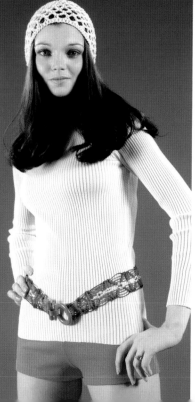

▲Granny dresses

Dresses with empire waistlines, an ornate fabric bodice and exotic sleeves were popular in a feminine, Earth Mother way, as was the granny dress with a high frilled or lace neckline and floral prints on brushed fabric. Laura Ashley contributed to the fashion with her romantic floral cotton prints and deliberately old-fashioned dresses reminiscent of the Victorian era.

Punk

Led by Malcolm McLaren and Vivienne Westwood, the punk movement was deconstructive and anti-establishment; it was characterized by bondage, safety pins, ripped edges and chaotic, irregular stitching. By 1977 Zandra Rhodes was using punk elements – gold safety pins and chains to connect and decorate uneven hems and slashed holes edged with gold thread.

▲Disco fashion

Strongly influenced by 1977's *Saturday Night Fever*, disco was characterized by shiny, metallic and glittery materials such as sequins, Lurex and Spandex. The pieces, including bandeau tops and stretch skirts, were often adaptations of dancewear that made its way into discos. Gold lamé, leopardskin and white clothes that glowed in UV lights captured the disco era.

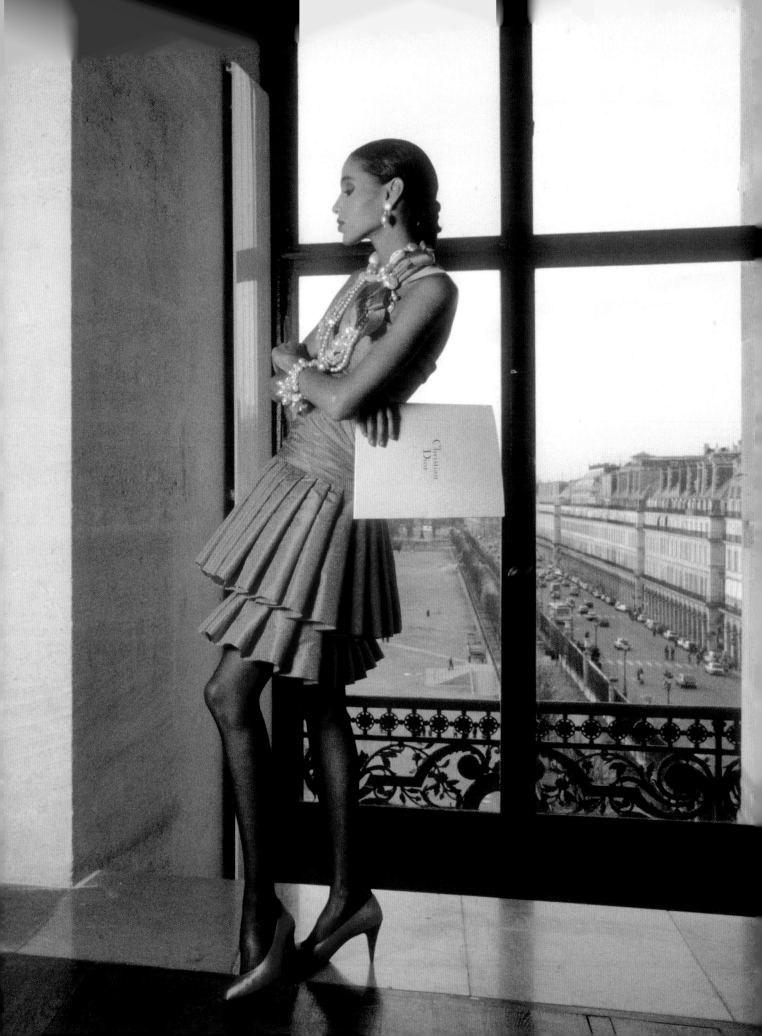

1980s

The 1980s was the decade of 'Hard Times'; not just a song by the Human League and a popular London nightclub, 'Hard Times' was a way of life for many. Money, as Mick Hucknall sang, was literally 'too tight to mention'. This was the dawning of the age of Thatcher and Reagan, and the working classes were feeling the pinch. Street fashion, born out of broke fashion students' imaginations and a few ingenious musicians, was adopted as the uniform of the trendy. Those who could afford upmarket designer fashion from names like Gianni Versace, Louis Féraud, Claude Montana or Chanel were wealthy, but not fêted for their sense of style. Until clever designers like Jean Paul Gaultier picked up on street accents and adapted them, designer clothing remained a separate entity.

By the middle of the decade, things were looking up. The financial capitals of the world witnessed a boom and there was a sudden surge of interest in designer shoes, bags and jewellery – it was the birth of the label. New York became a fashion mecca. Calvin Klein, Donna Karan and Ralph Lauren were the big names, while on another level, hip-hop music began the passion for bling and sportswear tracksuits by Nike, Adidas and Reebok, teamed with gold chains, medallions, rings and the latest training shoes, became street fashion's most enduring look.

Nightclubbing was big news on both sides of the Atlantic and fashion was strongly influenced by the latest club looks. Stephen Sprouse and Norma Kamali dressed New York's clubbers, while individual designers including Antony Price and John Richmond with Maria Cornejo made names for themselves on London dance floors. Young, single heiresses, including Francesca Thyssen in London and Cornelia Guest in New York, dominated the people pages of style magazines like Andy Warhol's *Interview* in New York and Lord Lichfield's *Ritz* in London.

Tailoring Trends

Tailoring and menswear took off as a major trend, inspired initially by Diane Keaton's *Annie Hall* character and other unisex looks of the 1970s.
Androgynous-looking women, including Annie Lennox of the Eurythmics and model-turned-singer Grace Jones, inspired a new wearable and classic look. Lennox wore a tutu when she sang as a punk with the Tourists, but re-emerged in a dapper black 'mod'-style suit and brogues as a Eurythmic in 1982 – and in doing so quickly became a fashion icon.

Menswear Influences

Early in the decade, trousers were left with nowhere to go. Narrowed into oblivion by punk and installed in the ultimate style ensemble as Yves Saint Laurent's Le Smoking tuxedo, designers focused on the man's jacket instead. Worn on a woman, a male jacket shape made an important and assertive statement. Padded shoulders, pioneered towards the end of the 1970s by Perry Ellis, Thierry Mugler and Karl Lagerfeld, to name a few, made the box-shaped, longer-line jacket the shape of 1980s.

Giorgio Armani, Gianni Versace and Calvin Klein took up the slack, creating wearable, mannish suit shapes in soft wools, cashmeres and plaid fabrics in the early part of the decade. A feeling of classic luxury combined with the power of simple tailoring quickly catapulted them to the top of many most-wanted lists. By 1983, Giorgio Armani had established himself as the number one purveyor of menswear-inspired classical looks. His 1983 collections featured lightweight wool suits in monotone shades with blouson jackets and softly draped trousers, along with boxy, square-shaped coats teamed with simple berets and heels. His designs for the fashion house Erreuno were more grown-up, featuring broad-shouldered monotone tweed coats, shaped in at the waist and tapering to just above the knee.

Armani, Luciano Soprani, Gianfranco Ferré and Gianni Versace in Milan – and Donna Karan for Anne Klein, Calvin Klein and Ralph Lauren in New York – created tailored styles tinged with glamour. In 1986, Calvin Klein's summer collection epitomized the new classic with cream flannel trousers, cashmere sweaters and lightweight wool coats and blazers. Now synonymous with Ralph Lauren, the edged blazer was a strong Klein feature in the early 1980s.

It took a British designer to dilute all this grown-up chic with some humour. For autumn/winter 1984, Betty Jackson, who started her own label with husband David Cohen in 1981, reworked Armani-style tailoring into chunkier shapes. Subtle colouring was replaced by bright red, yellow and blue checks. Shirts were teamed with matching scarves in purple, yellow and black boxy prints or dark mustard and red stripes.

PAGE 182 A Christian Dior dress by Marc Bohan, 1987. Bohan's tenure lasted from 1960 until 1989, and he reworked classic Dior shapes and styles for current times, always in discreet, elegant and simple designs.

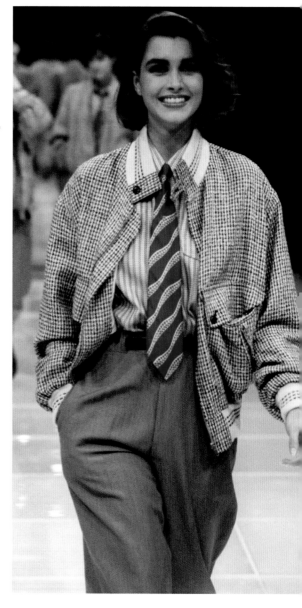

RIGHT Giorgio Armani's mastery of soft tailoring is evident in this menswear-influenced suit, 1984. Early Armani pieces were made in very expensive, luxury fabrics but his mid-1980s Mani and late 1980s Emporio ranges were developed for a wider market.

OPPOSITE Wool Chanel suits in navy, white and red, 1983. During the 1980s Lagerfeld revitalized the house of Chanel, producing many variations on the classic tweed suit and introducing the gilt chain belt and other glitzy details.

1980S MENSWEAR INFLUENCES:

- ❖ Oversized men's-style suit jackets, single- or double-breasted
- ❖ Checks, plaids and tweeds
- ❖ Belted-in waists and peg-topped gathered trousers
- ❖ Brogues or flat lace-up Dr Marten shoes
- ❖ Blouson-style jackets in tweed or wool
- ❖ Men's shirts in traditional pale cotton stripes or checks
- ❖ Berets or flat caps, braces (suspenders) and cufflinks
- ❖ Ties, either fat and long or skinny

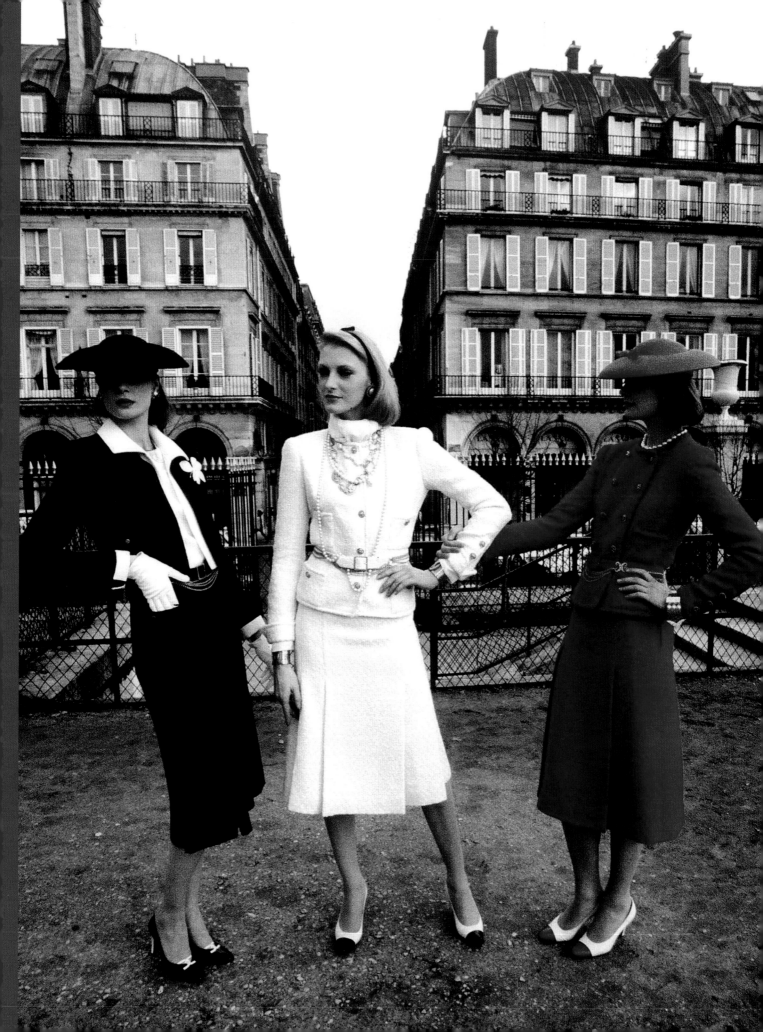

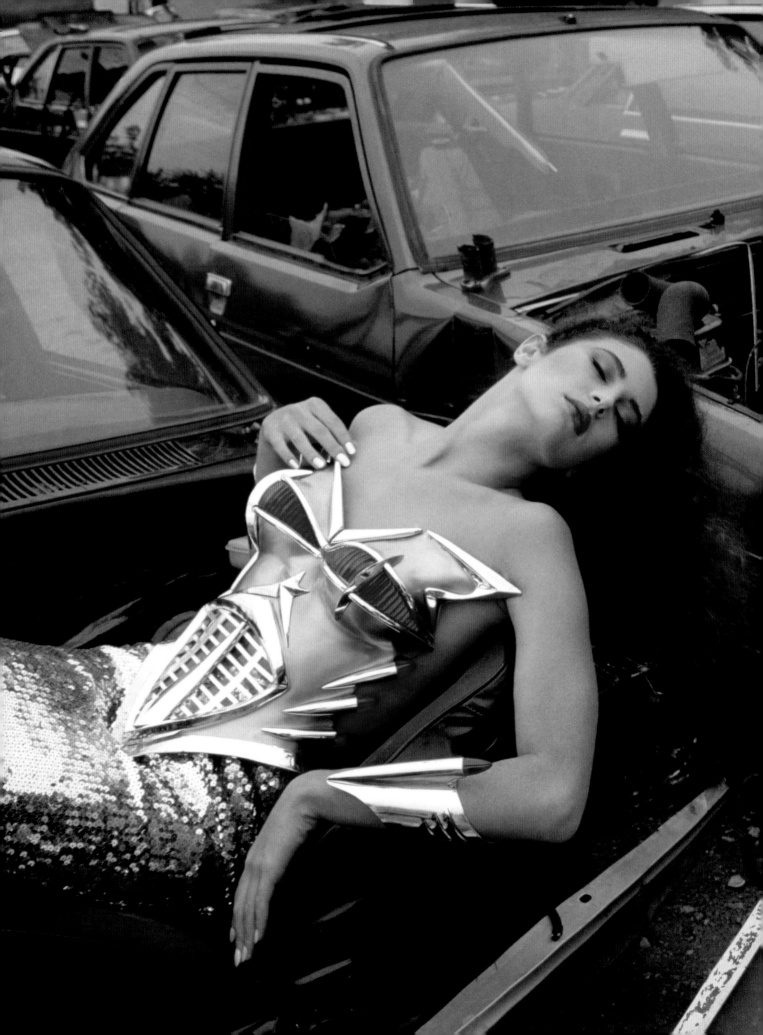

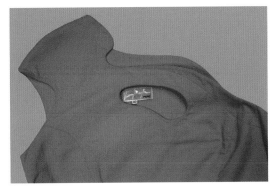

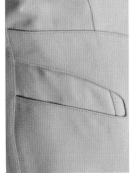

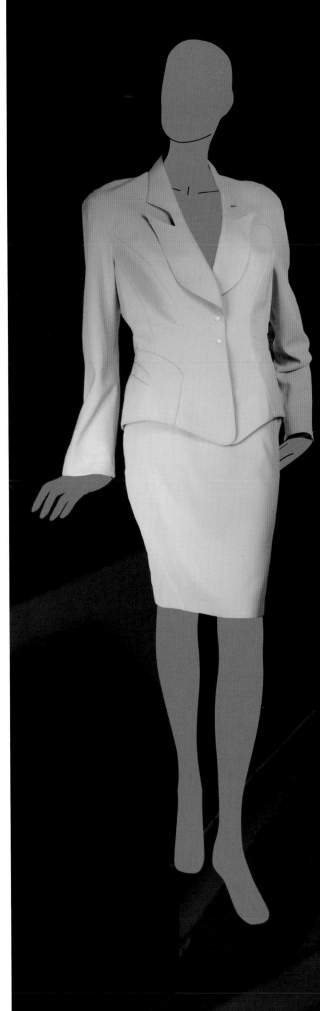

Unsurprisingly, it was a French man who reworked tailoring once again. Jean Paul Gaultier's 1985 autumn/winter menswear collection Wardrobe for Two featured androgyny as a theme, and he went on to design spectacularly feminine-shaped tailoring. Corseted jackets in dark pinstripes with sharp double-breasted fastenings were worn over tapered trousers and pencil skirts. A notable piece was his 1987 dogstooth-check lightweight suit with wide trousers and a long, double-breasted, fitted jacket. Other Gaultier tailored classics included tartan suiting and denim jackets in leopard prints.

The working girl's suit

This was the decade when working women sought to break through the glass ceilings of banking and industry and the image of the modern career woman was born. The film *Working Girl* (1988) starring Melanie Griffiths as Sigourney Weaver's beleaguered secretary echoed the feelings of women working for the female superboss. The uniform was the 'power suit', a fitted, tailored jacket worn over a neat knee-length skirt, an off-shoot of the mid-1980s trend for tailoring. Designers were inspired by John T Molloy's 1977 book, *The Woman's Dress for Success*, which suggested that straight skirts, tailored jackets and feminine takes on the male's office attire was the way forward. Thierry Mugler's form-fitting but stern shapes transmitted the combined air of professional authority and femininity across the boardroom.

New York designers were especially clued-in on the look. By the end of the decade, Richard Tyler and his wife Lisa Trafficante had become the city's coolest cutting duo, creating a 1989 womenswear collection of business suits that had the immaculate detailing of British Savile Row. While New Yorkers worked on masculine styles, Parisians pioneered a more feminine version of the suit. The end of the decade saw 1987 suits from Christian Dior in lightweight polka-dot charcoal wool fabrics, with single-breasted jackets and knee-length skirts. Karl Lagerfeld reworked the classic Chanel boucle suit with brass buttons in navy and cream and it quickly became the media/fashion boss's favourite. In the UK, Roland Klein and Bruce Oldfield created feminine versions of the power suit in lighter wool fabrics, dropping waists on jackets for a blouson effect, as with Klein, or softly gathering skirts for a more feminine effect, as Oldfield.

ABOVE LEFT Red 1980s dress with one-shoulder neckline and oblong keyhole opening, by German designer Thierry Mugler. Mugler worked in a variety of different materials, from taffeta, lace and raffia to chrome, Latex and plastic.

ABOVE AND RIGHT Lime Thierry Mugler suit, 1980s. The designer's overtly sexy, fetishistic silhouette was defined by broad shoulders and a defined waist, making his extreme proportions almost body distortions. His body-fitted designs were controlled and highly structured.

OPPOSITE A 1989 automotive-inspired dress by Thierry Mugler. Mugler took delight in industrial styling, which he displayed in his geometries of detailing and his references to such themes as 1950s cars.

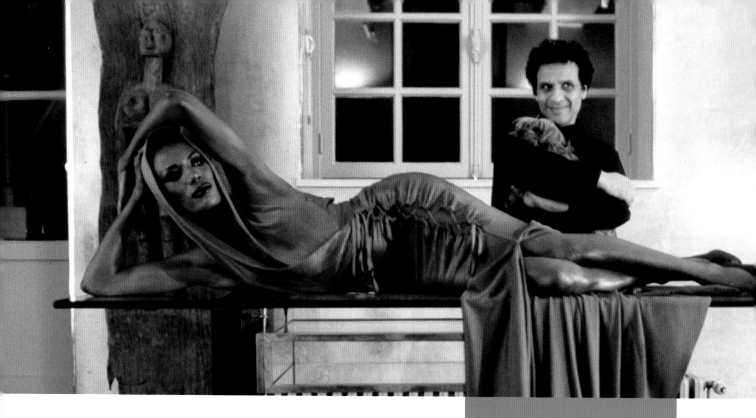

Body-conscious Fashion

Body-conscious styling crept into fashion toward the end of the 1980s, when most women had exhausted the androgynous and clumsy oversized looks of the first half of the decade. Wool, jersey, cotton drill, velvet and denim all appeared on the market in stretch versions and designers had no trouble styling sexy, form-fitting garments in the new fabrics. By the end of the decade Jean Paul Gaultier was dressing models in fitted corsets with pointed conical breasts, sparking the trend for underwear as outerwear.

Thanks largely to the development of Lycra, and its use as an outerwear fabric, not just for lingerie and swimwear, many new fashion shapes were born in the decade. Azzedine Alaïa, sold through Joseph Ettedgui's stores, created dresses in thick cream, chocolate brown and black stretchy fabrics for spring/summer 1987 that sold out in days. He arrived on the fashion scene via side-laced, sexy creations in 1985, and went on to produce form-fitting fashion's most iconic looks. In 1987 he teamed sleeveless tank-style and long-sleeved, scoop-necked dresses with matching opaque tights and shoes creating a streamlined overall look fashionistas went crazy for. Opaque tights have stayed in style, though they remain considerably easier to lay one's hands on than an Alaïa original. A famous look from 1988 featured models in black Lycra minidresses with white shirting details, waist-cinching black leather belts, slicked back hair and red lips.

Jean Paul Gaultier's 1983 Dadaiste collection heralded the arrival of the corset dress. Fitted in satin or thick, stretchy lycra with built-in corset top and lacing, the dress sparked a million copies. The Russian

ABOVE Grace Jones and Azzedine Alaïa, 1985. Grace wears a corset-strapped dress in Lycra stretch. Called the 'King of Cling' Alaïa mastered the spiral and crisscross seaming that lengthens the leg and lifts the bosom and bottom, while the stretch fabric clings to the curves of the body. His designs are often constructed from many smaller interlinking pieces.

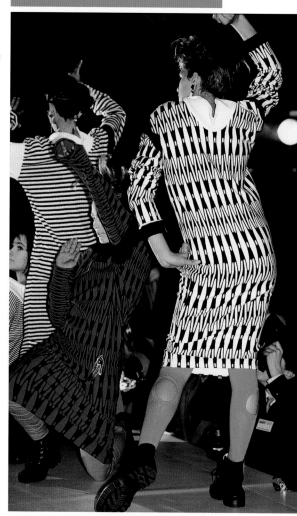

RIGHT Bodymap's The Cat In The Hat Takes A Rumble With The Techno Fish collection in 1984 shows dresses with graphic patterns by Hilde Smith. The concept of Bodymap was to restructure fabric around the body, creating areas that reveal and conceal the body. The designers were clearly influenced both by Japanese avant-garde and Vivienne Westwood.

Biker collection of 1986 combined fitted garments with fun styling. A striped dress was reminiscent of a road cyclist's ensemble. It was sexy, fun dressing and the long, fitted stretchy skirt became a signature Gaultier piece. The Rock Star collection of 1987 showcased Gaultier's love of such iconic pieces as the denim jacket, reworked into fitted leopardprint or black leather. Most famously, his rock-star looks led him to a meeting with Madonna, the rest as they say is history.

Sportswear and dancewear Influences

In New York, sporty, stretchy and jersey fabrics were pioneered in the designs of Perry Ellis during the late 1970s. Hot on the heels of disco, body-hugging fabrics became cool, not just for dancing and partying. In 1980 New Yorker Norma Kamali produced a collection fashioned entirely from sporty fleece-type fabric. In grey sweatshirting, a utilitarian fabric used for years in American active sportswear, Kamali produced drop-waisted full skirts, dresses, jumpsuits, long raglan-sleeved jackets and tops, rollneck dresses and leggings. Style with comfort was born, and soon a new trend was born.

Such looks followed on from stretchy, fun fashion pieces designed by groundbreaking duo Bodymap in 1981. David Holah and Stevie Stewart were London fashion graduates who enjoyed brief fame with their immensely fun and wearable fishtail skirts, cropped trousers, short jackets and long or large-looped knits. Other London designers including Helen Robinson's PX label developed the trend, producing wraparound jersey skirts, turbans and tops that became a fashion staple during the first half of the decade.

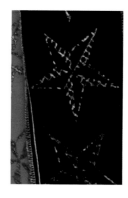

ABOVE AND LEFT Bodymap cardigan and skirt with textile detail, mid-1980s. Designed to shape the body, the pieces had holes in unexpected places, as on the sleeves and shoulders here. Designers David Holah and Stevie Stewart used multiple layered prints in their textile designs.

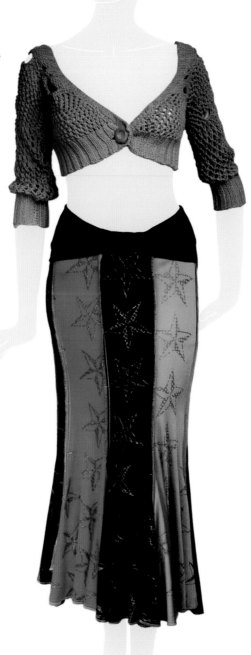

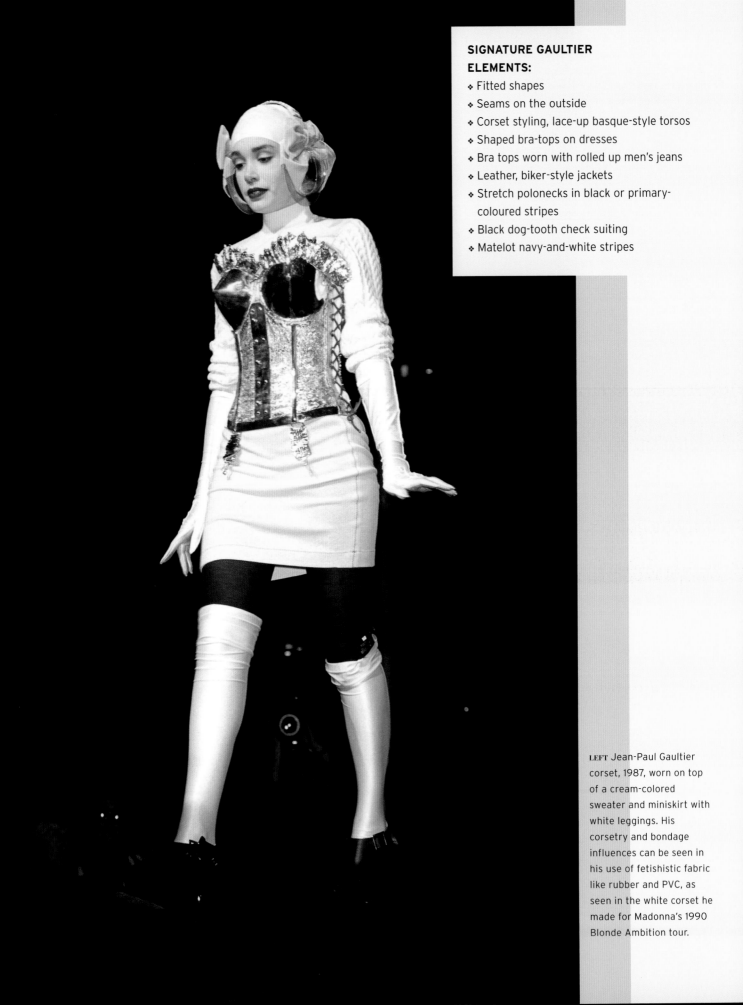

LEFT Jean-Paul Gaultier corset, 1987, worn on top of a cream-colored sweater and miniskirt with white leggings. His corsetry and bondage influences can be seen in his use of fetishistic fabric like rubber and PVC, as seen in the white corset he made for Madonna's 1990 Blonde Ambition tour.

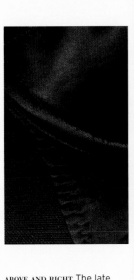

ABOVE AND RIGHT The late
1980s Jean-Paul Gaultier
corset dress defined the
'inner wear as outer wear'
moment in fashion history.

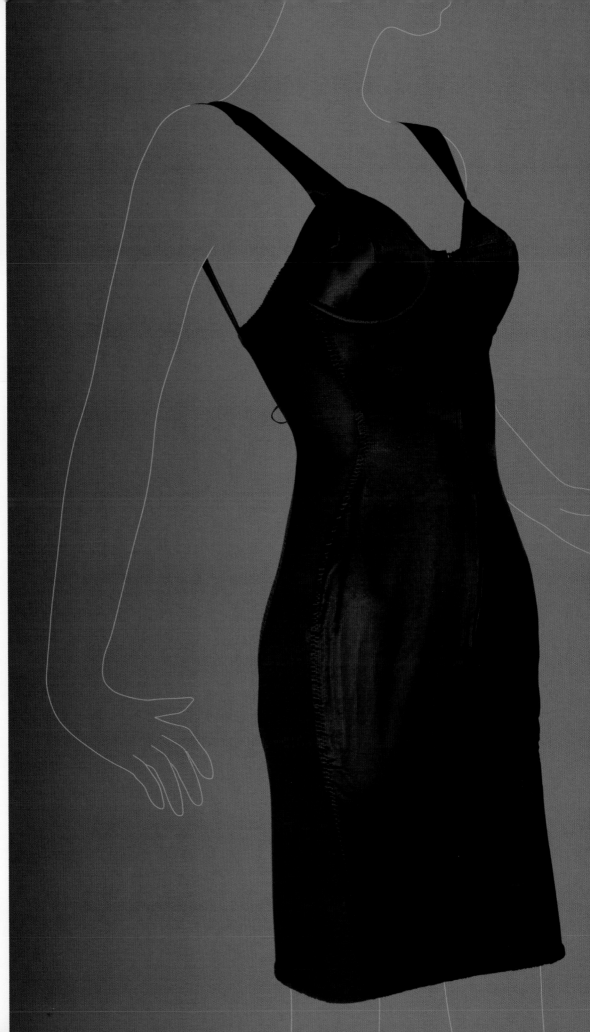

Bustles in Hedgerows

Skirt shapes went wild in the 1980s. After decades of A-lines and soft drapes, it was time for a change. Enter the puffball, ra-ra and mini-crini, the look that put Vivienne Westwood firmly on the international fashion map. As the 1970s faded out, skirt shapes became pretty tired. Softly draped tulip shapes or pencil skirts were sold on the high street, while designers dabbled with fluid shapes following in the footsteps of successful New Yorkers like Roy Halston and Geoffrey Beene. Then, in spring 1983, the masterful Yves Saint Laurent shook everything up with new, neat, feminine shapes featuring nipped-in waists, fuller skirts and shorter jackets. As so often happens in fashion, other international design houses produced similar looks, including Calvin Klein in New York, Missoni with full skirts in Milan and Chantal Thomas in Paris. Thomas's delightful collection featured cinched waists, puffed sleeves and grown-up, buttoned-up pinafore dresses.

Vivienne Westwood created a series of wacky collections following on from the largely London-based success of her Pirates/Buccaneer and Buffalo collections in 1981 and 1982 respectively. Featuring layered shapes, and underwear as outerwear in the case of the Buffalo Gals, who wore bras over the top of woolly sweaters and full, hitched-up skirts, there was some semblance of female shaping. But it was to take the introduction of Westwood's mini-crinoline in 1985 to really cement the full skirt shape and send fashion reeling off in a brand new direction. The 'mini-crini' was a short, hooped skirt based on Victorian outlines, worn with cotton over-the-knee stockings and flat or clumpy shoes. Teamed with short fitted blazers in lightweight wool patterns and stripes, the look was immediately seized upon by chainstore retailers. However, the quality and cutting of the fabric was difficult to copy, so lots of cheaper versions hit the streets with appalling results!

After the mini-crini came the puffball, designed by Christian Lacroix in 1986 for his 1987 spring/summer collection, and earning him the Golden Thimble prize, couture's highest award. The crini and puffball were swiftly followed by the ra-ra, a two-or-three-tiered short skirt, which became the national costume for the average girl in 1986 and 1987. Tutus also reemerged in collections by Lacroix, Moschino and Chanel towards the end of the decade.

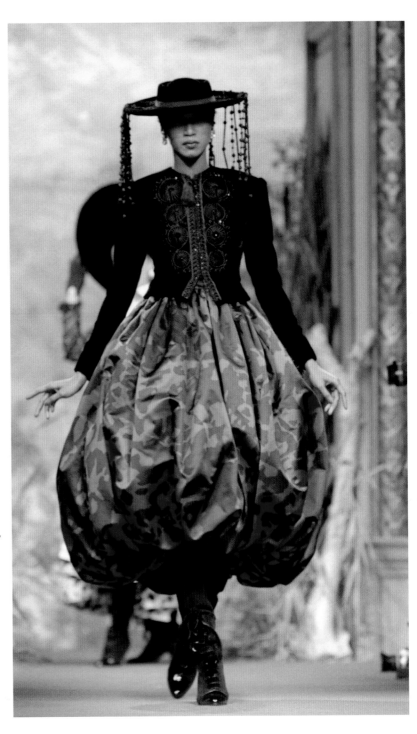

ABOVE A model displays a styled Spanish ensemble, black jacket embroidered over a balloon-dress and Castilian hat for Christian Lacroix 1987. His puffball (pouf) skirt was a thigh-high version of this dress.

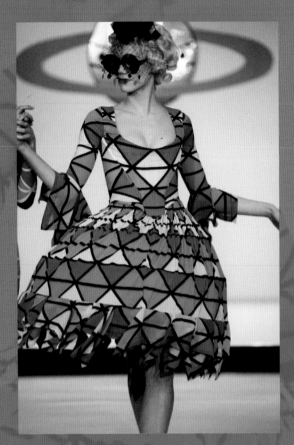

ABOVE In 1985 Vivienne Westwood launched her mini-crini – a short hooped skirt inspired by the Victorian crinoline and made in tweed or cotton. The shape brought back an hourglass silhouette, rather than the inverted triangle so popularized by the power suit trend.

RIGHT A polka-dot mid-1980s mini-crini by Vivienne Westwood. The mini-crini designs incorporated prints in harlequins, stripes and dots, which were cartoonish and child-like in feel; the one here directly references Minnie Mouse. Westwood would continue to look to historical costume for years to come.

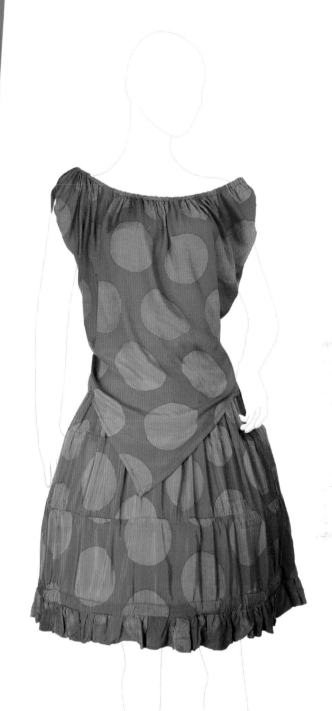

On the Street

Streetwear took on new dimensions as designers operating entirely separately from couture and high fashion created arty, super-trendy looks fuelled by politics and passion. In London, street fashion was inspired by clubs and nightlife. In New York, it had roots in a number of different movements, from hip-hop and world music, to punk-rock and Pop Art. Jean-Charles de Castelbajac was a Parisian who loved the work of New York artists such as Andy Warhol, Robert Indiana and Keith Haring, and he incorporated Haring's graphic human prints into garments towards the end of the decade. Haring had been a graffiti artist, but his trademark prints also appeared on jackets by Vivienne Westwood in her 1983 collection.

Other trend-setting New Yorkers included Norma Kamali, whose sporty, stretch clothes were inspired by the street sportswear of hip-hop fans. Their brightly coloured professional sportswear had yet to filter into mainstream fashion, but the stretch and stripes of Adidas, Nike and Reebok worn on the street proved inspirational for Kamali. Away from the catwalks, a punkier attitude pervaded New York. Stephen Sprouse began his career assisting Roy Halston in the 1970s, but broke away to design pop fashion classics. Finally setting up his own label in 1984, he went on to dress such icons as Debbie Harry in his signature brightly coloured '60s-style leatherette minidresses.

Graphic word-prints made dramatic statements on the catwalk for Katharine Hamnett in her autumn/winter 1984 collection. Politics were the issue with 'Worldwide Nuclear Ban Now' a key slogan and Hamnett's over-sized T-shirts became the trendy choice for young Londoners. Hamnett herself famously attended a Downing Street fashion reception with Margaret Thatcher, wearing a T-shirt bearing the anti-war slogan '58% Don't Want Pershing'. The image and message were taken on board by rock band Frankie Goes To Hollywood, with their 1984 hit song 'Relax'; part of their gimmick was to wear oversized Hamnett T-shirts bearing the word 'Relax', which became an enduring image of the decade.

Street fashion was just that, so it was hard to buy the look off the peg. Successful British designers who moved from designing street looks to selling the odd piece and even, occasionally, whole collections to boutiques, included Bodymap, Wendy Dagworthy, Rachel Auburn and Dexter Wong, to name a few. Wong dressed Boy George and sold his funky, big jackets, long dresscoats and tartan trousers. Other street trends included rockabilly, ragamuffin and goth, but the looks were created by kids in their bedrooms or rock band stylists and were never really available in fashion boutiques.

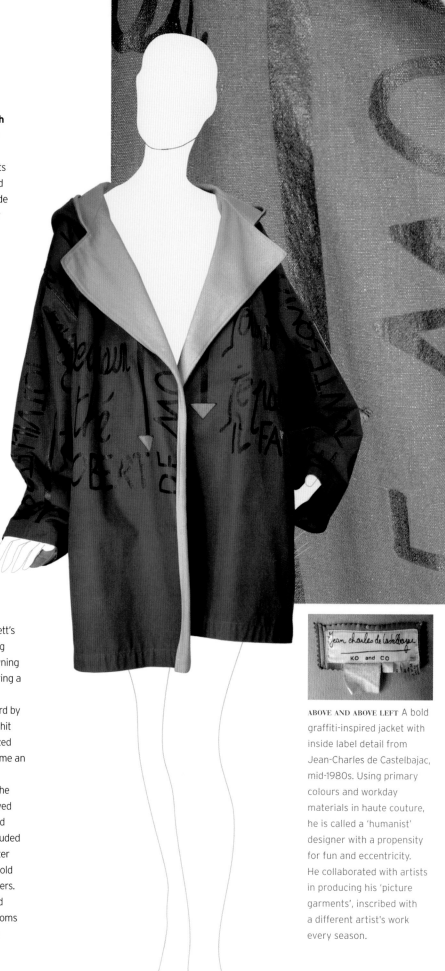

ABOVE AND ABOVE LEFT A bold graffiti-inspired jacket with inside label detail from Jean-Charles de Castelbajac, mid-1980s. Using primary colours and workday materials in haute couture, he is called a 'humanist' designer with a propensity for fun and eccentricity. He collaborated with artists in producing his 'picture garments', inscribed with a different artist's work every season.

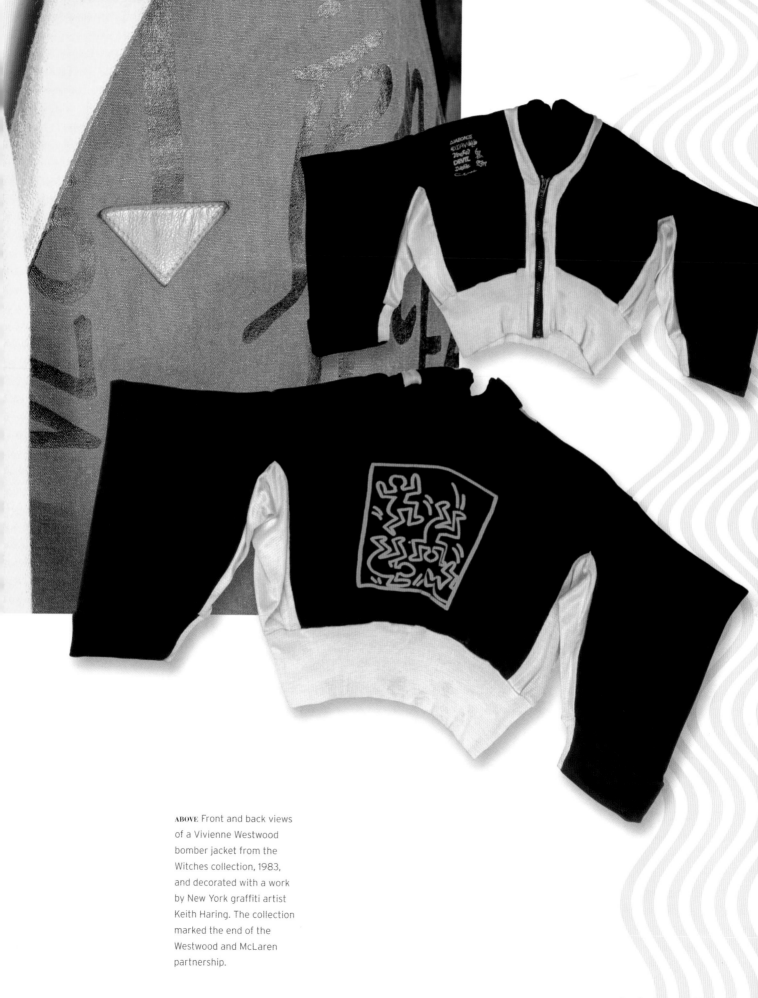

ABOVE Front and back views of a Vivienne Westwood bomber jacket from the Witches collection, 1983, and decorated with a work by New York graffiti artist Keith Haring. The collection marked the end of the Westwood and McLaren partnership.

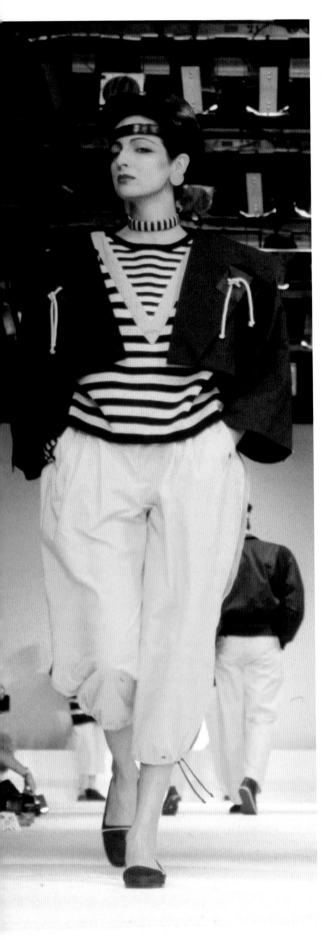

Colours and Prints

The 1980s was the decade when colour came into fashion. Bright primaries and bold monotones, vivid prints, dots and stripes dominated. This was no time for shrinking violets. Designers went fabric mad. Many collections were led by the fabric, the styling following as a sort of afterthought. Nobody looked particularly great in giant polka dots or deckchair stripes, but that didn't stop Claude Montana, the Emanuels and a host of others putting them on the scene.

Bold colours

As the decade dawned, fuchsia pink had made its way to the forefront of fashion. After the muted purples, browns and beiges of the 1970s, this was a welcome arrival. The Italian fashion houses of Milan loved colour, particularly Gianni Versace and knitwear guru Missoni. Versace cofounded the label with his brother Santo in 1978; flamboyant, luxurious colour was a staple from the start and the Versace house style evolved to become the most glamorous label in the world by 1990. In 1982, royal blue, red and gold swirls decorated a sexy bodice, while blue and black chiffon stripes with a peak of red beneath made up a slashed up-the-front skirt.

Gianfranco Ferré, meanwhile, produced black-topped dresses with skirts that resembled huge satin sashes in primary blues, reds and yellows in 1982. Primary colours became key elements for many designers. Claude Montana mixed them with navy for a nautically themed collection in 1983. In New York, Norma Kamali sent models out in vivid yellow plastic skirt suits with oversized blazers. Less traditional shapes, but even brighter colours came through from Thierry Mugler; his 1984 collection featured lime-green stretch velour dresses with raglan sleeves, his trademark skullcaps in white, and oversized canvas macs in a combination of bright colours.

Neutrals and simplicity

A welcome antidote to bright colours and overtly feminine styling came from Japanese designers, notably Issey Miyake, Rei Kawakubo of Commes des Garçons and Yohji Yamamoto. Always favouring monotones or neutrals, Yamamoto brought the black poloneck into fashion in 1986, teaming it with black hoisery, Dr Marten boots and simple wool coats. In 1982 Kawakubo's black 'lace' wool sweater, oversized and full of holes, followed on from the 'rags' of her 1981 neutral, bare-seamed separates. By 1987, Commes des Garçons had changed direction slightly, producing more formal, black tailoring of oversized pinafores, jackets and trousers worn with crisp white shirts. Issey Miyake, meanwhile, focused on pleated silks in neutral colours, wrapped around the body into tube shapes. In 1985 he produced the famous bamboo bodice, part of his *Body Works: Fashion Without Taboos* exhibition at London's Victoria & Albert Museum.

LEFT Nautical offerings from Claude Montana, 1983. Best known for his leather work and extreme broad shoulders, the striped top, jacket and pantaloons give a New Romantics shape.

OPPOSITE Karl Lagerfeld's graphic print knitwear, 1984, shows the bold gestures and black-and-white themes that defined textiles in the 1980s.

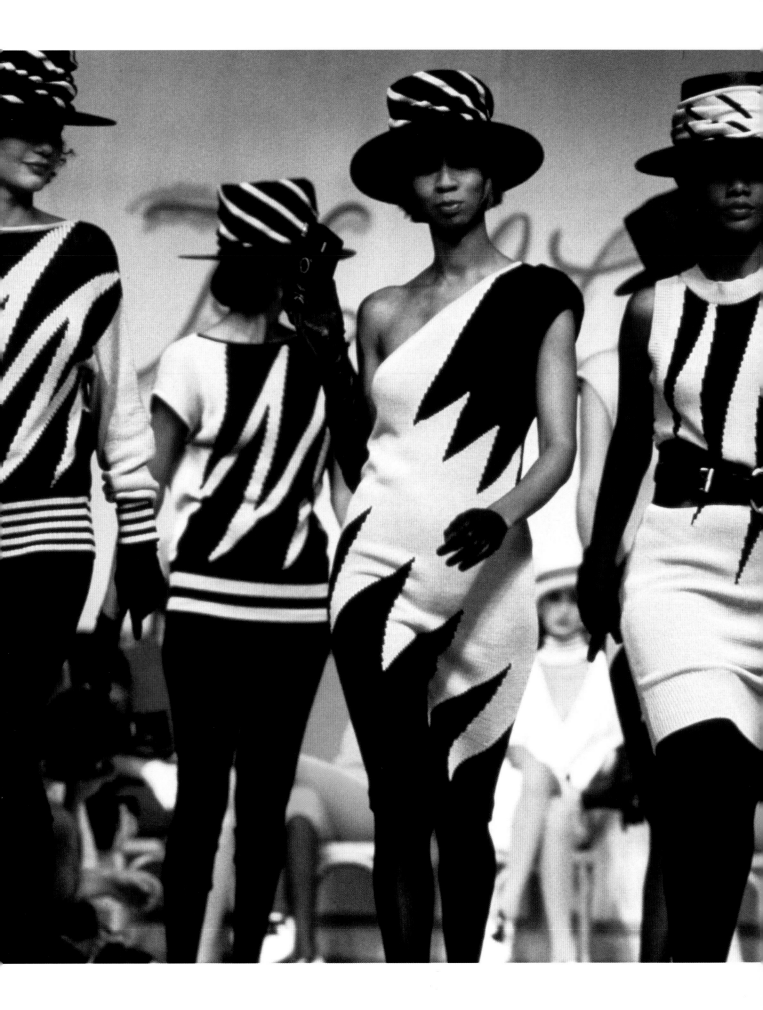

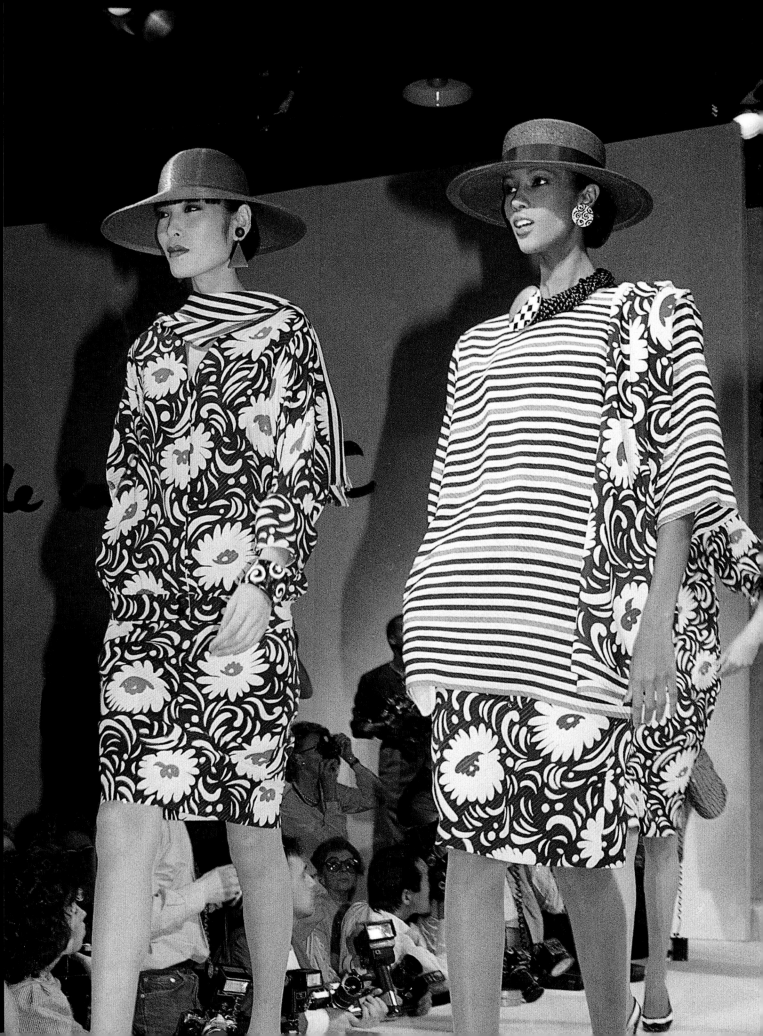

Fabrics and Textiles

Never before in fashion history did so many fabrics compete for centre stage. Post-punk, leather and tartan were adapted into mainstream looks and many designers attempted to move denim upmarket. The 'stretch' movement, brought about by the developments in Lycra and dancewear fads, had a huge impact, as did sportswear jersey (see pages 188–9), but the textures of denim, leather, parachute silk and tweed were also liberally apparent.

Denim and jean fashions

Although denim was fashioned into every kind of garment during the 1980s, jeans remained a fashion stalwart. At the start of the decade, 'designer jeans' by Calvin Klein had just been introduced. Gaultier took denim design a step further, stretching the denim jacket into a tailored, hourglass shape in 1986. Made of dark-coloured denim with otherwise traditional fastenings, it sold out in stores almost immediately. Yet this remains one of the only designer denim success stories of the decade. Mid-market, companies including Guess, made a huge noise with their 1987 campaign featuring a Bardot-esque Claudia Schiffer in a basque, gold hoop earrings and Guess jeans, but on the whole, denim stayed downmarket.

Leather styling

Claude Montana and Thierry Mugler had the most impact on leather as a fashion fabric. Mugler honed his skills in the 1970s, creating bronzed leather space-age catsuits with matching skullcaps. Montana is credited for turning women on to high-fashion leather. Using lambskin dyed to purple, black, fuchsia and royal blue, blouson jackets, fitted leather trousers or plain miniskirts were his most-wanted items. Throughout the 1980s, Montana's design silhouette of huge shoulders and nipped-in waist became synonymous with his name. In 1983, military detailing added a new dimension, and suits with long-line skirts and jackets in beige or black were decorated with epaulettes, studded belts and metal details. A black-and-red swimsuit line featured matching black leather jackets with red leather turnback cuffs and detailing. Some of Montana's most wearable designs emerged in the 1987 to 1988, such as knee-length black stretch dresses featuring leather inserts that fitted in at the waist around sexy front zips, or miniskirts and zip-up jackets with leather detailing. In Italy, Versace produced cropped, oversized black leather biker jackets for autumn 1984, which are highly wearable today.

Textures

Parachute silk was one of the decade's most-used and prettiest fabrics, featuring in Katharine Hamnett's 1984 collection in vivid red, green and yellow, cut into simple vests, parachute pants or oversized sleeveless dresses with matching duster coats. Tartan appeared in Vivienne Westwood's and Betty Jackson's tailoring, 'growing up' from punk influences into a favoured suiting fabric.

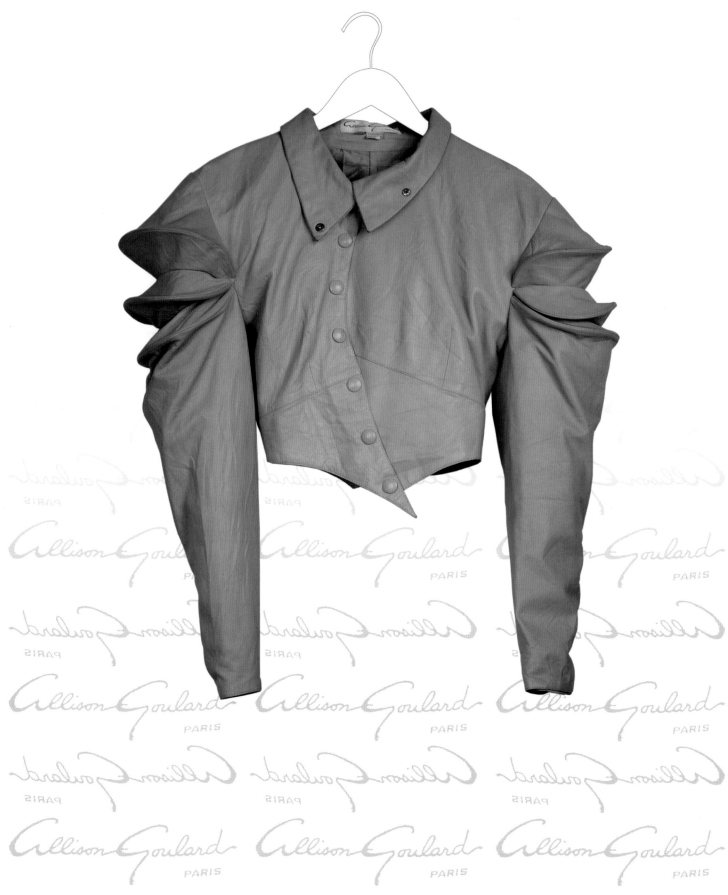

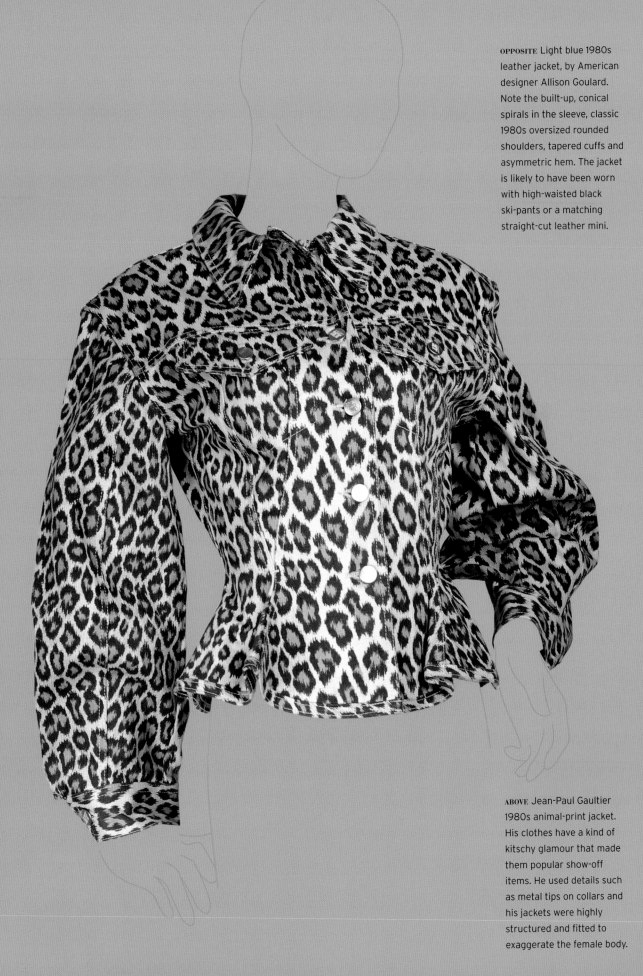

OPPOSITE Light blue 1980s
leather jacket, by American
designer Allison Goulard.
Note the built-up, conical
spirals in the sleeve, classic
1980s oversized rounded
shoulders, tapered cuffs and
asymmetric hem. The jacket
is likely to have been worn
with high-waisted black
ski-pants or a matching
straight-cut leather mini.

ABOVE Jean-Paul Gaultier
1980s animal-print jacket.
His clothes have a kind of
kitschy glamour that made
them popular show-off
items. He used details such
as metal tips on collars and
his jackets were highly
structured and fitted to
exaggerate the female body.

Evening Glitz

The 1980s evening gown is a classic that works for two reasons: first the sleek, feminine lines accentuate all a woman's curves, no matter what her size or shape, and second the fabrics are also female friendly – no woman can fail to look good in a gleaming black crepe de chine. Dresses from the era were varied, the best versions having draped or cowl necks, or slashed or boat necklines. Batwing sleeves were stunning, as were full long sleeves with cuffs. Other typical features were deep V-necks, high poloneck collars and cutaway backs.

Eveningwear master Antony Price began as a menswear designer creating looks for rock star Bryan Ferry in the 1970s. At the 1985 Fashion Aid, a huge event staged at the Albert Hall in London by Bob Geldof, Price dressed his muse, Jerry Hall, in a peplum-waist creation in red, orange and gold sparkling brocade that stole the show. This was not typical Price, who was famous for boned, fitted bodices, simple lines and sexy satin fabrics. As well as famous 'mermaid' fish-tailed evening dress, he is credited for bringing men's tailoring to women's eveningwear. His dresses were named 'resultwear' because they always got the right results!

Christian Lacroix created the decade's newest evening outlines in 1986, with fitted bodices and short, puffball skirts. For years, women had stuck to classic floor-length ball gowns, but the black-tie event 'came out' as a fashion parade ground in the 1980s. Heady with the success of the cocktail and eveningwear explosion, which came hand-in-hand with the mini-economic boom, the Parisian designers went over the top design-wise. Jean-Louis Scherrer created the ruched satin mini-evening dress in 1987. With huge frills around strapless tops, drop-waist tutu-style skirts, back bustles, bows and ribbons, these pastel-coloured, short dresses were copied everywhere. In 1987 Yves Saint Laurent and Emanuel Ungaro took evening dresses even shorter. Ungaro's version featured ruched satin skirts in plain chocolate brown, teamed with pink details that included rose corsages or an ankle-trailing sash. Saint Laurent produced cream ostrich-feather confections.

Some American and Italian designers had a different approach to eveningwear. Luxurious satins and velvets came in black, brown or beige. Donna Karan's black Lycra 'body' of 1984 was worn with a simple wrap-around full skirt as an antidote to the 'hysteria' in Europe. Giorgio Armani produced floor-length, sequinned sheaths in neutral colours. Other designers, including Michael Klein, experimented with much simpler, graphic designs – a 1989 piece in black viscose features a slash, knee-length super-simple sheath, built on to a conical bra shape.

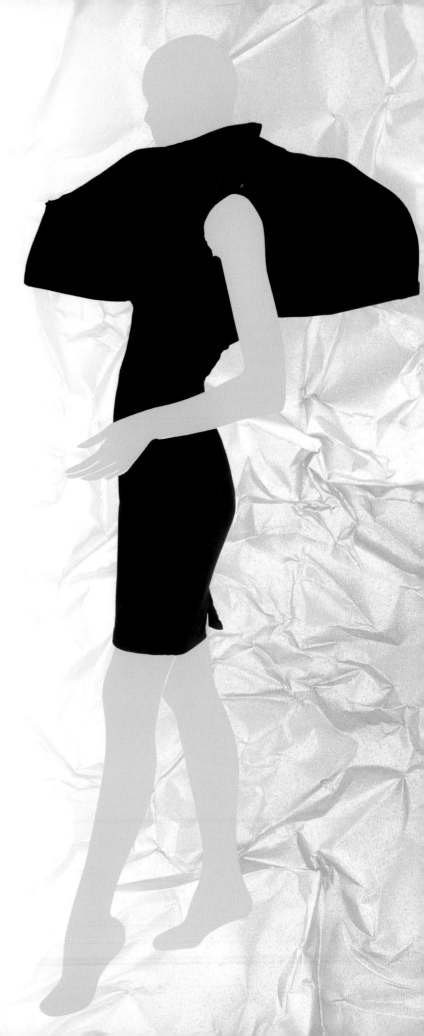

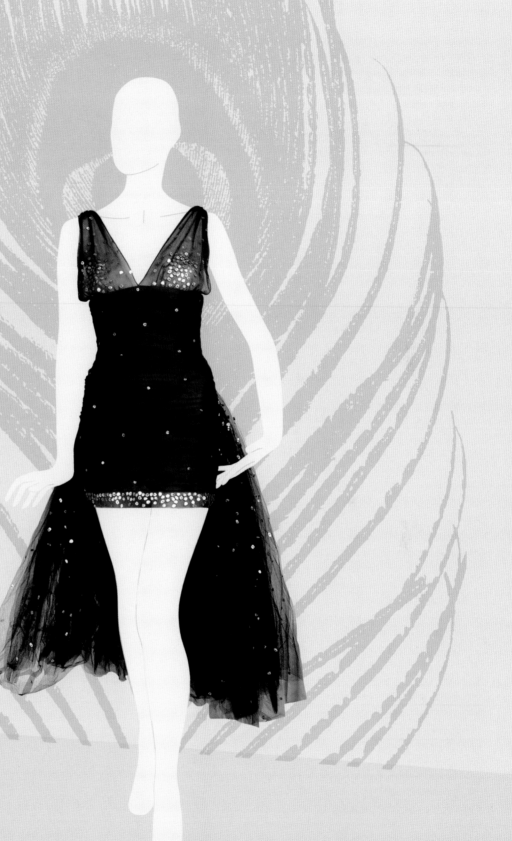

OPPOSITE Anthony Price black velvet evening dress, mid-1980s. Price's evening gowns had intricate corsetry and interfacing to achieve the remarkable shapes, which created an old-style Hollywood glamour that reverberated with his rock-star clients. Here his magnificent show-stopping dress is all about over-the-top '80s excess.

RIGHT As Henry Ford said, you can have 'any colour so long as it's black', and this can be said of fashion in the 1980s when black was the only colour the fashion pack wore. Here a tulle train and broken sequin decoration adds brilliance to a 1980s Chanel evening gown designed by Karl Lagerfeld. Lagerfeld, already successful as the name behind fashion house Chloé, became artistic director for Chanel in 1983, taking traditional Chanel shapes and fabrics and adding his own dynamic twists.

The Avant-Garde

If 'back to nature' was the fashion theme of the 1970s, 'into the future' was the mood when 1980 dawned. Oddities, quirky shapes, heterosexual looks and sculpted fabrics provided the materials for the new avant-garde. Many artists turned to fashion as a vehicle for expression; many fashion designers in turn were inspired by art. New fabrics, cutting techniques and manufacturing methods made it easier to create flimsy, cut-out fabrics, as in Rei Kawakubo for Comme des Garçons' knitwear or Issey Miyake's laminated polyester breastplate from his 1982 collection. Miyake's 1980s designs are dramatic: multistitched, layered cloaks with deep hoods and space-age pink satin mini dresses with stand-away yolk collars worn with chiffon fingerless gloves and stockings were two of his more wearable 1983 masterpieces.

The avant-garde in fashion existed on two levels. On the street, New Romantics spent the beginning of the decade heading out for the evening dressed in perhaps a black shroud with a totally shaved, white-powdered head with one purple eyebrow. Extreme dressing was a mode of self-expression. Naturally, extreme looks suited very few, so the real collector's pieces were created by either Japanese or a few young British designers, who recognized a woman's need to wear as well as display clothes.

John Galliano produced his first collection at the end of his fashion degree at St Martin's in London in 1983, Les Encroyables, which introduced a new word to fashion: deconstructionist. The process of producing garments that look almost-finished or fit the wearer in new or unconventional ways marked his collection and became a movement in the 1980s. Inspired by the clothes of the French Revolution, Galliano's frock coats with exposed seams, upside-down looking skirts and stiff organdie shirts decorated with broken-up chandelier necklaces were an immediate success.

Galliano's collection heralded the return from Victorian times of the frock coat, a garment much beloved by deconstructionist designers, including Yohji Yamamoto, whose black 1987 version featured a red tulle bustle. Yamamoto's early 1981 collection was called 'oplique chic' by *Vogue*, referring to his misshapen, asymmetrical lines. He worked draping and wrapping around the body and took the ideas for the shaping from the fabric itself.

Yamamoto and Kawakubo paved the way for a new wave of deconstructionist designers. Martin Margiela, a young Belgian, made his debut in 1989 with appealing, tailored separates that seemed to fasten incorrectly, or simply be the wrong size – yet once on, fitted perfectly. After the powered-up leather, multicolours and aggressively feminine shaping of tailoring, deconstructionism provided a welcome alternative.

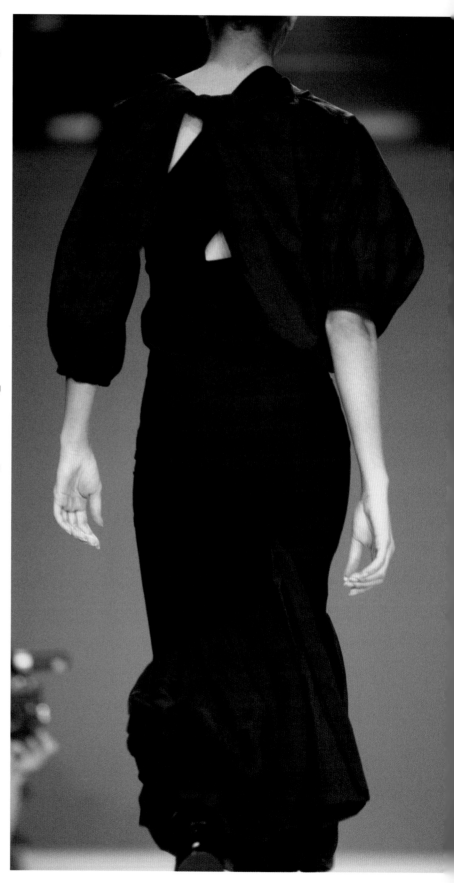

FAR RIGHT Lace knitwear
by Rei Kawakubo for
Comme des Garçons, 1982.
Her deconstructed jumpers,
incorporating rips, holes and
tears that recall intricate
webs, were labelled 'post-
Atomic' by the press.
Kawakubo was known for
her complex cut, random
ruching, asymmetrical
seams and hems, crinkled
surfaces and unfinished
edges. This piece seems to
recall Vivienne Westwood's
Hangman's jumper
(see page 172).

RIGHT A fluidly asymmetrical
1980s dress by John
Galliano, showing his
inventive cutting and
draping qualities. The
complicated cut and
asymmetrical draping
are only fully revealed
once on the wearer.

OPPOSITE A 1980s Comme
des Garçons dress that
exhibits the distinctive
masterly cutting, knotting
and draping techniques of
Rei Kawakubo.

Androgyny

Style setters who included Annie Lennox and Grace Jones made the androgynous look big news with men's suits, ties and close-cropped hair, combined with the ultimate feminine touch – red lips or a corset-style basque.

▶Streetwear

Letters, numbers and graphics made the oversize T-shirt the most popular single item in the 1980s. New York artist Keith Haring, his work shown here in a design for Vivienne Westwood, created simple graphic drawings that popped up everywhere.

Full skirts and layering

Vivienne Westwood's multilayered full skirts and sweaters worn with bras over the top, completed with chunky boots, epitomized the street urchin look.

White prairie skirts

Pioneers and prairie girls at Ralph Lauren and English roses at Laura Ashley wore white lace and broderie anglaise skirts and dresses. Full tiered skirts with peasant tops, accessorized with brown leather belts and purses, finished the look.

Key looks of the decade

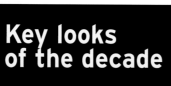

1980s

▲Stripes and tartan

Colour was riotous; Betty Jackson and Wendy Dagworthy sent models down runways in bulky, multicoloured tweeds. Short kilts and other traditional clothing returned, albeit in subverted styling.

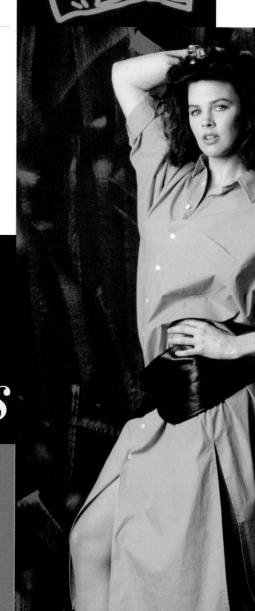

Wide cinch belts

The cinched-in waist was the keypoint of 1980s dressing. A curvaceous silhouette came back into style with belts making a huge impact.

▶Suits and shoulders

The television programme *Dynasty* helped the power suit catch on worldwide, but couture had led the way: black-and-white dogstooth pencil skirts with a nipped-in jackets by Marc Bohan for Christian Dior and Giorgio Armani's 'Donna' ad campaign from 1984–85 were notable. Here a black-and-white 1983 Jean-Louis Scherrer suit exhibits the extreme styling of the silhouette.

◀Oversized

Oversized looks featured in many catwalk collections, from Catharine Hamnett to Issey Miyake to Kenzo. This oversized shirtdress, based on a man's work shirt, but with deep side splits, is worn with an oversized black leather belt.

Puffball skirts

Christian Lacroix brought this little gem into style in 1986, hot on the heels of Vivienne Westwood's 'mini-crini'.

Asymmetrics

Slashed shoulders and halfway hems, one-sleeve wonders and black Lycra with cut-outs were prevalent. Couture versions included Comme des Garçons designs, especially as they appeared on Kim Basinger in the film *9 ½ Weeks* (1986).

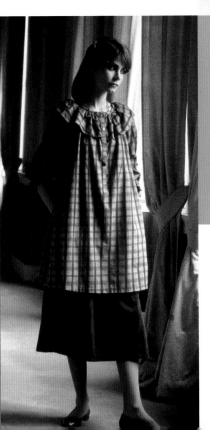

◀Laura Ashley dresses

Reaching its apogee in the early 1980s, Laura Ashley brought a sweet femininity to women's dresses that worked as a counter to the power suit, as shown left. The clothes had a neo-Victorian, old world romanticism that seemed to find relevance in the conservative tastes of the time.

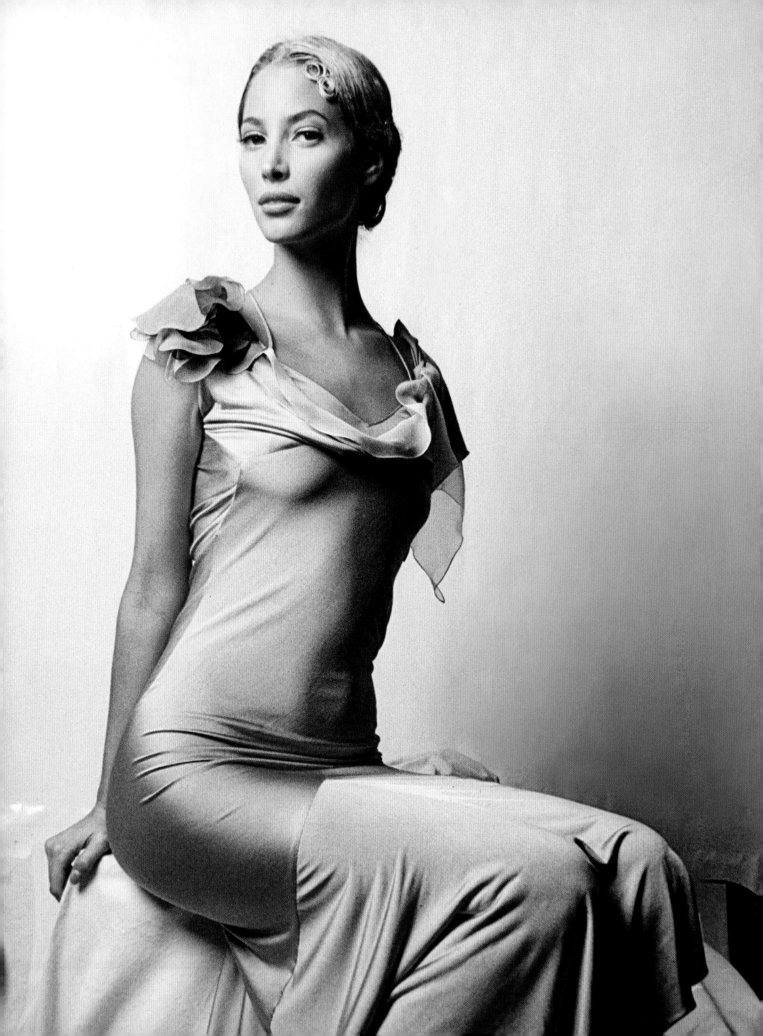

1990s

The final decade of the century was a time for both reflection and forward thinking. Designers drew inspiration from the past while embracing new technology and ideas. The fun and freedom of previous eras was replaced with a more serious mood and the fear of being underdressed was replaced by the fear of being overdressed. Fashion itself became less fashionable. Calvin Klein's advertising slogan 'Be Yourself' encouraged consumers to approach fashion with a less slavish attitude and the emphasis was moved from 'fashion' to 'style'.

At street level, there came a ubiquitous teenage rebellion. Just as the 1960s gave birth to the mod, the 1970s created the hippy and the 1980s bore punk, so too the 1990s had its own dissident uniform – Grunge. One of the defining looks of this era may have originated around the underground alternative rock scene of Seattle's disengaged youth, but its influence was far wider reaching. Marc Jacobs was labelled the 'Guru of Grunge' and his New York contemporary Anna Sui wasn't far behind.

But if this downbeat look wasn't for everyone, relief came in the form of Prada and Jil Sander's minimalism, proving that thrift fashion wasn't the only way to reject the ostentatiousness of the 1980s. The varied colour palettes of previous decades were replaced with more sombre tones of white, beige, brown, grey and black. The 1990s were also the decade when visionary designers such as Alexander McQueen, Martin Margiela and John Galliano shook up the fashion world and established radical new design concepts. Jean Paul Gaultier and Dolce & Gabbana were also on hand to offer more irreverent forms of sexuality and Tom Ford's re-invention of the house of Gucci was a perfect injection of luxurious glamour in an otherwise more restrained time.

Deconstruction

Deconstruction in fashion arrived at a time when grunge and minimalism were in full swing, and it captured the mood of the moment perfectly. Clothes were literally being dismantled in order to destroy the very concept of fashion. A rebellion against artifice, deconstruction was against everything that was traditional and taught. Its aim was to break the accepted codes of garment construction and offer an alternative to mainstream style and ways of thinking.

Production techniques were deliberately exposed. Shoulder pads, for example, might be attached to the outside of the garment, or stitching would be exaggerated. Defined by characteristics such as raw unfinished edges, revealed linings, fraying, exposed zippers and unusually sewn seams, deconstruction was as much a philosophical statement as it was a fashion one. Fabrics were layered, recycled and even

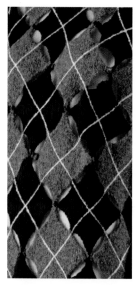

PAGE 208 Christy Turlington modelling John Galliano 1997. Along with Calvin Klein, Galliano's spaghetti-strap slipdresses, cut to slinky perfection on the bias, sparked a trend for lingerie dressing.

LEFT AND RIGHT Two deconstructed sweater dresses in Argyll and black cotton from Yohji Yamamoto's spring/summer 1993 collection.

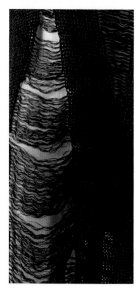

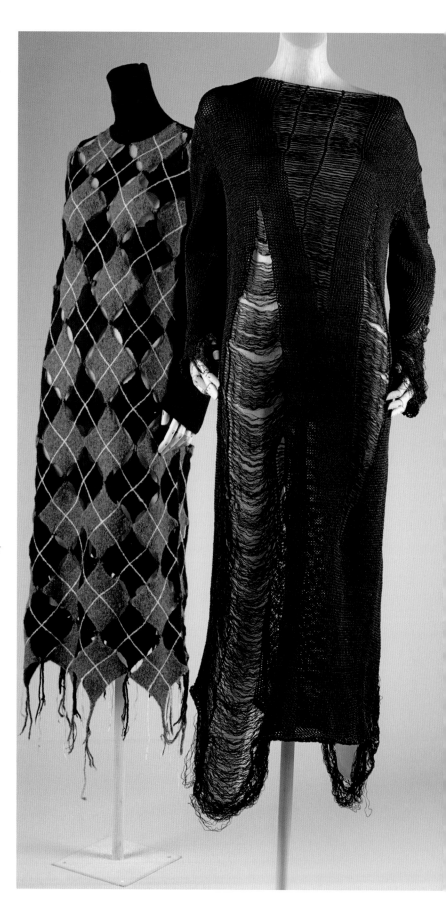

decomposed to offer a post-modern sartorial outlook that reflected the thinking of the French philosopher Jacques Derrida. Deconstruction fashion designers gave new relevance to garment components that would previously have been concealed. Yet, instead of merely destroying the heritage of garment construction, this new wave of design was a gesture that also acknowledged and effectively celebrated heritage and innovation. It looked to the past and future of fashion simultaneously, in a way that paralleled Derrida's philosophical deconstructive thinking.

If the Japanese designers Yojhi Yamamoto, Rei Kawakubo for Commes des Garçons, and Junya Watanabe were the first to dabble with deconstruction in the 1980s, it was the Antwerp Six – Ann Demeulemeester, Walter van Beirendonck, Dirk van Saene, Dirk Bikkembergs, Marina Yee and Dries van Noten – who took the torch and ran with it throughout the 1990s. Together with fellow Belgian Martin Margiela, often thought of as the seventh member of the Antwerp Six, they dominated the movement.

Margiela was widely known as the 'King of Deconstruction'. Showing in venues such as cemeteries and fire stations, his work transcended fashion, and his shows often came closer to performance art exhibitions than traditional ready-to-wear presentations. He worked non-fashion materials such as broken porcelain, bottle tops and coat hangers into his garments. His autumn/ winter 1991 collection was a fine example of his ideas, featuring sweaters patched together from cut-open and resewn raglan socks – the sock's heels were intentionally placed to form the bust line and elbows.

RIGHT More restructure than deconstructure, this bulbous gingham top by Rei Kawakubo for Comme des Garcons spring/summer 1997 plays with the ideas of form and shape in fashion, disregarding the normal lines and fit of the human body. Decidedly anti-fashion, her pieces are often asymmetric, frayed, unfinished or crumpled.

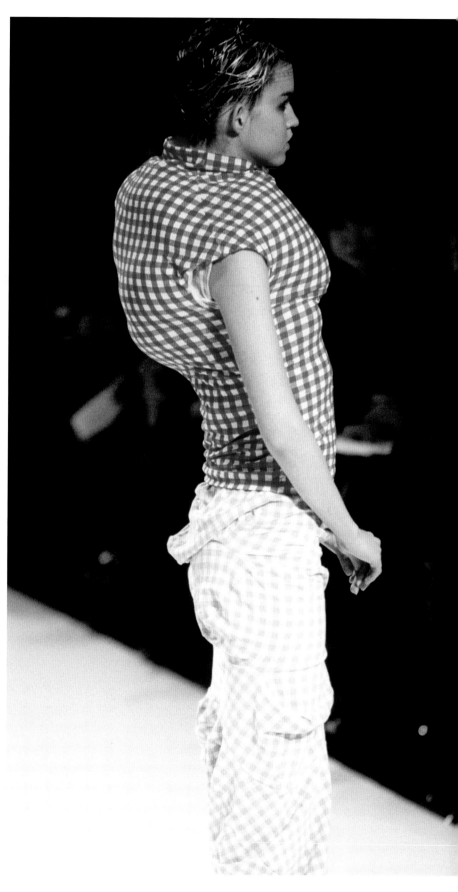

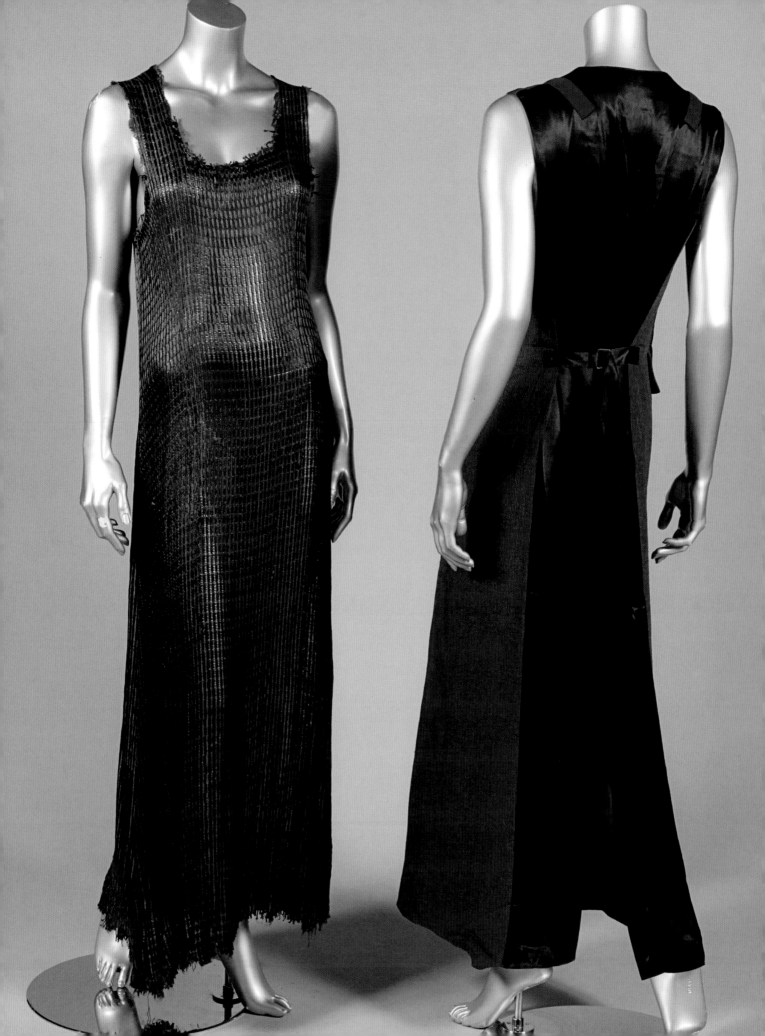

Ann Demeulemeester made her womenswear debut in Paris in 1993 with a collection that promptly put her on deconstruction's fashion map. Her garments were intentionally left unfinished, and although her shredded fabrics may have harked back to the punk era, when street fashion embraced razor-slashed T-shirts, they lacked any of punk's aggression, and her predominantly black colour palette gave her an instant cult following.

In the same year, British/Turkish-Cypriot designer Hussein Chalayan unveiled his graduate collection 'Tangent Flows'. This comprised garments that had been buried beneath the earth and then later dug up after they had partially decomposed.

Deconstruction swept through fashion for the whole of the '90s, and even less avant-garde names began to embrace the theme. Gianni Versace, a designer associated with more traditional glamour, gave a high-octane nod to deconstruction with his 1994 collection featuring slashed dresses, which appeared to be held together with out-sized safety pins. By the middle of the decade, high-street brands such as All Saints and Diesel were delivering deconstruction fashion to the mainstream, with their collections featuring pre-aged garments and distressed denims. What had begun as something of an anti-fashion statement had now gone full circle, entering the wardrobes of the masses as a widespread trend.

OPPOSITE Two dresses, circa 1990s, by Ann Demeulemeester – an open-weave mesh with distressed hems and an open-backed pinstriped jerkin.

RIGHT A romantic gypsy-themed ensemble from Dries van Noten's autumn/winter collection. The red bias-cut dress with fur-lined black overcoat is worn by model Esther Canadas.

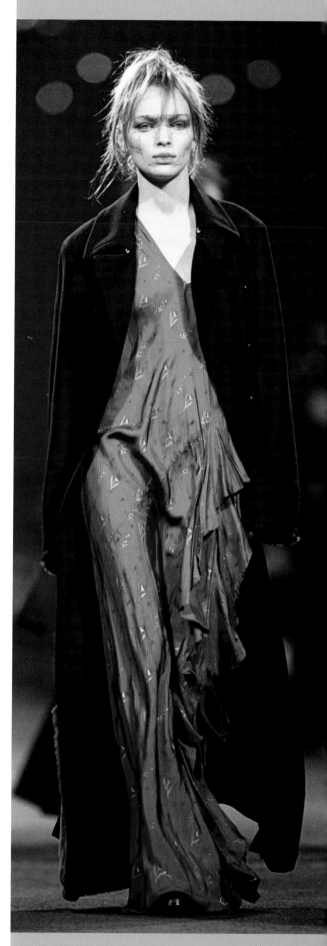

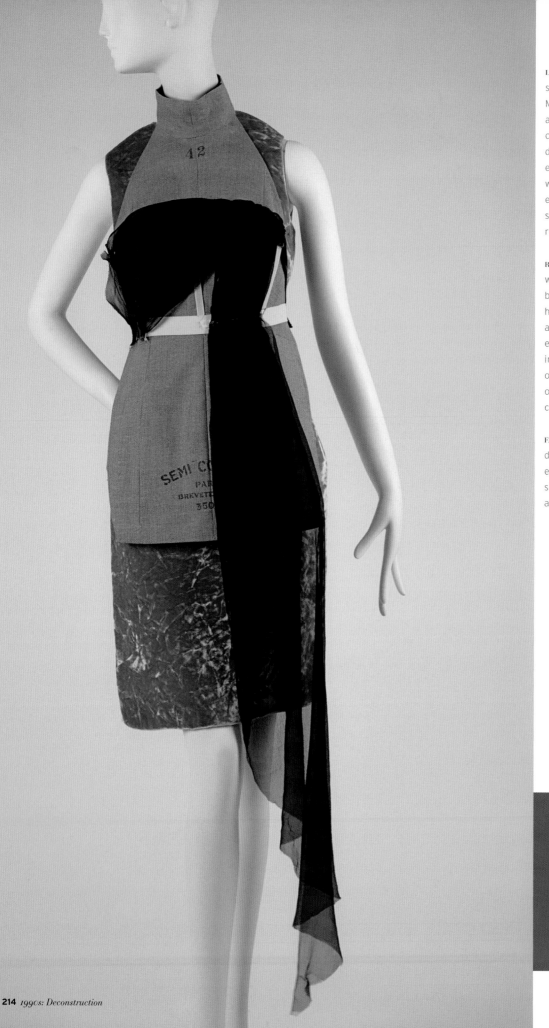

LEFT A drapery study from spring/summer 1997 by Martin Margiela. Known as one of the most conceptual and eccentric designers, and famously elusive, Margiela works with oversized volumes, exposed hems, visible stitches, draping and recycled materials.

RIGHT Patchwork knitwear with embellished elbows by Martin Margiela from his first collection in autumn/winter 1989. An early adopter of recycling in fashion, his pieces are often created by reworking objects and remnants into couture garments.

FAR RIGHT An open-weave distressed knit with exaggerated neckline and sleeves from Margiela, autumn/winter 1990.

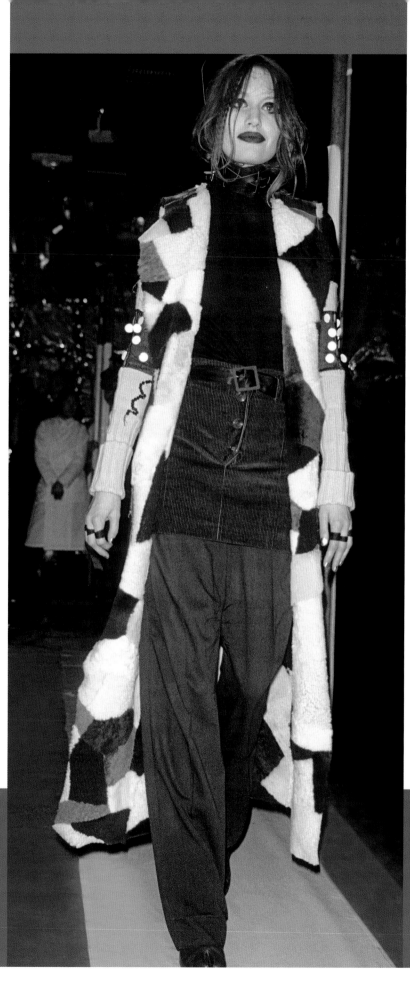

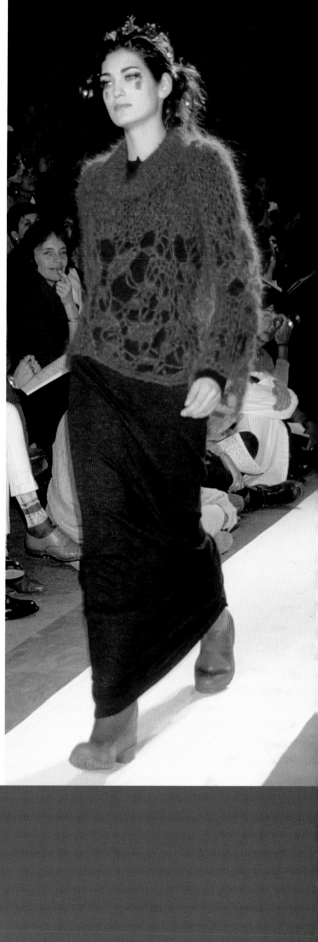

Minimalism

After the bright and booming 1980s, the 1990s got off to a darker start. The Gulf War began in August 1990, the global economy took a downward turn, and the fashion world responded accordingly. Minimalism was the new buzzword as the flounce and flare of recent years were replaced with a starker look. Power dressing became stealth dressing. Tailoring was reduced to its simplest form, hemlines dropped modestly to below the knee, and plain white T-shirts were given cult status.

Fashion was no longer the forum for grand displays of wealth and privilege; the smart way to dress was with educated restraint. Luxury labels such as Prada, Jil Sander and Martin Margiela intentionally marketed themselves with a lack of prestige – 'anti-status' was the ultimate goal, and even brand logos became spare and unassuming. Martin Margiela may have leant closer towards the concept of deconstruction but his ultra-discreet logo of four little white pick stitches on the outside of garments was also the perfect understated symbol of '90s minimalism.

Clean lines, quality fabrics and basic colours such as black, brown, olive green, beige, navy and white became the wardrobe staple. Fur was long gone. Low-heeled, elastic, knee-high boots were a smart choice throughout the mid- to late '90s, and Prada's black nylon totes, with their discreet silver triangle logos, were the ultimate accessory. For those who couldn't afford the real thing, high-street versions quickly followed. Acknowledging the adulation that Miuccia Prada received for her bags from international fashion editors, the Council of Fashion Designers of America gave her its award for accessories in 1993.

RIGHT Known for the power trouser suit that catered to the executive business-women, Jil Sander's luxury fabrics, muted colours and precise cuts made her pieces wearable and effortlessly stylish. She has been described as the 'Queen of Less'.

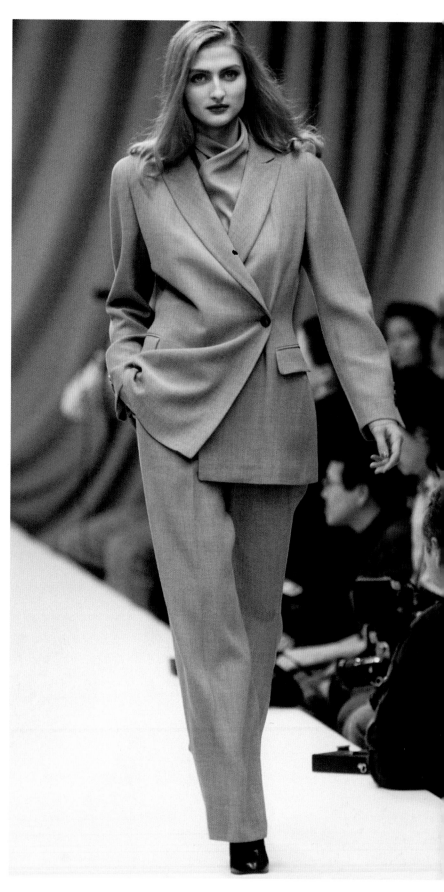

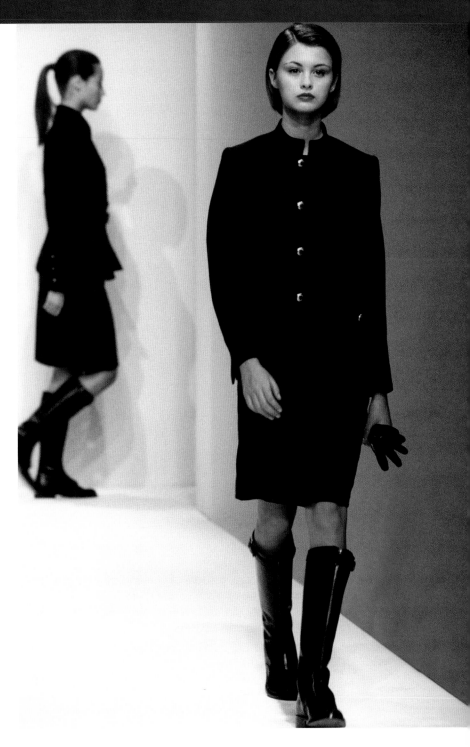

RIGHT Prada's pared-back pieces without visible branding became status symbols for those in the know in the 1990s. Suits in simple silhouettes and bland, neutral colours, such as these from autumn/winter 1994, were in stark contrast to the 1980s obsession with ostentation.

Prada's autumn/winter 1993 advertising campaigns featured black-and-white images of Christy Turlington with cropped elfin hair, wearing clothes that were so simple and unassuming that they almost went unnoticed. Throughout the decade, Prada's catwalk shows continued to epitomize a more streamlined femininity: simple, understated, with a hint of androgyny. Her spring/summer 1996 collection exemplified this look, featuring sleeveless white shirts and low-waisted, mid-calf-length, black pencil skirts.

Meanwhile, German designer Jil Sander, who also showed her collection on the catwalks of Milan, was widely accepted as one of the most respected minimalist fashion designers of the time. Although her first collections were shown in the 1980s, it wasn't until the 1990s that her style really became a hit. Her signature pieces were sharply cut trouser suits, slim-fit shirts and tailored coats in luxurious yarns.

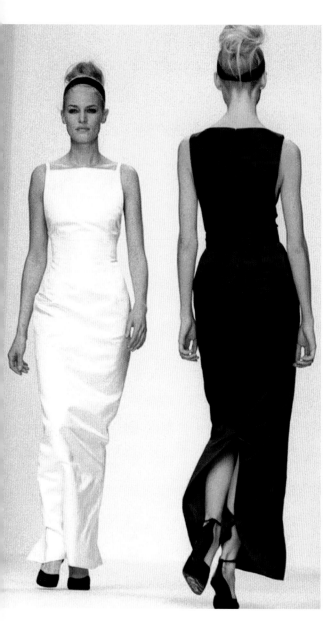

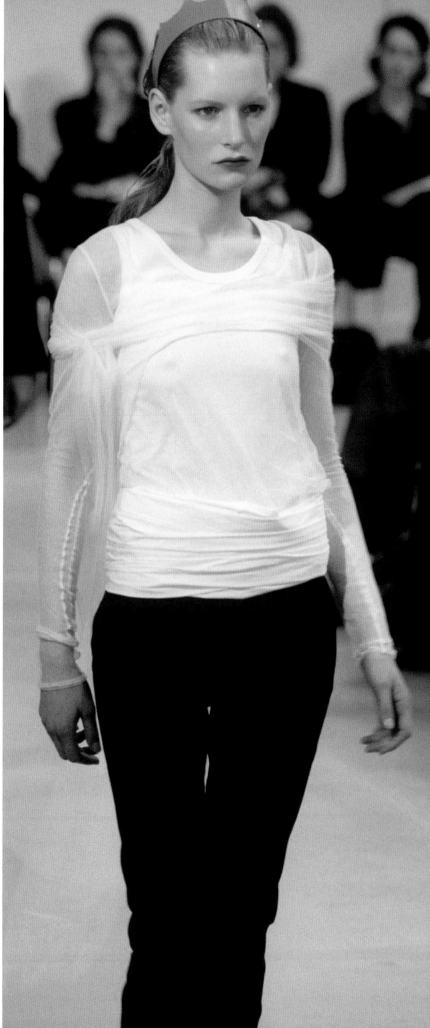

Sander's early advertising campaigns in the '90s pushed the boundaries of minimalism even further. When Peter Lindberg photographed a make-up-free Amber Valetta wearing nothing but a semi-sheer white cotton shirt and shiny black wide-legged trousers, the only accessories to the look were the creases left intentionally unironed at the sleeves. Although minimalism was in one sense sharp and deliberate, it also strongly reflected the '90s mood for effortless style.

Numerous other designers embraced minimalism throughout the decade, with Calvin Klein, Helmut Lang and Giorgio Armani all key players. Even Japan, traditionally relied upon for its difficult to wear avant-garde offerings, served up its own minimalist commercial hit. In 1993, Issey Miyake's Pleats Please was born. In a pioneering new technique called 'garment pleating', basic oversized cloth patterns were cut to shape as a full garment and then sandwiched between two layers of washi paper and fed into a heat press. These pleats remained permanently in the fabric's memory. Miyake's aim was to create clothing that would suit the needs of women everywhere and become as universal as jeans and T-shirts. His concept was simple and his clothes achieved the rare feat of being admired for both their originality and wearability, and arriving at just the right time.

Minimalism maintained a firm grip on fashion throughout the decade. It was defined perfectly by Amy M Spindler in the *New York Times* in June 1993 as 'best described not by what it is, but by what it lacks'.

FAR LEFT Models present matching white and brown long evening dresses at the Calvin Klein autumn/winter 1995 fashion show in New York, 1995.

LEFT Sheer, white, bandage-style, long-sleeved top is layered over a white tank top and worn with simple black trousers, from the Helmut Lang 1997 autumn/winter collection.

RIGHT A vibrant dress from Issey Miyake's 1994 spring/summer ready-to-wear collection. Functional and practical, Miyake's pleats designs came in simple shapes and diverse colourways and store and travel easily.

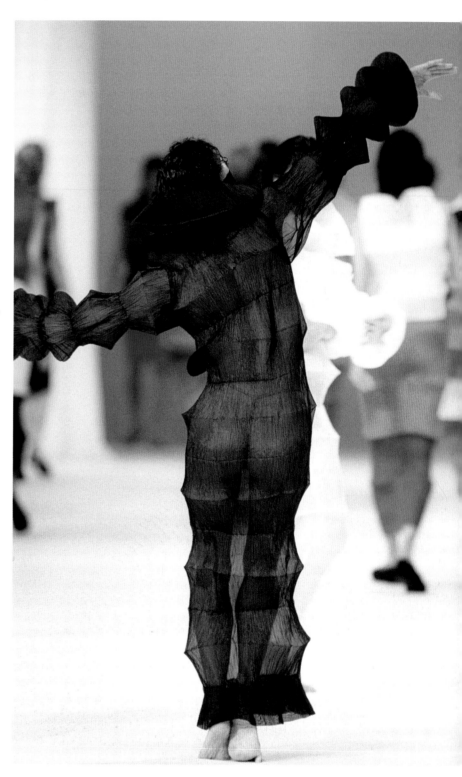

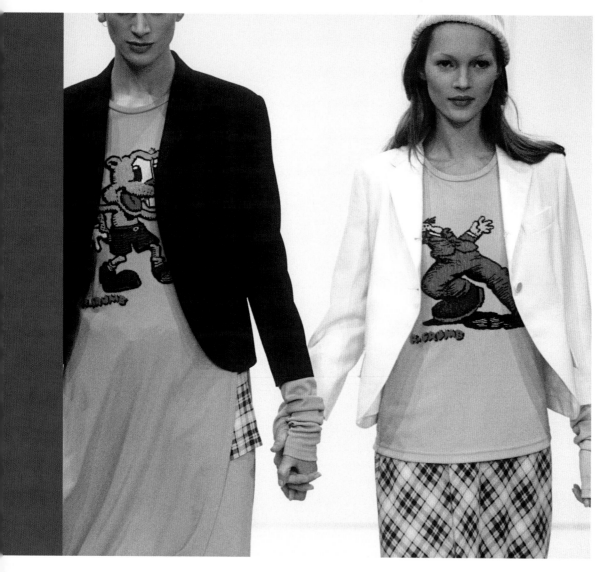

LEFT Marc Jacobs for Perry Ellis, spring/summer 1993, saw Jacob's groundbreaking grunge look hit the catwalk, striking a tone with twentysomethings but without creating the high-fashion buzz needed to go into production.

Grunge

Until the 1990s, 'grunge' was a word that meant dirt, filth and rubbish. All that changed when a musical subculture from Seattle screeched into mainstream consciousness under the title of Grunge, bringing with it not just a new sound but a new look, too.

Rock bands such as Soundgarden, the Melvins, Pearl Jam and, most importantly, Nirvana transformed the musical tastes of a new generation, and by the summer of 1991, the fashion press were obsessing over the deliberately unkempt, charity-shop style of these new music icons. The perfect backlash against the blinged-up, pithy pop fashions of the 1980s, grunge was a rebellion against the vulgarity of the previous decade and represented a quest for new values. There was a general feeling that ecological awareness and social responsibility were more fashionable than fashion itself. Anti-fashion had found its moment, and grunge captured the zeitgeist perfectly within the economic and cultural landscape of the time. Ripped jeans,

threadbare flannel shirts, bobbly cardigans, Converse trainers and Doctor Marten boots were the foundations of the grunge dress code. Kurt Cobain became an unlikely pin-up with his greasy hair and secondhand clothes, and his girlfriend Courtney Love, front-woman of Hole, was the ultimate grunge princess – her tattered babydoll dresses, tiaras and ripped stockings redefined femininity for '90s youth.

The appetite for grunge was huge and this new teen spirit took no time in leaving the streets of Seattle for the catwalks of New York. In November 1992, Marc Jacobs, who had never even visited the Pacific Northwest, was hailed as 'the guru of grunge'. His thrift-inspired collection for Perry Ellis was such a hit with the fashion critics that he was awarded Womenswear Designer of the Year. The look was relaxed, androgynous and unkempt, but although his lumberjack shirts, leggings, baggy dresses and sleeveless jackets had the fashion editors drooling, they failed to impress the US sportswear label. Not a single piece from the collection went into production, and Perry Ellis and Marc Jacobs parted ways soon after.

Jacobs wasn't the only designer to take this street-fashion look and deliver it to an international high-fashion audience. According to American *Vogue*, Anna Sui became 'the darling of downtown fashion' when she unveiled her spring/summer 1993 collection featuring floral print granny dresses, army fatigues, chunky boots, floppy hats, chokers and plenty of embroidered butterflies. That same season, young American designer Christian Francis Roth also offered up his version of the look, with baggy shirts tied around waists and layered over stretch cotton leggings.

Even the likes of Karl Lagerfeld, Christian Lacroix and Calvin Klein brought elements of the trend to their own collections. Elsewhere, the healthy vibrant supermodels of the 1980s were replaced with pale-skinned, emaciated young waifs who embodied the new aesthetic for heroin chic.

Corrine Day's grungy black-and-white images of a then unknown 16-year-old Kate Moss, for the cover of *The Face* magazine, became iconic, helping bag Moss the 1992 Calvin Klein jeans campaign and making her the ultimate super-waif. The photography of the Sorrenti brothers, Mario and Davide, represented and glamourized a gritty reality and was published in magazines such as *i-D*, *Surface* and *Detour*. Davide's girlfriend, model Jamie King, became one of the main poster girls for heroin chic.

It was a cheap and easily attainable look that endured well on the streets, however, in the ranks of high fashion, its appeal was relatively short-lived – there was limited enthusiasm from consumers of luxury brands to pay high prices on 7th Avenue for a look that could be better achieved with charity-shop finds. In 1999, *Vogue* launched Gisele's career under the headline 'The Return of the Sexy Model'. The fashion industry turned its back on grunge and heroin chic, and a new healthy look began to emerge.

RIGHT Goth sensibilities in a black velvet lace bell-sleeved minidress from Anna Sui's 1993 autumn/winter collection is modeled by Kate Moss.

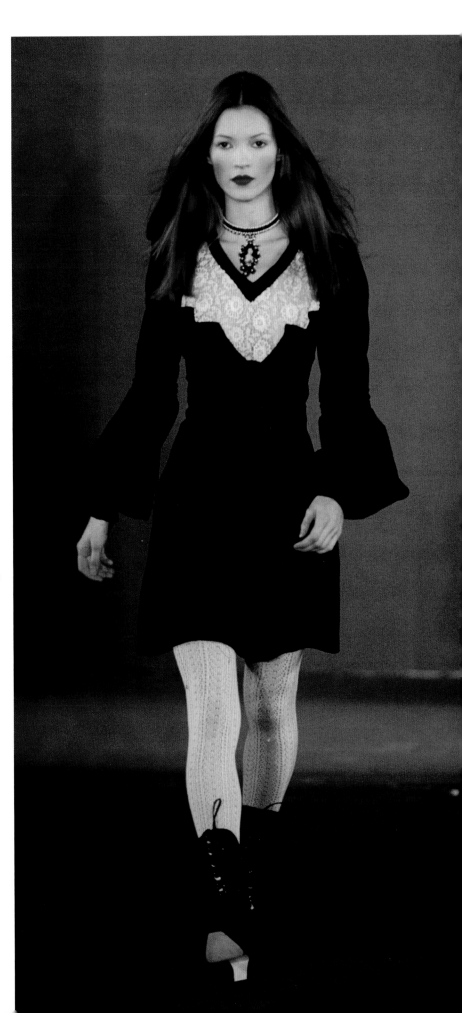

American Casual

Effortless elegance for the elite leisure classes, as seen in an advertisement for Ralph Lauren in the 1990s. Grounded in classic sportswear design, his clothing was associated with a preppy lifestyle that had somewhat surprising wide-spread appeal.

Peter Lindbergh's first *Vogue* cover of the 1990s featured Naomi Campbell, Linda Evangelista, Tatjana Patitz, Christy Turlington and Cindy Crawford looking the epitome of casual chic. Bare-faced with clean-cut hair, they wore cotton Lycra bodies, blue jeans and not a scrap of jewellery. It was an iconic image that signalled a total change in taste and values for the decade ahead. If the 1980s were all about dressing up, then the 1990s were about dressing down. Casual was the new byword for style; the aim was to look effortlessly cool.

'Dress down Fridays' became prevalent in American corporations and soon the concept went global. Office workers hung up their formal wear, and power dressing became a much-derided notion. This new end-of-week freedom was a passport for self-expression yet the sartorial comment made by most was that of comfort and relaxation. Companies allowed and encouraged workers to sport jeans, chinos, T-shirts, hoodies, casual shirts and even trainers, while brands such as Gap, Old Navy, Banana Republic and Abercrombie & Fitch deliberately marketed themselves to appeal to this new casual consumer. The US sitcom *Friends* debuted in 1994, with a wardrobe that also channelled the casual mood of the time. Jennifer Aniston's character Rachel became a style icon, and her scoop-neck, shrunken sweaters, high-waisted jeans, dresses worn over T-shirts and preppy dungarees epitomized the casual look.

Luxury brands also embraced the new mood. Known for his streamlined aesthetic, Calvin Klein was the perfect ambassador for the new casual dress code, and his cK Jeans helped prove that high-end labels could sell low-key style, too. His mainline collection with its easy elegance set the standard for many other brands.

RIGHT Clean-lined luxury in a Michael Kors ensemble worn by Christy Turlington on the catwalk for his spring/summer 1992 ready-to-wear show. His timeless, season-appropriate clothing was superbly tailored and made in quality fabrics.

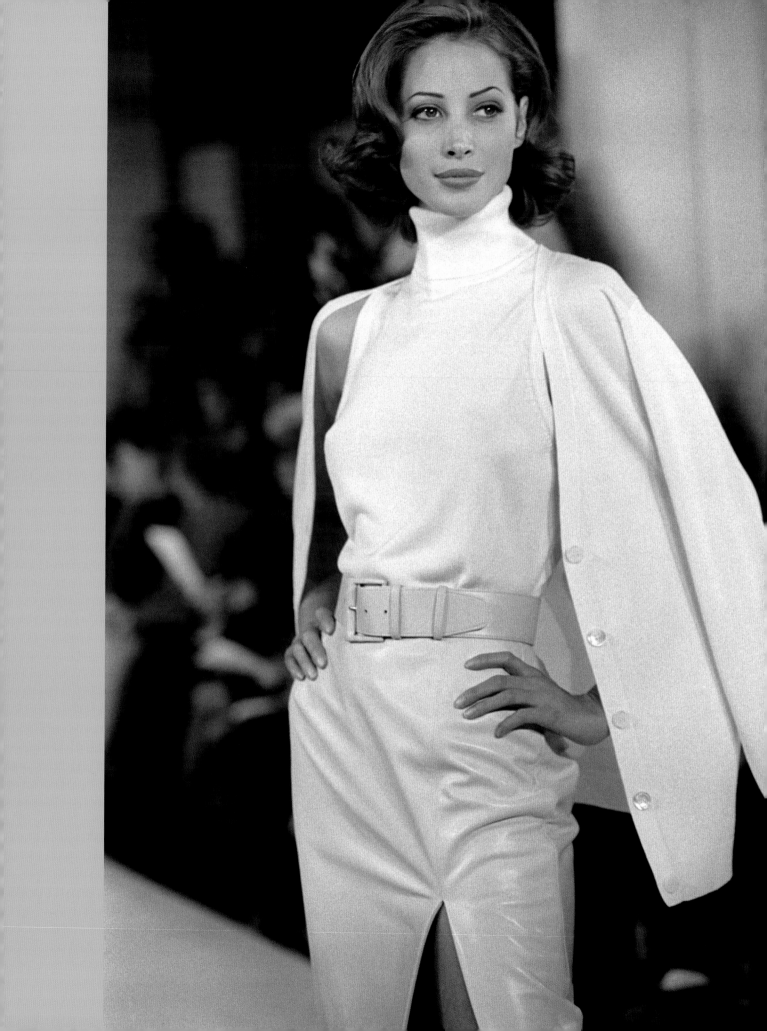

Michael Kors was another designer to find favour with a new generation of wealthy customers seeking simple, well-cut clothes. Steeped within the American sportswear traditions, his clothes offered comfort and luxury while maintained a level of sophistication. The real appeal of his clothes was based on their versatility: a Kors dress or trouser suit could be worn day or night, and never look over- or under-dressed. Since the launch of the Michael Kors Collection line in 1991, the designer has been a major influence in American fashion – the success of his own collections led the French fashion house Céline to pick him in 1997 as their creative director and first-ever women's ready-to-wear designer.

Ralph Lauren continued to thrive throughout the 1990s as the brand went global. Aimed primarily at elite Americans, his clothes and homeware lines became synonymous with casual East-Coast style and won him several prestigious awards throughout the decade, including Womenswear Designer of the Year in 1995 and Menswear Designer of the Year in 1996 from the Council of Fashion Designers of America. His collections, which featured tweed jackets, jodhpurs and luxurious knits, evoked a look of upmarket yet sporty elegance. Meanwhile, his signature polo shirts, which came in a wide spectrum of colours, all featuring his woven, polo-player logo, became an essential part of the preppy wardrobe.

BELOW The 1990s, when Calvin Klein was still at the helm of his extensive clothing, fragrance and homeware empire, was the heyday for the brand and similarly affordable designer labels like DKNY. His underwear, slipdresses and cK sportswear (comfortable, interchangeable separates), were accessible for all.

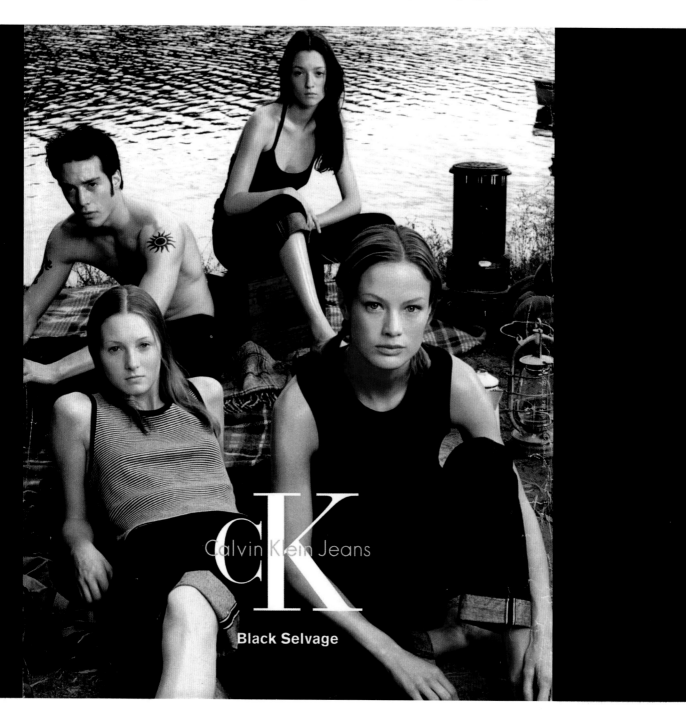

Calvin Klein Jeans

CK

Black Selvage

RIGHT Known for its easy, slouchy pieces, Gap mastered the T-shirt and khaki look, as seen in this advertisement from 1999. The brand went upmarket during the decade, graduating from a jeans-based enterprise to a lifestyle company, firmly based in the American sportswear mode.

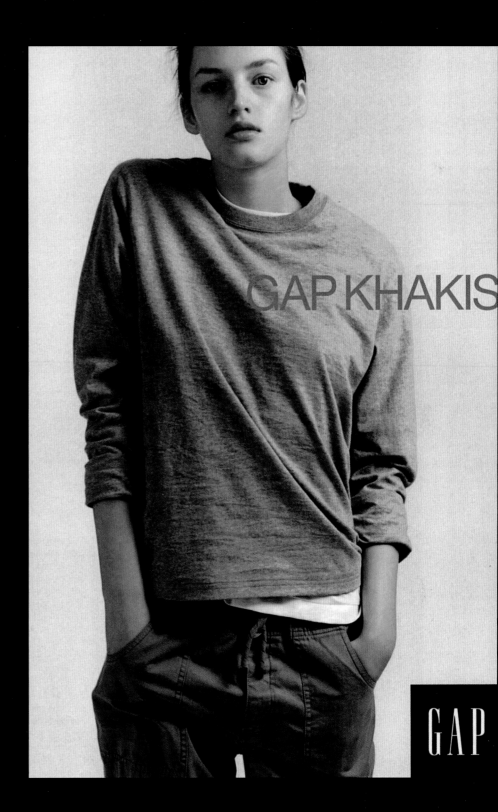

Hip Hop and Streetwear

Hip-hop fashion was heavily influenced by traditional African dress during the early 1990s. Red, black and green, the colours of the Pan-African flag, were popular hues for many rappers, as were the ornate headdress and bright, printed head-wraps favoured by the likes of Queen Latifah and, later, Erykah Badu. Black Nationalism was also popularized by artists such as KRS-One, Public Enemy and X-Clan, who wore African trends such as fez hats, kufis decorated with the Kemetic ankh, kente cloth hats and African chains. Baggy African-style harem pants were another favourite. MC Hammer became a global star with his 1990 super-hit 'U Can't Touch This' and the outsized trousers he wore became known as Hammer pants.

Sportswear became even more of a mainstream fashion feature. British Knights, a New York footwear company, produced chunky-soled, large-tongued sneakers, which were hugely popular until the Crips street gang adopted them, taking the BK logo to indicate 'Blood Killer'. Nike sponsored Air Jordan to produce highly desired sports shoes throughout the decade, bringing out a new style every year. Other popular athletics labels included Reebok Pro-Keds, Adidas, Champion, Stussy and Nautica, as well as workwear labels such as Carhartt, Timberland and Caterpillar.

Designer names from the luxury sector catered for the urban streetwear market, too. Polo Ralph Lauren, Calvin Klein, DKNY and Tommy Hilfiger were all

BELOW Colour-block 8-ball jackets, popularized by the hip-hop trio Salt 'n' Pepa, were an 1980s trend that continued into the 1990s.

RIGHT Urban hip-hop fashion from Tommy Hilfiger, October 1996. The designer courted the market with black models in the advertising campaigns and Sean Combs (aka Puffy) and Coolio on the catwalk.

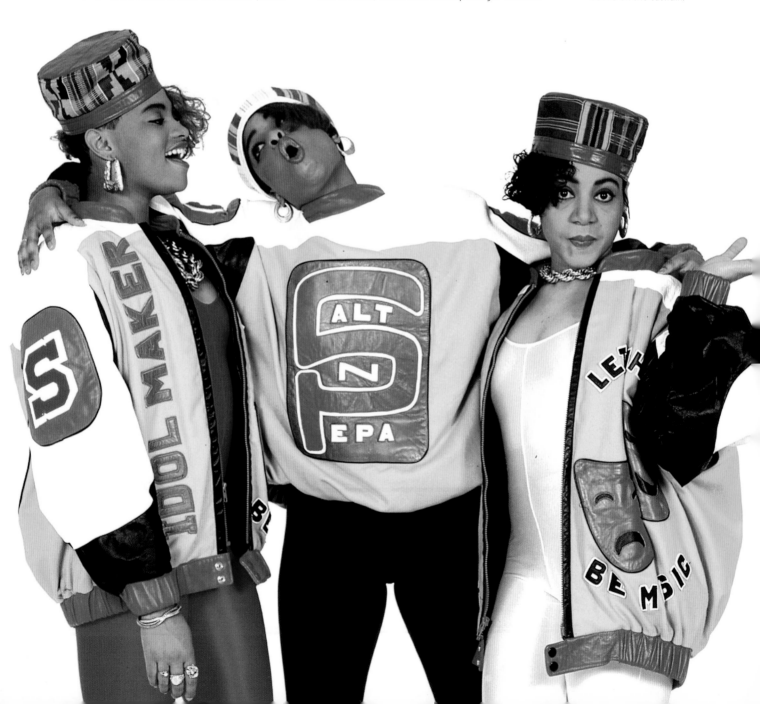

considered aspirational and when Snoop Doggy Dogg appeared on *Saturday Night Live* wearing a red, white and navy Hilfiger rugby shirt, it sold out of New York stores the very next day. The designer capitalized on his popularity by featuring black models and hip-hop and R&B artists such as Puffy, Coolio and Aaliyah in his campaigns and catwalk shows. The Beastie Boys, an all-white American hip-hop band, had their own version of the style taken from black street culture, which featured baggy low-slung jeans, side-turned baseball caps, gold chains and high-top sports shoes by brands such as Fila.

Starter jackets were something of a status symbol for men and women. Made by the Starter Clothing Line, the shiny satin jackets, often in bright colours, were designed to endorse various sports teams and reports of widespread robberies of the jackets led to their cult status. '8-Ball' leather jackets, manufactured by North Beach Leather Brand Michael Hoban, held onto their popularity through the early 1990s, thanks to artists such as Salt 'n' Pepa, who frequently wore them.

The hip-hop look was in many ways unisex, as women strived to make it in a male-dominated music genre. Female rapper Da Brat epitomized the look with her baggy jeans, workwear boots, bandanas and braided hair. Neneh Cherry brought a more British twist, favouring fur-trimmed parka jackets, leggings and high-tops. On the flip side, Lil Kim and Foxy Brown were popularizing a trashier and more sexualized image with plenty of flashy jewellery and 'ghetto fabulous' clothes that drew on pornstar influences. All these looks eventually made it to fashion houses, with Chanel, Louis Vuitton, Gucci and Isaac Mizrahi sending their models down the catwalk wearing versions of the street style and adorned in blingtastic accessories.

As the 1990s continued, 'gangsta' style became ever more the mode and MCs such as Ice T, Dr Dre, Tupac Shakur and Jodeci often channelled looks that were representative of prison style. Baggy low-slung jeans, bandannas and tattoos were all embraced, as were heavy silver or platinum chains and jewellery. Other rappers, most notably The Notorious B.I.G but also Puff Daddy and Jay Z were taking a more ostentatious approach to 'gangsta style'. Inspired by films like *Scarface*, they wore double-breasted suits, bowler hats, silk shirts and alligator-skin shoes.

By the late decade artists capitalized on their images, bringing out their own clothing lines. Puff Daddy launched his sportswear label Sean John in 1998. The following year, Damon Dash and Jay Z co-founded Rocawear and Kimora Lee Simmons, model and wife of hip-hop magnate Russell Simmons, launched Baby Phat in 1998.

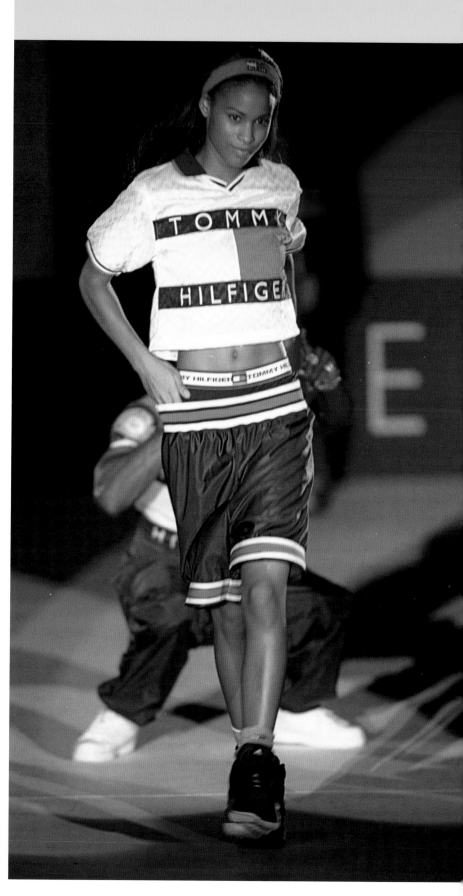

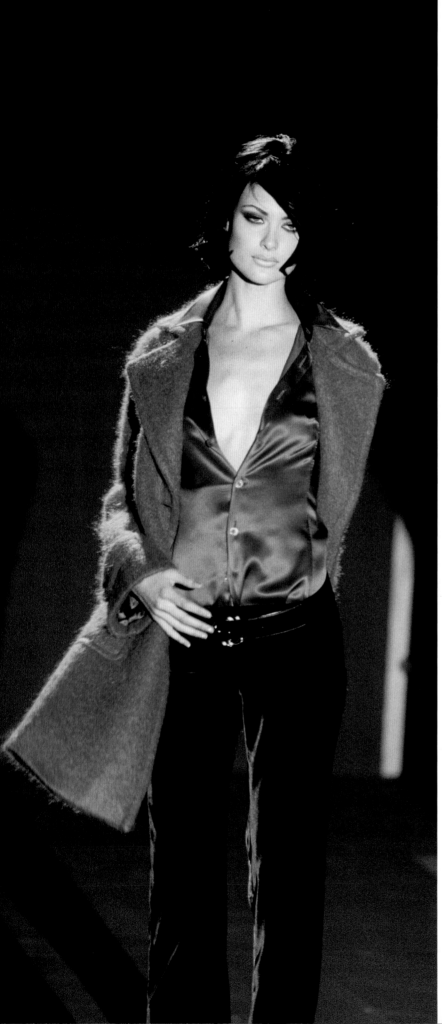

Cool Britannia and the New Mods

If the 1990s began with the domination of America's grunge and hip-hop styles, by the mid- to late decade, fashion had taken a geographical shift and there was no place on earth more happening than Britain. 'Cool Britannia', a term coined by the media, was used to describe the thriving cultural landscape of Great Britain, a culture that involved music, art, politics, films, sport and fashion.

Vivienne Westwood was awarded the Order of the British Empire in 1992, and a year later British supermodel Naomi Campbell, wearing a pair of Westwood 30-cm (6-in) blue platform heels, a giant pink feather boa and a tartan kilt, took a catwalk tumble. It was an image that set the mood for all things bright, fun and unequivocally British.

Via MTV, Britpop bands such as Oasis, Blur, Pulp and Suede were propelled from the streets of London and Manchester to global stardom, and how they dressed was as important as the music they made. The look was rooted in urban fashion, but Britpop was sharper, brighter and sportier than anything the Seattle street scene had previously offered. Damon Albarn summed up the changing attitude in 1993 when, after being asked if Blur were an 'anti-grunge band', he replied, 'Well that's good. If punk was about getting rid of hippies, then I'm getting rid of grunge.'

With a hint of irony, Jarvis Cocker became an unlikely style icon – his penchant for thick-rimmed spectacles and crimplene slacks crowned him the king of geek chic. Cocker also brought geek chic to the house of Gucci when Tom Ford dressed him in a snake-hipped trouser suit and matching skinny shirt. The Gucci look was a passport to Britpop style and snapped up by the likes of Victoria Beckham and Oasis's Gallagher brothers.

In March 1997, *Vanity Fair* published a special edition on Cool Britannia, with Liam Gallagher and Patsy Kensit on the cover and the title 'London Swings Again!' Accordingly, the mod styles of the early 1960s found themselves revisited. Mini-skirts, pop-bright colours, sleek graphic silhouettes, zippers and monochrome were back in fashion – and so, too, were classic British leisure brands like Fred Perry, Pringle and Ben Sherman. As ladies became ladettes, polo shirts, diamond-knit sweaters and parka jackets were essential additions to the new-mod wardrobes of both men and women.

If one element truly became symbolic of Britpop style, it was the Union Jack. When the Spice Girls stormed the Brit Awards in February 1997, it was Geri Halliwell's skimpy Union Jack mini dress that made all the headlines. Over night, the patriotic print became the ultimate fashion statement and soon it was everywhere, from bikinis and T-shirts to jackets

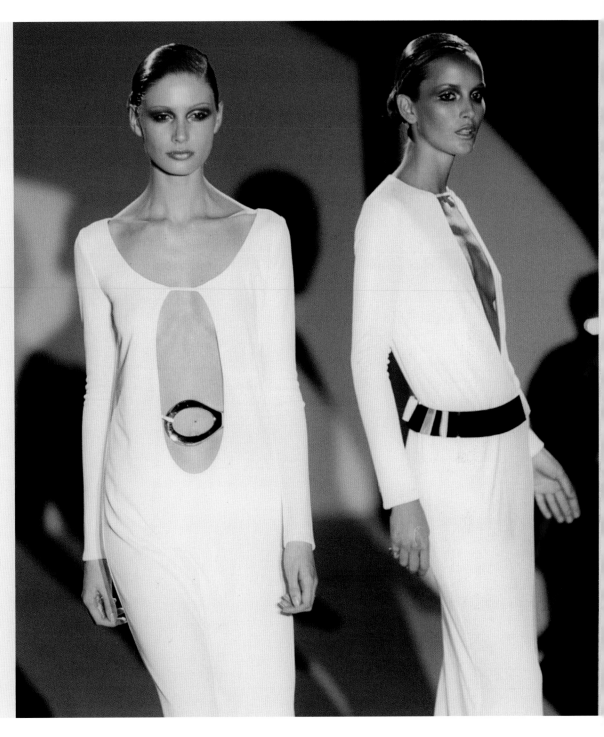

LEFT Silk blouses and velvet hip-huggers by Tom Ford at Gucci – two of the most desirable vintage pieces to collect from this time period, for men or women, from autumn/winter 1995–6.

RIGHT After becoming creative director in 1994, Tom Ford launched the look that evoked the 1960s mod and simultaneously captured the the mood in the UK. Here Gucci dresses from 1996 are high-octane sexy: long, lean and with delicately placed slashes for showing off hardware and erogenous zones.

and jeans. Paul Smith, a British designer known for his classic tailoring with an English eccentric twist, featured the Union Jack throughout his collections, ensuring that by the mid 1990s his export sales accounted for two-thirds of his business – countries such as Japan couldn't get enough of the British look.

In May 1997, Tony Blair was elected as prime minister, putting the Labour government back in power. In keeping with the new left-wing political mood, '90s British style was accessible, easy to wear and designed for everyone to enjoy. Red or Dead, a label that began as a stall in Camden Market, became a popular brand, winning the British Fashion Council's Streetstyle Designer of the Year Award from 1995 to 1997. Wayne Hemingway, the company's founder, said his goal was 'to be the first designer company that sold to everyday people'. This statement perfectly exemplified the Cool Britannia attitude.

Red Carpet Glamour

Red-carpet fashion took on new levels of importance, as dressing appropriately for major events became an art form in itself. In the past celebrities and film stars had chosen their own outfits and dealt directly with designers, now powerful fashion stylists stepped in and awards ceremony dressing became a cleverly orchestrated affair.

Stylists such as Deborah Waknin and Philip Bloch started introducing a more discerning look to the red carpet. High-fashion labels like Valentino, Alexander McQueen and Galliano began to replace local Hollywood dressmakers. In 1995 Philip Bloch's career took off after dressing Uma Thurman in a much-admired violet Prada gown. He repeated his success a year later by dressing Nicole Kidman in an equally popular empire-line lilac gown. When Halle Berry appeared at the 68th Annual Academy Awards in 1996 in an on-trend lilac Valentino gown, it was Deborah Waknin who had chosen it.

Some critics mused that stylists took away some of the flair and excitement of red-carpet dressing, with stars looking uniformly groomed and fashionable. But with ever more scrutiny being placed on who wore what, fewer celebrities were prepared to take risks. Fashion editors and media pundits scrutinized and celebrated what the stars wore, with the result that getting it right could enhance the careers of celebrities and designers alike.

In general, eveningwear during this period was an exercise in restrained elegance. Hemlines sat somewhere around knee length for a cocktail dress and full-length gowns had a slimline silhouette. Elsewhere 1990s eveningwear reflected the existing trends of the time. In 1996, the white tunic and matching cropped trousers, which Nicole Kidman wore to the Los Angeles premiere of *Mission Impossible* were a perfect reflection of 1990s minimalism. Similarly, the long green chiffon gown, which Kidman wore in 1997 to the premiere of *The Portrait of a Lady* was a floor-length version of the grungier baby-doll looks that were still popular.

Giorgio Armani was one of the first international fashion houses to hire a Hollywood public relations team. By the end of the 1980s, the Milanese designer had begun loaning dresses to selected stars for red-carpet occasions and through the 1990s many other fashion houses followed suit. Jodie Foster repeatedly wore Armani throughout the decade – a move that helped transform her from a fabulous actress with dubious sartorial taste into a fashion icon.

Princess Diana, one of the most photographed women of the 1990s, also enhanced her fashion credentials with the strong relationship that developed between herself and Gianni Versace. She regularly wore his dresses to high-profile events, most notably the little black dress she wore in 1995, the asymmetric-shouldered, slimline blue gown in 1996 and the purple dress with matching

accessories which she wore the same year. But perhaps the most significant red-carpet moment of the decade was in 1994 in the form of Elizabeth Hurley's Versace safety-pin gown. The dress caused a media frenzy and was proof that a red-carpet outfit could turn an unknown actress into a global star overnight.

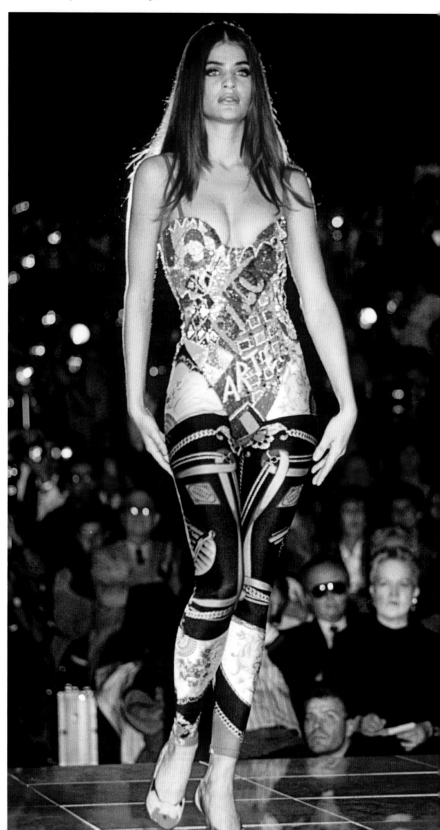

OPPOSITE Helena Christensen in a corset-styled bodysuit from Versace's spring/summer 1991 collection, ticking off two of the decade's trends: neon brights and the corset. Bright colours, often heavily outlined in black, were a hallmark of his early pieces.

RIGHT AND DETAIL BELOW Widely influenced by the florid shapes and colours of artists such as Sonia Delaunay and Raoul Dufy (both of whom collaborated with fashion designers during their careers), Gianni Versace frequently referenced historical art and culture. This piece, in silk jersey, beads and rhinestones from 1991, is printed with the iconic faces of Marilyn Monroe and James Dean, and alludes to the designer's fascination with Andy Warhol and celebrity culture.

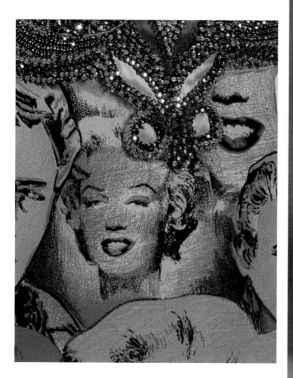

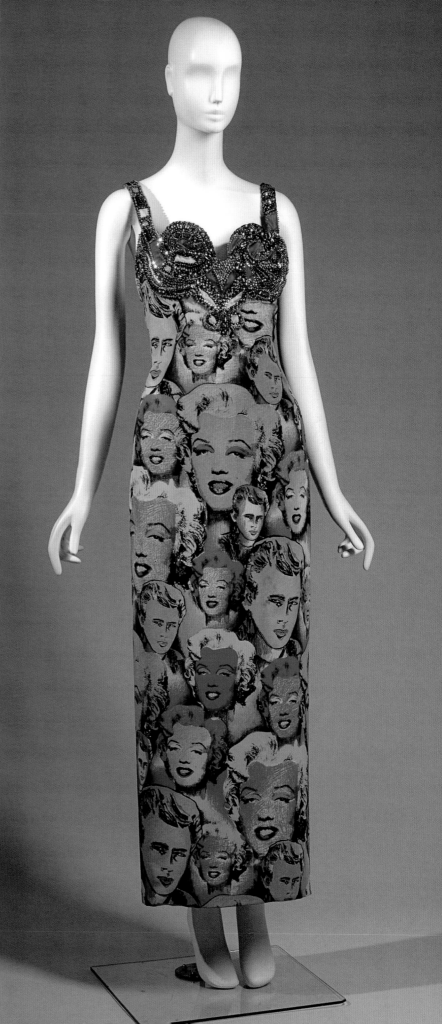

Eurotrash

With much of the fashion industry kicking off the decade in a rather understated and serious mood, light relief was promptly served by the flamboyant French designer Jean Paul Gaultier. Grunge and minimalism were the perfect backdrops against which Gaultier's colourful and irreverent collections could shine out. Dressing women in pinstriped tailoring and men in skirts and glittery bodysuits were just some of the tools he employed to subvert the clichés of masculinity and femininity; his androgynous aesthetic and use of unconventional pierced and tattooed models of varying ages and physiques attracted him media attention from the tabloids to the high-end glossies.

His ability to shock ensured that when Madonna was looking for a designer to create the costumes for her 1990 Blonde Ambition tour, Gaultier was the only man for her to turn to. The conical cupped bustiers teamed with slashed pinstriped trouser suits ensured Gaultier's name reached an even wider audience. He soon found himself in the unique position of being both a respected international fashion designer and a household name all at once. The success of the collaboration was consecrated further when in 1992 Madonna strutted down the Paris catwalk, arm in arm with the peroxide-haired designer. Looking every inch the Gaultier muse, wearing a gold tooth, black beret and outsized boyfriend blazer, the real *pièce de résistance* came

OPPOSITE Dolce & Gabbana was another of Europe's flamboyant designers to rise to prominence in the 1990s. Domenico Dolce and Stefano Gabbana became known for their flashy, erotic fashions and the idea of the 'Sicilian widow', an uninhibited, erotic woman, with lingerie on show, wearing expensive materials such as lace, snakeskin and fur. Animal print has long been one of the pair's signatures, as seen here in a zebra-print jacket from autumn/winter 1994–5, worn by model Linda Evangelista.

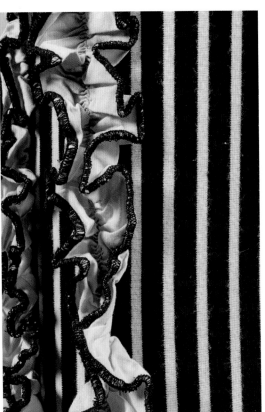

LEFT DETAIL AND RIGHT Jean Paul Gaultier's French Can-Can ready-to-wear collection from autumn/ winter 1991–2. Iin this collection the designer mutated and subverted traditional Parisian icons – the beret and the trench, the cigarette, the Eiffel Tower, the Pigalle showgirl.

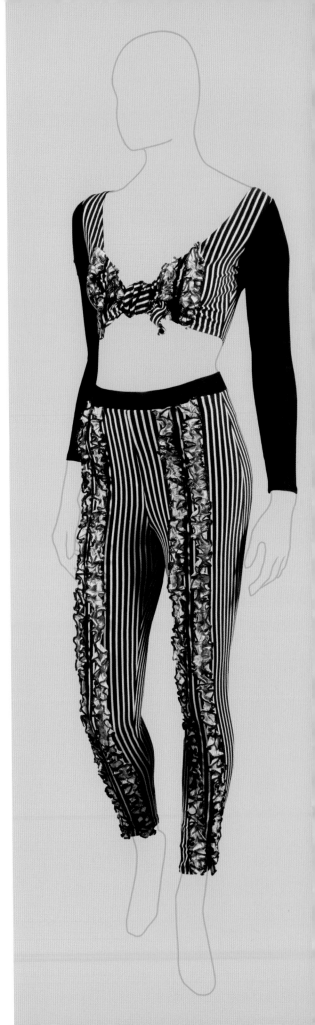

when at the end of the show she slipped off her jacket to reveal her bare breasts, perfectly framed in a brace-topped tight black dress. The audience roared with delight and the media lapped up this controversial finale.

But it wasn't just Gaultier who enjoyed the Madonna effect. Dolce & Gabbana offered their own Italian version of sexed-up androgynous dressing. Masculine pinstripes were offset with cleavage-enhancing corsets and a heavy dose of their signature leopard print.

Meanwhile Jean Paul Gaultier was busy carving out his own showbiz career when in 1993 he was chosen to host the late-night British TV show *Eurotrash* alongside Antoine De Caunes. Dressed in his signature Breton striped tops he delivered a show filled with popular culture, sexual innuendo and outrageous fetishes – all the subjects Gaultier loved. But while all this was great entertainment, some cynics commented that his reputation as a master tailor was being jeopardized. After the seventh series he quit, putting his focus fully back onto his fashion lines. In 1997, disappointed that he hadn't been chosen as the new creative director at Christian Dior, Gaultier launched his first couture line to great acclaim. The collection featured all his trademarks – pinstriped suits, perfect tailoring, rich embroideries, feathers, fur, silk and velvet, all brought together under an exotic umbrella of restrained fetishism and ethnic influences.

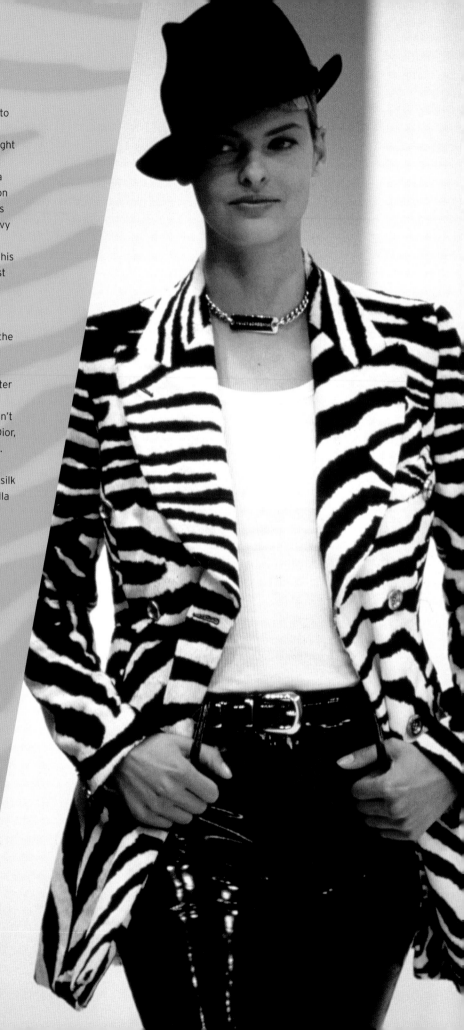

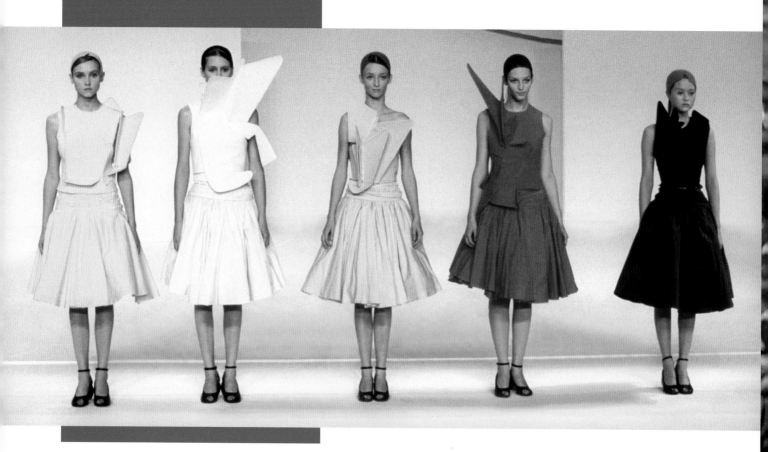

Visionairies

British fashion enjoyed something of a renaissance during the 1990s as Central Saint Martins College of Art and Design continued to nurture a steady output of exciting new talent that included the likes of Alexander McQueen, Stella McCartney and Hussein Chalayan. John Galliano, who had graduated the decade earlier in 1984, put the turbulent start to his career behind him and in 1990 set up a studio in Paris where he brought a sense of wild excitement to the slightly stale French fashion scene. His collections continued to reflect his obsession with history and romanticism, with collections given grand titles such as Napoleon and Josephine and Princess Lucretia to reflect his inspirations. His collections were created around narrative themes, but while he let his imagination run riot, his focus on technique and garment construction was unparalleled and he became known for his 1930s-inspired bias-cut dresses, crinolines, pyjama suits and mastery of fabric and tailoring. He was appointed creative director at Givenchy in 1996 and the following year, Galliano, the great romanticist of 1990s fashion, was enlisted to revive the house of Christian Dior. His first collections at Dior featured a mixture of ideas such as belle époque, Maasai princesses, birds of paradise, 1920s Berlin nightlife and African Maori costumes – winning him a steady stream of international awards and a list of fans that included Princess Diana, Madonna and Nicole Kidman.

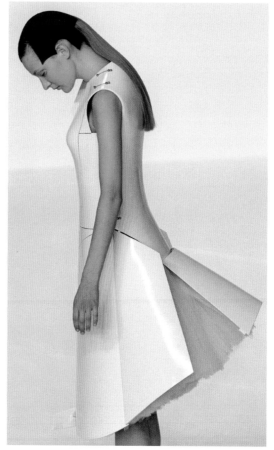

ABOVE Chalayan's work is often architectural, transformational and cross-platform, exploring breakthroughs in design, technology and multimedia, such as in his Along False Equator wooden bodice from autumn/winter 1994–5, the chair dress from Geotropics spring/summer 1999 and the airplane dress, first seen in Echoform 1999 and then developed in Before Minus Now, spring/ summer 2000, above.

OPPOSITE John Galliano's first haute couture collection for Christian Dior, spring/summer 1997, featured gowns worn with beaded Maasai neckpieces and exotic, exaggerated feathers. *The New York Times* ran the headline: 'Among Couture Debuts, Galliano's is the Stand Out'.

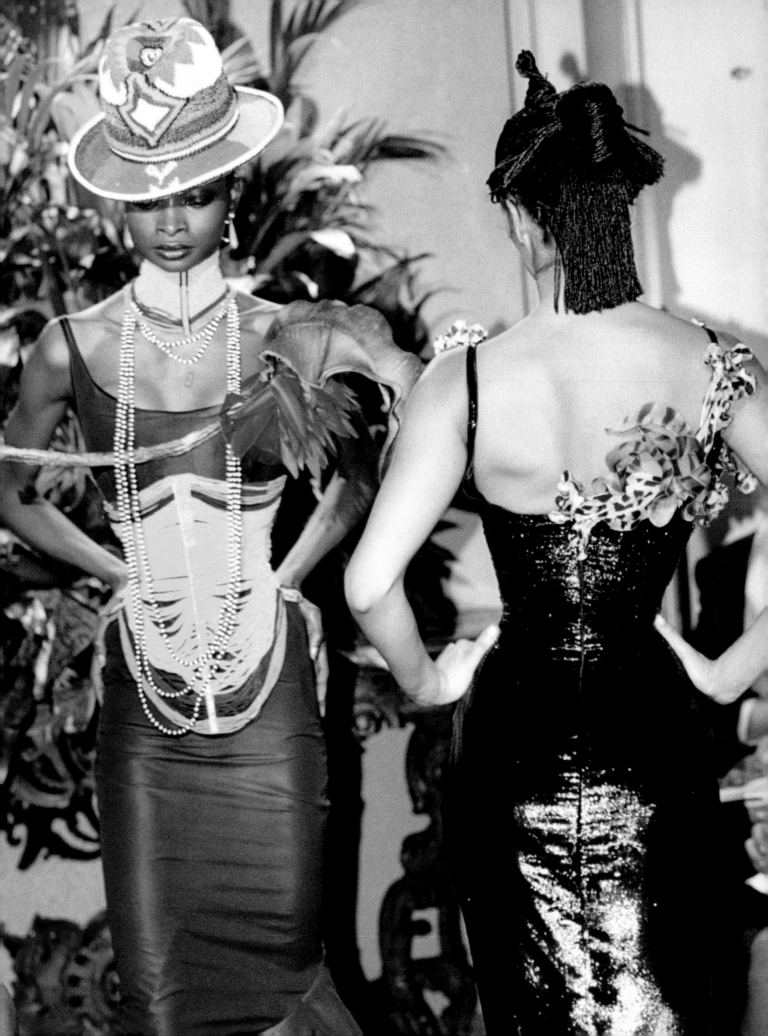

Back in London, Hussein Chalayan and Alexander McQueen were creating their own harder-edged versions of avant-garde fashion. Chalayan explored themes such as cultural identity, displacement and migration but the underlying focus was his obsession with new technology and meticulous pattern cutting.

Alexander McQueen's collections, like Galliano's, followed a narrative approach and while his shows were every bit as extravagant as his predecessor, they were undeniably darker and more savage in their mood. Graduating in 1992 with a collection entitled Jack the Ripper Stalks His Victims, the designer's fascination with history, and more specifically Victorian culture, was clear to see. Like Galliano, his creations stood in strong contrast to the casual, minimalist fashions that were the dominant mode of the time.

The first show after his graduation collection was inspired by the film *Taxi Driver*, and models were wrapped in cling film and made up to look bruised and battered, while his second show, Nihilism, featured blood- and dirt-splattered clothes and shredded Edwardian jackets. His real breakthrough came in 1995 with Highland Rape. The collection, which included bodices torn to reveal models' breasts, commemorated the slaughter of his Scottish ancestors by the English. The show was considered a triumph by fashion editors but was scandalized by the wider media as being a misogynistic display of brutalized femininity.

Not one to shy away from controversy, the following season, his Dante collection featured his legendary 'bumster' trousers. With most of the models' upper derrières on show, the garments were hailed as obscene. Soon, however, low-rise hipsters went mainstream as the look made its mark on the street.

In 1997, the *enfant terrible* of London fashion followed in Galliano's footsteps and replaced him at Givenchy. Here his creativity really took flight and his shows, which featured dramatic concepts such as robots spraying paint over Shalom Harlow in a white dress, were considered a must-see event. He was radical, a shock master and totally original. His respect for traditions of the past fused perfectly with a rebellious approach to fashion's future.

RIGHT Model Shalom Harlow has her dress spray-painted by robots during the Alexander McQueen show for the autumn/winter 1999-2000 collection entitled The Overlook.

BELOW Low-cut 'bumsters' at The Birds, Alexander McQueen's spring/summer 1995 show – well over a decade of low-slung trouser fashions followed.

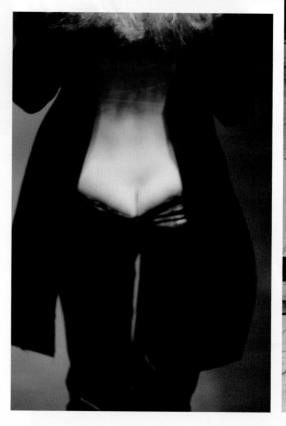

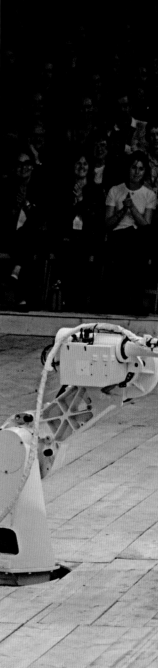

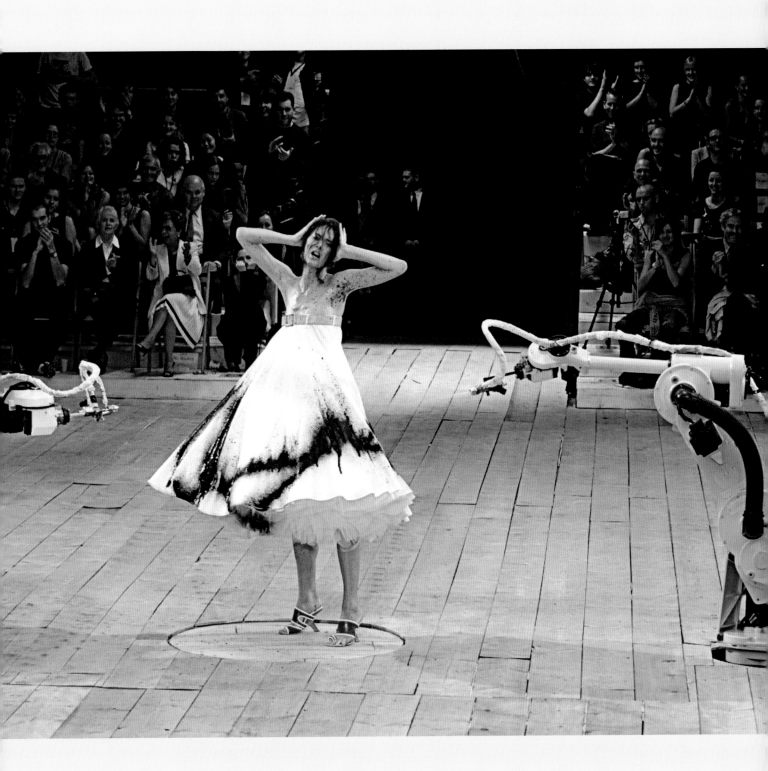

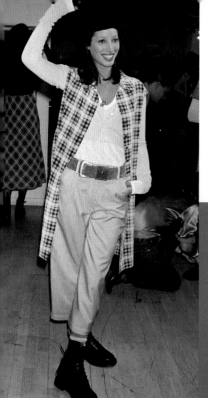

◀ Grunge
Originating from Seattle, bands such as Pearl Jam and Nirvana became poster models for the Grunge look: baggy ripped jeans, threadbare flannel shirts, bobbly cardigans, Converse trainers and Doctor Marten boots. The trend was quickly translated to the catwalks by designers such as Marc Jacobs and Anna Sui. This version is Marc Jacobs for Perry Ellis from 1993.

Utilitarian chic
First worn by the British and American military in the Second World War, the cargo surged onto the fashion scene in the mid 1990s and by 1998 Ralph Lauren was presenting silk versions on the catwalk. This utilitarian-chic trend was an example of the decades 'trickle-up' fashions – developing from streetwear to high fashion.

▼ Babydolls and slipdresses
Frilly chiffon babydoll dresses and delicate tiaras were often worn with thigh-high socks and Mary Jane shoes; the ironic look was popularized by the likes of Courtney Love, who in many ways was far from sweet and girly. The very short empire-line dresses were often accented with lace trim, oversized collars and embroidery. Kitschy-cute Anna Sui babydolls in 1993, below.

Key looks of the decade
1990s

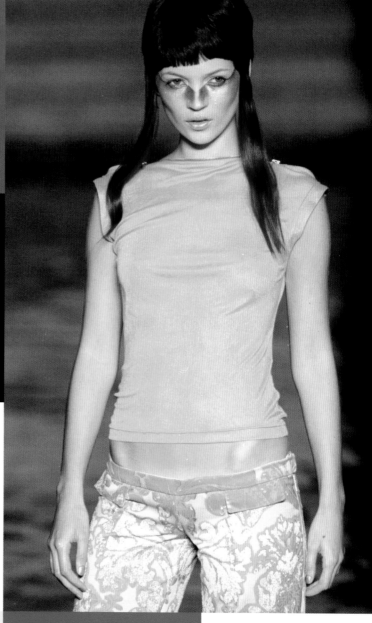

▼ Hip-hop
Hip-hop fashion went mainstream, with baseball jackets, bombers and tracksuits worn with oversized jeans and chunky trainers. Streetwear labels such as Phat Farm and Rocawear and sportswear brands such as Kangol and adidas were key to the original look, but hip-hop soon infiltrated classic preppy brands like Tommy Hilfiger and Polo Ralph Lauren.

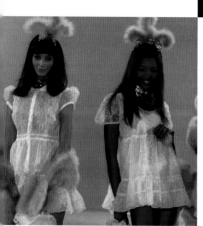

Cool Britannia
Bands such as Oasis, Blur and Suede popularized a number of British labels such as Pringle, Ben Sherman and Fred Perry while Jarvis Cocker's Geek Chic style was feted throughout the fashion industry. The look included aviator sunglasses, green parkas, harrington jackets, velvet suits, and polo shirts, as well as Union Jack motifs.

▲ Bumsters and bootcuts
Alexander McQueen's bumsters, which appeared in 1996 (worn by Kate Moss, above) were considered obscene when they first appeared but spawned the decade's trend for super low-slung jeans and trousers. Soon all jeans, including the decade's popular bootcut, were low-riding hipsters.

Preppy casual

the 1990s, East Coast preppy
shion came back into style
th designers like Ralph Lauren,
mmy Hilfiger, Marc Jacobs and
ella Bartley. Khaki chinos, navy
ue blazers, accordion-pleat
irts, mini-kilts, oxford shirts
d argyle and tartans were
me key looks that were widely
cumented in the 1995 fashion-
sessed film *Clueless*.

Deconstruction

Deconstruction brought
new techniques and ideas
to the fashion industry with
clothes being deliberately left
unfinished or made improperly.
Stitching would be exposed or
exaggerated, seams were left raw
and unfinished and zippers were
intentionally exposed. Martin
Margiela was a champion of
this trend.

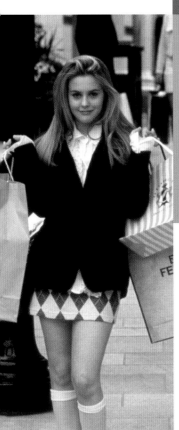

▼New Mod

Tom Ford was credited with
putting the glamour back
into fashion in the mid 1990s,
introducing Halston-style velvet
boot-cut hipster suits (1996,
below), skinny satin shirts and
car-finish metallic patent boots
and thus making Gucci a byword
for aspirational and hedonistic
fashion. Britpop bands Pulp, Blur,
Oasis and the Verve also rocked
the 1960s Mod look.

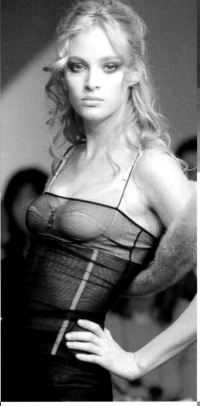

▲Neutral minimalism

After the flashy fashions of the
1980s there was an appetite
for a more restrained aesthetic.
Designers such as Prada
(1998, above), Jil Sander and
Calvin Klein channelled a more
streamlined look with simple
tailoring and a neutral colour
palette of black, white, beige and
brown. Plain white t-shirts and
Prada's black nylon tote bags
were given cult status.

oho chic

oral dresses or skirts worn
th combat boots and tights
ere some Grunge-crossover
daptations but pretty sprigged
rints were also more feminine
ersions. Flowing, floral minis or
axis, paired with crochet vests
d trainers, were adaptations of
e Boho look.

▲Underwear as outerwear

In the 1990s Dolce & Gabbana
(above) began putting lingerie
on the outside of the clothing, a
look spearheaded by Jean Paul
Gaultier's corset for Madonna's
Blonde Ambition tour in 1990,
but which then became part of
mainstream fashion. Sexy bra
tops, bustiers and corsets were all
paired with jeans and high heels
for a night out.

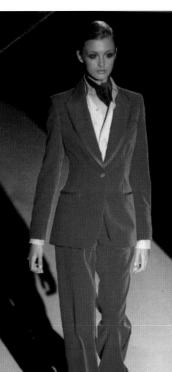
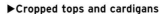

▶Cropped tops and cardigans

Initially an athletics-inspired
trend, midriff-exposing tops were
everyday casualwear during this
decade. Often worn with low-slung
cargoes or oversized jeans, the
tiny-on-the-top trend appeared on
celebrity and schoolgirl alike. In
keeping with the emphasis on the
mid-section, cardigans and shrugs
were undersized and shrunken.

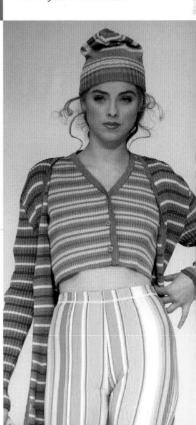

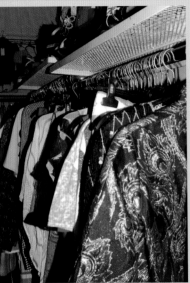
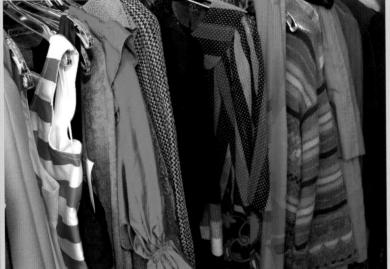
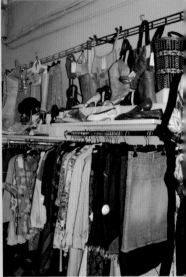

Shopping Guide *by Mark and Cleo Butterfield*

Most people who collect and wear designer fashions do so simply because of the sheer pleasure involved. The hunt for a good piece, the knowledge you gain in the process and the personal stories you hear along the way can be as compelling as finding and purchasing a highly desired, sought-after piece. Whether your aim is collecting a specific designer or within a particular time period, or finding a unique piece you know no one else will have or wear, there are a few ground rules and tips to keep in mind, which will help you locate the best pieces for you.

First of all, know what you are buying. There really is no substitute for the experience gained from seeing and handling vintage pieces.

Where to buy
Specialist vintage fashion fairs and markets are a great opportunity to meet a lot of dealers and see a huge variety of classic vintage clothing gathered together in one place. Specialist shops and viewings at major auction houses are also excellent places to see a high concentration of quality pieces. Here you can familiarize yourself with clothes from different periods and the work of specific designers.

Online auctions such as eBay can be full of pitfalls for the unwary. First, the seller is unlikely to be a

vintage dealer and may know very little about the garment they are auctioning. Without any deliberate attempt to mislead, items are quite frequently incorrectly assigned to periods or accredited to designers. Second, there's no way of seeing the item to check its condition. Always email the seller about stains, repairs, alterations, etc, and ask to see the label if it hasn't been shown.

Buying tips
❖ Never buy a stained garment with the hope that it will come out with washing or dry cleaning. If the mark's been there for a long time, it probably isn't going to shift. Get a full description of stains, such as rust, mildew or sweat, as well as any odours.

❖ Always check the item thoroughly for condition. Hold it up to the light to reveal any moth holes. Check both sides of the fabric for scorches, tears, mended areas, missing beadwork or embellishments and for disintegration of any type. Any professional seller will automatically point out tears or other signs of damage, but always ask.

❖ Focus on a particular time period or designer; you will gain deeper knowledge about a specialized subject and meet like-minded buyers and sellers who will further your experience and be able to give you

> *'Fashion is not something that exists in dresses only… fashion has to do with ideas, the way we live, what is happening.'*
> *Coco Chanel*

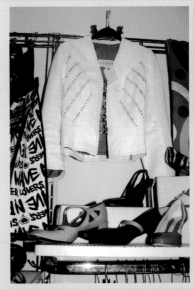 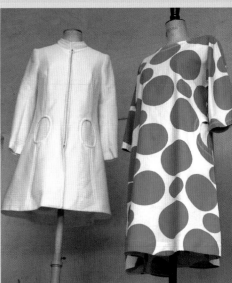

more information on the subject. This will also help you focus on your aim, rather than trying to pick from what you like of a century's worth of designs.

❖ If you are buying for a collection or investment, look for pieces that typify a designer's work and always buy the best pieces that you can afford.

❖ If you are buying for wearing the clothes, follow the sizing tips on page 210 so that you choose the era that best suits your body shape and inherent style; otherwise you may feel uncomfortable, or as if you are wearing a costume rather than a piece that makes you look and feel great.

❖ Couture dresses claim the highest prices, but the price also depends on the designer, age, workmanship, condition and size; if you are keen for a specific designer, for example, you may compromise on size or condition to own it. Likewise you may accept an unauthenticated piece if the detailing is remarkably rare or beautiful.

❖ Many sellers use standard descriptions to indicate the condition of the garment: **mint** is rare and perfect, probably never worn; **near mint** indicates light wear, as in evening dresses; **excellent** means it is sound with some wear but no flaws; **very good** indicates minor flaws or stains but otherwise high quality; **good** means that it is wearable but shows some deterioration.

Dating garments

Once you have some experience handling period garments, you will develop an intrinsic sense of the time period. A knowledge of the fabrics, haberdashery and stitching techniques typical of the time will also give you good indications of the era. Familiarize yourself with fabric and trimming terms from past eras, and learn the difference between them and when they were in common use. The glossary on pages 217-19 will help, as well as the further reading on page 223. Construction methods and the silhouette of the garment are also good indicators – for example, garments were much more fitted before 1960. The underlying structure of the piece will also offer clues on whether the piece is couture or ready-to-wear, in the case of missing labels, and the value and age of the piece.

If the designer or label is known, this may help you identify the date by the time period the designer was active. Many designers changed the style of their name or label over time, or were affiliated with various brands – see pages 214-16 for the glossary, which lists the labels designers worked under.

When attempting to date garments, here are a few additional guidelines to help you pinpoint the date.

❖ Washing care labels only came into popular use in the 1970s.

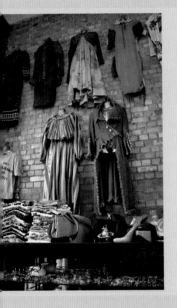

'The truly fashionable are beyond fashion.'
Cecil Beaton

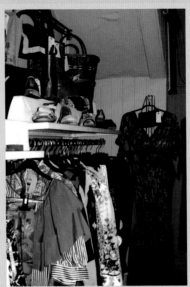

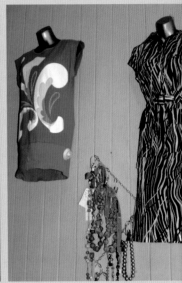

❖ Zips were in use in the 1920s for heavy-duty fastenings, boots, and so on, but are not common in dresses until the postwar period. You will find some 1930s dresses with zips, but these were stopped during wartime because of utility restrictions.

❖ Plastic zips were introduced in the 1930s, but constructed along the same lines as metal zips, with individual teeth.

❖ Zips usually appeared in sides seams up until the 1950s, and later appeared in the centre back of dresses and skirts and the centre front of trousers.

❖ Most pre-war clothes were dressmaker-made and won't have labels.

❖ Machine overlocking of seams became widespread in the 1960s, so this can help you tell a modern copy from an original.

Sizes

As most clothing up to the 1960s was home- or dressmaker-made, there will be no size labels in pieces before this period. Each piece was bespoke, made for a specific person's shape, so for that dress to fit you perfectly you also have to be that same size. Standardization of sizes only came in with mass production. A 1960s or 1970s size would be expected to be one or two sizes smaller than a modern one, but waist measurements were proportionately smaller, so make sure you can try it on, or get all the measurements.

Thanks to better nutrition and exercise habits, however, women today are taller and bigger than ever before, so there's no substitute for trying the item on. If this isn't possible, ask for the seller to provide exact measurements, not only including length, waist and bust measurements but also the hip, cuff, sleeve length, neck opening, from nape to waist, back shoulder to shoulder, waist to hem, shoulder to hem, the circumference of the hemline, and any potentially restrictive areas, like under the upper arm.

In general, 1920s fashions generally suit the small and slight of figure; 1950s clothes are created along the hourglass line so they fit the curvaceous, though waists are very small; 1960s fashions are best on the tall and leggy.

Couture items

Many couture pieces are works of art, highly hand-constructed or hand-embellished and made of the finest materials available at the time. Authenticating a couture item can be very difficult; often the lining of a garment would wear through and be cut away, and along with it the label. Additionally, the best pieces are those made to measure, as a great deal of labour and craftsmanship went into the pieces; the name of the individual client often appears on the dress label.

Because these items will never be created again, and the level of artistry involved can never be repeated

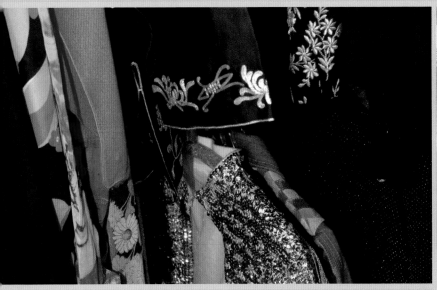

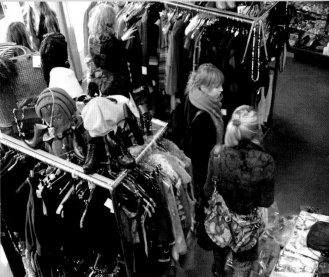

due to cost and expertise limitations, couture items are highly covetable. Pieces showing exquisite handworked beading or embroidery, unique hand-dyed colours, luxury fabrics or unique techniques, such as Fortuny pleating, are especially desirable. Keep these, and the below tips, in mind when looking for couture.

❖ Labels with the designers name, an ink number and the client's name.
❖ Stitching that is fine, neat and even.
❖ The garment is likely to have been well cared for, so should be in good condition.
❖ Careful sewing of buttons, buttonholes, hooks and other closures, and fabric-covered or concealed fasteners.
❖ Lining and interior structure that is as well-crafted as the exterior.

Care and storage

If you are ever in doubt about whether a piece should be washed, consult a professional conservator or ask a costume dealer for advice, especially if you suspect the piece may be rare or you are unsure of the fragility of its materials. Do not ever use a washing machine or dryer for vintage pieces, and think carefully about pressing any item as it can press stains into the fabric. Steaming is usually a good option for robust fabrics.

There is a risk that moth, carpet beetle or their eggs could be lurking in the fibres of your latest vintage purchase and they will happily destroy the rest of your wardrobe. Wrap the piece in acid-free tissue paper, place it in a sealed plastic bag and put it in the freezer for three days. Be gentle when removing it, especially with silk items, and allow it gradually to defrost. Here are a few general tips you can follow.

❖ Always clean any new item before storing. If the garment has a cleaning label that says it can be washed, it is always safer to hand wash. If it there is no label and you think that it ought to be washable (for example, if it's made of cotton), test an inconspicuous part first.
❖ Modern washing powders may be too harsh and cause colours to run, so use a pure soap powder such as Lux.
❖ Never wash a 1920s sequin dress, as the sequins are made of gelatine, and will dissolve in the water!
❖ Many older fabrics are not colour-fast and may discolour, shrink or distort, particularly any that are based on silk, acetate or rayon.
❖ Consider not only the fabric of the piece, but also any trims or linings.
❖ Dry cleaning is damaging to many fabrics, and may require the removal of labels or accessories, which will devalue the piece.
❖ Don't store anything in plastic. Natural fibres will hold moisture and once housed in the mini greenhouse of a plastic cover will release the water which may mark your garment. Wrap it in acid-free tissue and keep it in a cardboard box.

Collections & Stores

Museums & Collections

UNITED KINGDOM

Design Museum
Shad Thames
London SE1 2YD
Tel: 0870 833 9955
Email: info@designmuseum.org
Website: www.designmuseum.org
A showcase for all design genres,
including fashion.

The Fashion and Textile Museum
88 Bermondsey Street
London SE1 3XF
Tel: 020 7403 0222
Email: info@ftmlondon.org
Website: www.ftmlondon.org
Opened by Zandra Rhodes. Shows the
best of vintage and modern fashion
and textiles, with rotating exhibitions
featuring such designers as Vivienne
Westwood and Ossie Clark.

Gallery of Costume
Platt Hall, Rusholme
Manchester M14 5LL
Tel: 0161 224 5217
www.manchestergalleries.org
One of Britain's largest collections of clothing
and accessories, dating from the seventeenth
century to the present day.

Museum of Costume
Bennett Street
Bath BA1 2QH
Tel: 01225 477173
Email: costume_enquiries@bathnes.gov.uk
Website: http://www.museumofcostume.co.uk
Eveningwear from the 1900s to the 1950s,
as well as iconic 1960s and 1970s designs.
Annual exhibitions highlighting
a particular aspect of fashion.

Victoria and Albert Museum
Cromwell Road
London SW7 2RL
Tel: 020 7942 2000
Email: textilesandfashion@vam.ac.uk
Website: http://www.vam.ac.uk
Fashion and textile collection dating
from the seventeenth century to the
present day, with an emphasis on
influential European design. Also
showcases accessories such as gloves,
jewellery and handbags.

UNITED STATES

Cornell Costume and Textile Collection
Department of Textiles and Apparel
Cornell University
Ithaca, NY 14853-4401
Tel: 607 255 2235
Email: caj7@cornell.edu
Website (curator): www.human.cornell.edu
Website (online gallery):
costume.cornell.edu/greetingdb.htm
Cornell Costume and Textile Collection of
more than 9,000 items, a selection of which
are on public display during normal weekday
hours when the university is in session.
Online gallery also available.

The Costume Institute
The Metropolitan Museum of Art
1000 Fifth Avenue at 82nd Street
New York, NY 10028-0198
Tel: 212 535 7710
Email: thecostumeinstitute@metmuseum.org
Website: www.metmuseum.org
Vast collection of 80,000 costumes.

Hope B McCormick Costume Center
Clark Street at North Avenue
Chicago, IL 60614-6071
Tel: 312 642-4600
Webmail: www.chicagohs.org
A collection of 50,000 pieces, including
historical costumes and designer items by
such names as Charles Worth, Paul Poiret
and Issey Miyake.

The Kent State University Museum
PO Box 5190
Rockwell Hall
Kent, OH 44242-0001
Tel: 330 672 3450
Email: museum@kent.edu
Website: www.kent.edu/museum
A collection of mainly twentieth-century
garments, representing the work of most
major American and European designers,
including some of their archives and sketch-
books. Stages exhibitions from its collection.

Vintage Fashion Museum
212 N. Broadway
Abilene, KS 67410
Tel: 785 263 7997
Email: fashion@ikansas.com
Website: www.abilenekansas.org
Fashions from the 1870s to the 1970s.

CANADA

Costume Museum of Canada
Box 38
Dugald, Manitoba
Tel: 204 8532166
Freephone: 1866 853 2166
Email: info@costumemuseum.com
Website: costumemuseum.com
Intended as a national repository for
costume, textiles and accessories, the
collection includes designs by Chanel,
Norman Hartnell, Worth, Schiaparelli,
Vionnet, Scassi and Paco Rabanne.

AUSTRALIA

Powerhouse Museum
500 Harris Street Ultimo
PO Box K346
Haymarket, Sydney
New South Wales 1238
Tel: 61 2 9217 0111
Website: www.powerhousemuseum.com
Occasional exhibitions of contemporary
and vintage fashion and style icons, such
as Audrey Hepburn.

Stores and Boutiques

UNITED KINGDOM

Appleby
95 Westbourne Park Villas
London W2 5ED
Tel: 020 7229 7772
Email: jane@applebyvintage.com
Website: www.applebyvintage.com
Friendly and accommodating vintage
boutique run by Jane Appleby.

Blackout II
51 Endell Street
London WC2 9HJ
Tel: 020 7240 5006
Email: clothes@blackout2.com
Website: www.blackout2.com
Specializes in clothing from the 1930s
and 1940s.

Cenci
4 Nettlefold Place
London SE27 0JW
Tel: 020 8766 8564
Email: info@cenci.co.uk
Website: www.cenci.co.uk
Vintage fashion and accessories from
the 1930s onwards.

C20 Vintage Fashion
Email: enquiries@c20vintagefashion.co.uk
Website: www.c20vintagefashion.co.uk
Cleo and Mark Butterfield's inspirational
vintage garments are available for hire.

Decades
17–18 Dover Street
London W1S 4LT
Tel: 020 7518 0680
Email: info@decadesinc.com
Website: www.decadesinc.com

One of a Kind
253 Portobello Road
London W11 1LR
Tel: 020 7792 5284

Palette London
21 Canonbury Lane
London N1 2AS
Eclectic selection of vintage clothing.
Also a finder service.

Pop Boutique
6 Monmouth Street
London WC2H 9HB
Tel: 020 7497 5262
Email: info@pop-boutique.com
Website: www.madaboutpop.com
1960s, 1970s and 1980s originals as well
as its own retro Pop label.

Rellik
8 Golborne Road
London W10 5NW
Tel: 020 8962 0089
Website: www.relliklondon.co.uk
Clothing and accessories from the
1920s to mid-1980s.

Rokit
42 Shelton Street
Covent Garden
London WC2H 9HZ
Tel: 020 7836 6547
Website: www.rokit.co.uk

Steinberg & Tolkien
193 King's Road
London SW3 5ED
Tel: 020 7376 3660
Well-established shop owned by
Tracy Tolkien selling vintage clothing,
accessories and jewellery.

The Vintage Clothing Company
Afflecks Palace
Oldham Street
Manchester M4 1PW
Tel: 0161 832 0548
Website: www.vintageclothingcompany.com
Part of a chain of five retail outlets.

Virginia
98 Portland Road
London W11 4LQ
Tel: 020 7727 9908
Exquisite antique clothing.

UNITED STATES
Decades
8214 ¹/₂ Melrose Avenue
Los Angeles CA 90046
Tel: 323 655 0223
Website: www.decadesinc.com
Fabulous collection by Cameron Silver, who
has now opened his second shop in London.

Keni Valenti Retro-Couture
155 West 29th Street
Third floor, Room C5
New York, NY 10001
Tel: 212 967 7147
Website: www.kenivalenti.com

The Paper Bag Princess
8818 Olympic Boulevard
Beverly Hills CA 90211
Tel: 310 385 9036
Website: www.thepaperbagprincess.com

William Doyle Galleries
175 East 87th Street
New York, NY 10128
Tel: 212 427 2730
Email: info@DoyleNewYork.com
Website: www.doylegalleries.com
Auctioneers and appraisers of
haute couture and antique costume.

CANADA
Deluxe Junk Company
310 W Cordova Street
Vancouver, British Columbia V6B 1E8
Tel: 604 685-4871
Email: dlxjunk@telus.net
Website: www.deluxejunk.com
Vancouver's oldest vintage clothing store.
Great selection of vintage and contemporary
clothing, accessories and costume jewellery.

MaryAnn Harris
Ottawa Antique Market
1179 Bank Street
Ottawa, Ontario
Tel: 613 720 9242

AUSTRALIA
Vintage Clothing Shop
147–49 Castlereagh Street
Shop 5, CBD
Sydney 2000

Organizations
Vintage Fashion Guild
www.vintagefashionguild.org
An online resource set up by a collective
of vintage sellers. Offers information, news
and a virtual museum, plus guidance for
vintage vendors.

Costume Society
www.costumesociety.org.uk
The society includes collectors, curators,
designers, lecturers, students and informed
enthusiasts with the aim to explore all
aspects of clothing history.

Costume Society America
www.costumesocietyamerica.com
Dedicated to the history and conservation of
dress adornment and to interpreting culture
through appearance.

Online stores
www.antiquedress.com
www.antique-fashion.com
www.shockadelic.com
www.thefrock.com
www.tias.com/stores/decades
www.unique-vintage.com
www.vintageblues.com
www.vintagemartini.com
www.vintagetextile.com
www.vintagetrends.com
www.vintagevixen.com

Fashion websites
www.costumegallery.com
www.costumes.org
www.fabrics.net
www.fashionencyclopedia.com
www.fashion-era.com
www.pastpatterns.com
www.vpll.org

Glossary of Designers

Adolfo (1933-): Bergdorf Goodman; Emme; Adolfo

Adrian, Gilbert (1903-59): Paramount; Adrian Limited

Agnès, Madame (1910-40): Madame Agnès millinery

Alaïa, Azzedine (1940-): Christian Dior; Guy Laroche;
  Azzedine Alaïa

Amies, Sir Hardy (1909-2003): Lachasse; Hardy Amies

Armani, Giorgio (1934-): Nino Cerruti; Giorgio Armani

Ashley, Laura (1925-85): Laura Ashley

Augustabernard: founded by Augusta Bernard in 1919

Bakst, Léon (1866-1924): Ballets Russes

Balenciaga, Cristobal (1895-1972): Balenciaga couture house

Balmain, Pierre (1914-82): Robert Piguet; Edward Molyneux;
  Lucien Lelong; Balmain

Banton, Travis (1894-1958): Lucile Duff Gordon; Paramount;
  Twentieth-Century Fox; Universal Studios

Bates, John (1935-): Herbert Sidon; Jean Varon; John Bates

Beene, Geoffrey (1927-): Teal Traina; Geoffrey Beene Inc.,
  Beenebag

Berardi, Antonio (1968-): Antonio Berardi

Biagiotti, Laura (1943-): Roberto Cappuci, Laura Biagiotti

Biba: Founded by Barbara Hulanicki (1936-) in 1964

Bikkembergs, Dirk (1962-): Freelance designer for Nero, Bassetti,
  Gruno and Chardin, Tiktiner, Gaffa, K, and Jaco Petti;
  Dirk Bikkembergs

Birtwell, Celia (1941-): Ossie Clark and others;
  Celia Birtwell, London

Blass, Bill (1922-2002): Anna Miller and Company; Maurice Retner;
  Bill Blass Limited

Bodymap: Founded by David Holah and Stevie Stewart in 1982

Bohan, Marc (1926-): Jean Patou; Robert Piguet;
  Edward Molyneux; Patou; Christian Dior; Hartnell

Boué Souers, House of: Founded by Jeanne Boué in 1899

Bruce, Liza (1955-): Liza Bruce

Burrows, Stephen (1943-): Stephen Burrows' World

Byblos: Founded in 1973

Cacharel, Jean (1932-): Jean Jourdan; Société Jean Cacharel

Callot Soeurs, House of: Founded by sisters Gerber, Bertrand and
  Chanterelle in 1895

Capucci, Roberto (1929-): Emilio Schuberth; Roberto Capucci

Cardin, Pierre (1922-): Madam Paquin; Elsa Schiaparelli; Christian
  Dior; Pierre Cardin

Carnegie, Hattie (1889-1956): Macy's; Hattie Carnegie Originals;
  Hattie Carnegie

Cashin, Bonnie (1915-2000): Adler and Adler;
  Twentieth-Century Fox; Bonnie Cashin Designs

Cassini, Oleg (1913-): Jean Patou; Edith Head; Oleg Cassini;
  Jacqueline Kennedy

Castelbajac Jean-Charles de (1949-): André Courrèges;
  Jean-Charles do Castelbajac

Cavanagh, John (1914-): Edward Molyneux; Pierre Balmain;
  John Cavanagh

Céline: Founded in 1973

Cerruti, Nino (1930-): Nino Cerruti

Chalayan, Hussein (1970-): Cartesia Ltd; Hussein Chalayan

Chanel, Gabrielle 'Coco' (1883-1971): House of Chanel

Chéruit, Madeleine: Founded by Madeleine Chéruit in 1900

Chloé: Founded by Gaby Aghion and Jacques Lanoir in 1952

Clark, Ossie (1942-96): Quorum; Radley; Evocative

Clergerie, Robert (1934-): Charles Jourdan;
  Clerma Company; J Fenestrier

Colonna, Jean (1955-): Balmain; Jean Colonna

Comme des Garçons: founded by Rei Kawakubo (1942-) in 1973

Connolly, Sybil (1921-98): Bradleys; Richard Alan;
  Sybil Connolly Inc.; Tiffany's

Courrèges, André (1923-): Jeanne Laufrie; Cristobal Balenciaga;
  André Courrèges

Crahay, Jules François (1917-88): Nina Ricci; Jeanne Lanvin

Creed, Charles Southey (1909-66): Linton Tweeds; Bergdorf Goodman;
  Charles Creed

Daché, Lilly (1907-89): Reboux; Macy's; The Bonnet Shop;
  Travis Banton

De la Renta, Oscar (1932-): Cristobal Balenciaga; Lanvin;
  Oscar de la Renta

De Lisi, Ben (1955-): Saks; Penelope; Benedetto; Ben de Lisi

De Prémonville, Myrène (1949-): Myrène de Prémonville

Delaunay, Sonia (1885-1979): abstract painter and designer.

Demeulemeester, Ann (1959-): Ann Demeulemeester

Dessès, Jean (1904-70): Jean Dessès; Jean Dessès American Collection

Dior, Christian (1905-57): Robert Piguet; Lelong; Maison Dior;
  House of Christian Dior

Doeuillet, House of: Founded by Georges Doeuillet in 1900

Dolce & Gabbana: Founded by Dominco Dolce and
  Stefano Gabbana in 1985

Doucet, Jacques (1853-1929): Maison Doucet

Duff Gordon, Lucille (1862-1935): Lucile couture house

Edelstein, Victor (1947-): Alexon; Biba; Christian Dior; Victor Edelstein

Elbaz, Alber (1961-): Geoffrey Beene; Guy Laroche; YSL Rive Gauche

Ellis, Perry (1940-86): Miller & Rhoads; Perry Ellis International

Emanuel, David (1952-) and Elizabeth (1953-): Emanuel

Erté (Romaine de Tirtoff 1892-1990): Costume designs
  for ballet and theatre

Estrada, Angel (1957-89): Estrada

Ettedgui, Joseph (1936-): Chain of shops including Joseph,
  Joseph Tricot, Joseph Pour La Maison

Fath, Jacques (1912-54): Jacques Fath couture house

Fendi: Founded by Adele Casagrande in 1918

Féraud, Louis (1921-99): Louis Féraud

Ferragamo, Salvatore (1898-1960): Bonito;
Salvatore Ferragamo

Ferre, Gianfranco (1944-): Gianfranco Ferre Donna;
Christian Dior; Gianfranco Ferre

Ferretti, Alberta (1950-): Aeffe

Fiorucci, Elio: Founded by Elio Fiorucci in 1962

Flett, John (1963-91): Lanvin; Enrico Coveri

Foale & Tuffin: Founded by Marion Foale and
Sally Tuffin in 1961

Ford, Tom (1962-): Cathy Harwick; Perry Ellis; Gucci;
YSL Rive Gauche

Fortuny, Mariano (1871-1949): Fortuny couture house

Fox, Frederick (1931-): Otto Lucas; Mitzi Lorenz; Langée;
Frederick Fox

Fratini, Gina (1934-): Katherine Dunham dance group;
Hartnell; Gina Fratini

Galanos, James (1924-): Hattie Carnegie; Piguet; Davidow;
Galanos Originals

Galliano, John (1960-) John Galliano; Givenchy; Christian Dior

Gaultier, Jean Paul (1952-): Pierre Cardin; Esterel; Jean Patou;
Jean Paul Gaultier SA

Gernreich, Rudi (1922-85): Lester Horton Dance Company;
William Bass; GR Designs; Rudi Gernreich Inc.

Gibb, Bill (1943-88): Baccarat; Bill Gibb Fashion Group

Gigli, Romeo (1949-): Dimitri Couture; Romeo Gigli

Givenchy, Hubert de (1927-): Jaques Fath; Robert Piguet;
Lucien Lelong; Elsa Schiaparelli; Maison Givenchy

Godley, Georgina (1955-): Crolla; Georgina Godley Ltd

Greer, Howard (1896-1974): Paul Poiret; Edward Molyneux;
Paramount; Howard Greer

Grès, Madame (1903-93): Premet; Alix

Griffe, Jacques (1917-): Vionnet; Edward Molyneux,
Jacques Griffe

Gucci, Guccio (1881-1953): Gucci

Halston, Roy Frowick (1932-90): Lilly Daché; Bergdorf Goodman;
Halston Ltd

Hamnett, Katharine (1948-): Tuttabanken Sportswear;
Katharine Hamnett Ltd

Hartnell, Sir Norman (1901-79): Madame Desirée;
Norman Hartnell

Head, Edith (1907-81): Paramount Studios; Universal Studios

Heim, Jacques (1899-1967): Jacques Heim

Hermès: Founded by Thierry Hermès in 1837

Howell, Margaret (1946-): Margaret Howell

Jackson, Betty (1949-): Quorum Design Studio; Betty Jackson

Jacobs, Marc (1964-): Ruben Thomas Inc.; Perry Ellis;
Marc Jacobs; Louis Vuitton

James, Charles (1906-78): E Haweis James; Charles James

Johnson, Betsey (1942-): Paraphernalia Boutiques; Betsey, Bunky
& Nini; Alvin Duskin Co.; Alley Cat; Betsey Johnson; BJ Vines

Jones, Stephen (1957-): Fiorucci; Stephen Jones

Kamali, Norma (1945-): Kamili; OMO Norma Kamali boutiques

Karan, Donna (1948-): Anne Klein; Donna Karan; DKNY

Kelly, Patrick (1954-90): Le Palais club; Patrick Kelly, Paris

Kenzo (1939-): Freelance designer to Féraud; Rodier; Pisanti;
Jungle Jap; Kenzo

Keogh, Lainey (1957-): Lainey Keogh

Kerrigan, Daryl (1964-): Daryl Kerrigan

Khanh, Emmanuelle (1937-): Cacharel; Dorothée Bis;
Emmanuelle Khanh

Klein, Anne (1923-74): Varden Petites; Anne Klein

Klein, Calvin (1942-): Dan Millstein; Calvin Klein Co.

Kors, Michael (1959-): Michael Kors; Céline

Krizia: founded by Mariuccia Mandelli in 1954

Lachasse, House of: Founded in 1928

Lacroix, Christian (1951-): Hermès; Guy Paulin; Jean Patou;
Christian Lacroix

Lagerfeld, Karl (1938-): Balmain; Patou; Chloé; Krizia; Chanel

Lang, Helmut (1956-): Helmut Lang

Lanvin, Jeanne (1867-1946): Jeanne Lanvin couture house

Lapidus, Ted (1929-): Ted Lapidus

Laroche, Guy (1923-89): Jean Dessès; Guy Laroche couture house

Lauren, Ralph (1939-): Polo Fashions; Polo Ralph Lauren

Léger, Hervé (1957-): Fendi; Chanel; Lanvin; Chloé;
Charles Jourdan; Hervé Léger

Lelong, Lucien (1889-1958): House of Lelong

Lesage: Founded by Albert Lesage in 1868

Lester, Charles & Patricia: Founded by Charles and Patricia
Lester in 1964

Liberty: Founded by Arthur Lasenby in 1875

Loewe: Founded by Enrique Loewe in 1846

Louiseboulanger: Founded by Louise Boulanger in 1927

Lucas, Otto (1903-71): Otto Lucas

McCardell, Claire (1905-58): Emmet Joyce; Robert Turk;
Townley Frocks; Hattie Carnegie

McFadden, Mary (1938-): Mary McFadden

Mackie, Bob (1940-): Cole of California, Bob Mackie Originals

Mainbocher (1890-1976): Mainbocher couture house

Margiela, Martin (1957-): Jean Paul Gaultier; Martin Margiela

Matsuda, Mitsuhiro (1934-): Nicole Limited; Matsuda

Maxmara: Founded by Achille Maramotti in 1951;
encompasses 16 labels

Missoni: Founded by Ottavio and Rosita Missoni in 1953

Miyake, Issey (1938-): Laroche; Givenchy; Geoffrey Beene;
Issey Miyake

Mizrahi, Isaac (1961-): Perry Ellis; Calvin Klein; Isaac Mizrahi

Model, Philippe (1956-): shoes and accessories –
worked with Gaultier, Claude Montana, Issey Miyake
and Thierry Mugler

Molinari, Anna (1948): Blumarine

Molyneux, Captain Edward (1891-1974): Lucile; Molyneux

Montana, Claude (1949-): Idéal-Cuir; MacDougal Leathers;
Lanvin

Morton, Digby (1906-83): Digby Morton

Moschino, Franco (1950-94): Gianni Versace; Cadette;
Moschino

Mugler, Thierry (1948-): Gudule boutique; André Peters;
Thierry Mugler

Muir, Jean (1928-95): Jacqmar; Jaeger; Courtaulds;
Jane & Jane; Jean Muir Ltd

Norell, Norman (1900-72): Brooks Costume Company;
Charles Amour; Hattie Carnegie; Triana-Norell

Nutter, Tommy (1943-92): Donaldson, Williams & Ward;
Tommy Nutter; Austin Reed

Oldfield, Bruce (1950-): Bruce Oldfield Ltd

Oldham, Todd (1961-): L-7; Todd Oldham

Orry-Kelly, John (1898-1964): costume design for Warner
Brothers; Twentieth-Century Fox; Universal Studios; MGM

Ozbek, Rifat (1953-): Trell; Monsoon; Ozbek; Future Ozbek

Paquin: Founded by Jeanne Beckers and Isidore Jacobs in 1891

Patou, Jean (1880-1936): Jean Patou

Pertegaz, Manuel (1918-): Manuel Pertegaz

Piguet, Robert (1901-53): Paul Poiret; John Redfern;
Robert Piguet

Plunkett, Walter (1902-82): RKO; MGM

Poiret, Paul (1879-1947): Charles Worth; Jacques Doucet;
Paul Poiret

Porter, Thea (1927-2000): Thea Porter

Prada: Founded by Mario Prada in 1913

Price, Anthony (1945-): Stirling Cooper; Plaza; Antony Price

Pucci, Marchese Emilio (1914-92): Lord & Taylor; Pucci

Quant, Mary (1934-): Bazaar; Mary Quant Ginger Group

Rabanne, Paco (1934-): Givenchy; Dior; Balenciaga;
Paco Rabanne

Reboux, Caroline (1830-1927): Vionnet; Caroline Reboux

Redfern: Founded by John Redfern in 1881

Rhodes, Zandra (1940-): Zandra Rhodes Ltd

Ricci, Nina (1883-1970): Nina Ricci couture house

Rocha, John (1953-): John Rocha

Rodriquez, Narciso (1961-): Calvin Klein; Cerruti; Loewe

Rouff, Maggy (1896-1971): Drécoll; Maggy Rouff

Rykiel, Sonia (1930-): Laura Boutique; Sonia Rykiel

Saint Laurent, Yves (1936-): Christian Dior; Yves Saint Laurent;
YSL Rive Gauche

Sander, Jil (1943-): Jil Sander

Sant'Angelo, Giorgio di (1936-89): Sant'Angelo

Sassoon, Bellville: Founded by Belinda Bellville and David Sassoon in 1958

Scaasi, Arnold (1931-): Jeanne Paquin; Lilly Daché; Charles James; Arnold Scaasi

Scherrer, Jean-Louis (1936-): Christian Dior; Yves Saint Laurent;
Louis Féraud; Jean-Louis Scherrer

Schiaparelli, Elsa (1890-1973): House of Schiaparelli – worked
with Salvador Dalí, Christian Bérard and Jean Cocteau

Schön, Mila (1919-): Mila Schön

Sharaff, Irene (1910-93): Aline Bernstein; MGM

Sitbon, Martine (1951-): Chloé; Martine Sitbon

Sprouse, Stephen (1953-): Halston; Bill Blass; Stephen Sprouse

Stiebel, Victor (1907-76): Reville; Rossiter; Victor Stiebel; Jacqmar

Sui, Anna (1955-): Simultanee; Anna Sui

Tarlazzi, Angelo (1942-): Carosa; Patou; Angelo Tarlazzi; Guy Laroche

Thomass, Chantal (1947-): Dorothée Bis; Chantal Thomass

Trigère, Pauline (1912-2002): Hattie Carnegie; Pauline Trigère

Tyler, Richard (1946-): Anne Klein; Byblos; Richard Tyler Couture;
Richard Tyler Collection

Ungaro, Emanuel (1933-): Cristobal Balanciaga; André Courrèges;
Emanuel Ungaro couture house

Valentino (1932-): Jean Dessès; Guy Laroche; Valentino

Vanderbilt, Gloria (1924-): Gloria Vanderbilt

Van Noten, Dries (1958-): Dries Van Noten

Versace, Gianni (1946-97): Callaghan; Genny; Complice; Gianni Versace

Vionnet, Madeleine (1876-1975): House of Vincent; Kate Reilly;
Callot Soeurs; Jacques Doucet; House of Vionnet

Vittadini, Adrienne (1944-): Louis Féraud; Sport Tempo; Warnaco;
Kimberly Knits; Adrienne Vittadini

Von Furstenberg, Diane (1946-): Diane Von Furstenberg Studio;
Diane Von Furstenberg couture house

Walker, Catherine (1945-): Chelsea Design Company

Watanabe, Junya (1961-): Rei Kawakubo

Westwood, Vivienne (1941-): Vivienne Westwood

Workers for Freedom: Founded by Richard Nott and
Graham Fraser in 1985

Worth, Charles Frederick (1825-95): House of Worth

Yamamoto, Kansai (1944-): Junko Koshino; Hisashi Hosono;
Yamamoto Kansai Company Ltd

Yamamoto, Yohji (1943-): Yohji Yamamoto

Yuki (1937-): Louis Féraud; Michael Donellan; Norman Hartnell;
Pierre Cardin; Yuki

Zoran (1947-): Zoran

Glossary of Fashion Terms

Acetate: based on cellulose, this chemical fibre was first manufactured in 1864 and has been in mass production since 1920.

Ajouré: collective description of fine openwork, embroidered fabric.

A-line: created by Christian Dior, A-line describes a dress shaped in outline like the letter A. From narrow shoulders and a low waist, it flares out to a wide skirt.

American shoulder: an armhole obliquely cut to reveal the shoulder.

Argyll (also Argyle): often seen on woollen socks and sweaters, this diamond pattern was named after an area of western Scotland.

Armani sleeves: turned-up sleeves created from two different fabrics.

Baker's check: similar in pattern to gingham, but twice the size.

Ballerina length: hem length of a dress or skirt that falls just above the ankles.

Balloon skirt: wide skirt hemmed to curve inward at the knees. Fashionable in cocktail dresses until 1958; enjoyed a revival in the late 1980s and again as part of the late 1990s retro look.

Balloon sleeve: created in 1890, this very full sleeve is held in place by a cuff at the wrist. Later revived by Nina Ricci.

Bateâu sleeve: also known as a boat neck, this is a collarless, boat-shaped neckline that runs from shoulder to shoulder.

Batwing sleeve: set deep and wide in the armhole, this sleeve tapers toward a tight wrist.

Besom pocket: a pocket sewn inside the garment with a slit welt opening.

Bias cut: a technique of cutting across the grain of the fabric, introduced in the 1920s by Madeleine Vionnet.

Blouson: popular in the 1950s, a hip-length sports jacket with a drawstring around the base, which gathers at the hips.

Body stocking: close-fitting, one-piece garment of elastic material and covering the whole body.

Bolero: open, waist-length jacket adopted from Spanish national costume.

Bomber jacket: military-style, blouson jacket, usually made of nylon.

Bord-à-bord jacket: women's jacket in which the front edges abut rather than cross. Held together with toggles or frogs, etc.

Boule shape: similar to Paul Poiret's hobble skirt, this is a skirt that is full below the waist, becoming tighter at the hem.

Box skirt: a straight skirt with a waistband and two thick, often quilted monk's seams running along the front and back.

Bustier: corset-like, strapless top of variable length above the waist. First worn as an undergarment, corsets are now worn as outerwear.

Bustle: pad or hoops used as a base over which the rear of a skirt is draped to emphasize the derrière. First in fashion around 1785, it was later adapted by Christian Dior and more recently by Vivienne Westwood.

Camel hair: soft, short undercoat of the camel from which a soft, woollen fabric is made.

Capri pants: narrow, three-quarter length ladies' trousers with a small slit at the side of the hem. Created by Emilio Pucci in the 1950s, Capri pants were inspired by trousers worn by Italian fishermen.

Casaque: fashionable in the 1920s, 1930s and 1950s, this hip-length blouse is worn over a skirtor as a pinafore over trousers around 1965-70.

Cascade neckline: this neckline consists of narrow straps and a cascade of fabric at the front.

Cashmere: the hair of the Kashmir goat is used to make a soft, light wool.

Cauterization: acid is applied to a blended fabric to destroy part of one of the types of fibre and creates a pattern – for example, devoré velvet.

Chalk stripes: pale stripes set on a dark background but less defined and spaced wider apart than pin stripes.

Chantilly lace: fine black bobbin lace, often with Baroque or Rococo style motifs or swags of flowers.

Chasuble pleat: a pleat covering the top seams of sleeves, it broadens the appearance of the shoulders.

Chauffe-coeur: sleeve vest created from warm fabric with a low-cut, round neck. Barely waist-length, it was adapted from ballet clothes.

Chenille: cut in the warp of a fabric, the fibres of this yarn stand proud and produce a similar effect to velvet. Chenille yarn is used to make corduroy and velour; also towelling and carpets.

Chiffon: translucent, light fabric with an uneven surface and made from synthetic fibres or natural silk.

Circular skirt: based on a circular or semicircular cut, this skirt is narrow at the hips and frequently supported by godets.

Cocktail dress: a short dress, often with a low neckline. Suitable for a variety of occasions when worn with a bolero or short jacket, this dress dates back to the 1940s.

Colour blocking: contrasting expanses of colour on fabric give clothes a graphic quality, as in Courrèges designs.

Corsair pants: narrow trousers cut slightly wider than Capri pants with slits below the knees.

Cossack pants: ankle- or calf-length trousers, baggy with a wide waist held by a belt.

Cowl neck: this wide piece of fabric tubing is attached to the neck of a garment.

Crepe: heat and a crèpe weave give this fabric its wrinkled surface.

Crepe de chine: made from natural or synthetic silk, this is a delicate, sheer and crinkled fabric.

Crinoline: originally made of horsehair and later steel hoops, this rigid petticoat gave width to skirts. Reappeared in Vivienne Westwood's mini crinis in 1980s.

Cup collar: open at the front, this stand-up collar is set at the back so the fabric falls in cup-like arches.

Cutouts: can area cut out of dresses, trousers and tops.

Diana décolleté: first seen in the second half of the nineteenth century, this asymmetric neckline featured one bare shoulder. In the 1930s it was adopted by Elsa Schiaparelli and then later on by Madam Grès in the 1950s. It regained popularity in the late 1970s.

Dior vent or Dior pleat: a short vent created for Christian Dior's 1948 tight pencil skirt.

Dirndl: this full skirt is gathered into the waistband.

Dolman sleeve: cut as an extension of the bodice, this sleeve was probably copied from the Turkish dolman. Emanuel Ungaro created an angular version, known as the Ungaro dolman, in 1968.

Empire line: dresses and coats are gathered beneath the bust and fall loosely to the feet. This style frequently comes back in fashion.

Encrustment: fabric pieces, such as leather, lace or trimmings, inserted into another yet distinct from appliqué.

Epaulet: originally designed to prevent slippage of shoulder-slung rifles and later a symbol of rank, this shoulderpiece gives a military touch to clothes. It first appeared in 1930s female fashions.

Flapper dress: fashionable in the 1920s, this dress featured narrow shoulder straps and a low waist, often tied with a scarf or belt.

Folkloric: dress style that assimilates elements of national costumes from around the world.

French cuffs: double cuffs.

French pocket: a pocket set in the side seams of a skirt or trousers.

Garçonne: severe, masculine style of dress of the 1920s.

Gaucho pants: wide-bottomed, calf-length trousers based on those worn by South American cowboys (gauchos); fashionable in the early 1970s.

Georgette crepe: translucent crêpe fabric

Gigot or leg-of-mutton sleeve: tight-fitting from cuffed wrist to elbow, this sleeve puffs up from elbow to shoulder.

Godet: sewn into a skirt, this triangular piece of fabric is designed to produce fullness.

Greatcoat reverse: named after the lapel on the greatcoat, which is produced by undoing the top button, this is a wide lapel.

Halterneck: top or dress with straps tied at the nape of the neck to leave the back and shoulders exposed.

Herringbone: produced by a broken twill weave and often emphasized with yarns in a variety of colours, this diagonally lined pattern resembles the skeleton of a herring.

H-line: launched by Christian Dior in 1954-55, this slightly tailored line has a slender top and narrow hips.

Hobble skirt: created by Paul Poiret in 1910, this ankle-length skirt is cut and draped to narrow beneath the knee, allowing only small steps to be taken.

Houndstooth: traditional small check pattern of two colours, often black and white. Due to the pattern linking individual checks, it is distinguishable from pepita (*see below*).

I-line: a narrow line silhouette created by Cristobal Balenciaga in 1954-55.

Jabot: used to cover buttons on dresses or blouses, this decorative frill became popular with women from the late nineteenth century until the late 1950s, and then became fashionable once more in a modified form in 1980.

Jersey: a generic term for different types of knitwear, jersey is a fabric that feels soft to the touch and is pliable without losing its shape; first introduced in haute couture by Coco Chanel in 1916-17.

Jodhpurs: riding breeches that are narrow on the calves and very full from hip to knee. Since the 1970s they have enjoyed various revivals.

Jumpsuit: one-piece trouser-suit usually made of an elastic material such as jersey and with short legs. Introduced in 1969.

Kaftan: loosely cut, straight and buttoned dress.

Kangaroo pocket: often seen on the front of cagoules, this is a large patch pocket.

Kimono sleeve: like the Japanese kimono, this is a straight sleeve that is secured at right angles to a garment.

Knickerbockers: loose, full breeches gathered beneath the knee, but more narrow than plus fours; revived in the 1960s.

Lamé: fabric that is interwoven with metallic threads.

Leggings: footless leg covering created from elastic material in the 1980s.

Liberty: British fashion and textile firm famous for its cotton floral prints

Louvre pleats: pleats running horizontally.

Mandarin (or Chinese, or Nehru) collar: stand-up collar that is open at the front.

Maxi skirt: ankle- or floor-length skirt popular around 1970.

Midiskirt: calf-length skirt; although this term is no longer in use, the length itself has been dominant since 1973.

Military style: often in khaki, this look is inspired by military uniforms.

Miniskirt: a very short skirt, with the minimum distance between hem and knee being 10 cm (4 in).

Moiré: generally used for formal eveningwear, this is a watered effect on fabric; formerly silk and also acetate.

Nautical style: leisure- and sportswear style, usually in navy blue and white, and modelled on naval uniforms.

New Look (Corolle line): world-famous silhouette created in 1947 by Christian Dior. Very feminine with narrow, rounded shoulders, narrow waist, emphasized bust and wide, calf-length skirt.

Nylon: patented in the USA in 1937 and initially used in the manufacture of hosiery and underwear.

Op Art: art style typified by abstract, geometric patterns and bold colours, especially black and white; a major influence in 1960s fashion.

Organdy: lightweight, fine, sheer and stiffened cotton (now synthetic), usually in pastel shades.

Organza: similar to organdy, this fabric was originally made of silk.

Oversize look: garments that appear several sizes too large; fashionable in the 1980s.

Pagoda shoulder: launched in 1933 by Elsa Schiaparelli, this emphasized shoulder was inspired by Asian pagodas.

Paletot: single- or double-breasted coat with patch pockets and lapels.

Panniers: structured undergarment or hoops that extended the width of the dress to both sides while leaving the front and back flat. Popular in the eighteenth century, modified versions have appeared since then.

Parallelo: very fashionable in the 1950s, this is a horizontally knitted sweater or jacket.

Passementerie: generic term used to describe all kinds of garment trimmings, essential requirements for Coco Chanel's suits.

Passe-partout jacket: similar to a bolero.

Pencil line: figure-hugging style created by Christian Dior in 1948, whereby the skirt is cut from the hips in one straight line.

Pennant collar: triangular shaped collar.

Pepita: small, checked and woven pattern with diagonal connecting lines, usually in navy and white, or black and white.

Peplum jacket: short tailored jacket with flared flaps or flounces sewn into the waist.

Peter Pan collar: rounded, small flat collar.

Piqué: cotton fabric with a relief pattern; usually waffled or honeycombed.

Pinafore dress: collarless, sleeveless dress based on a chasuble.

Plissé: term used to describe pleats that are pressed into fabric.

Princess line: coat or dress without a waist seam; tailoring is achieved by working in the vertical seam. Launched in 1863 by Charles Frederick Worth, popular again 1900, in the 1930s and then again between 1955 and 1965.

Puff sleeves: gathered above the elbow, this is a balloon-like short sleeve.

Puffball or pouf skirt: created by Christian Lacroix in the 1980s, the skirt is doubled over at the hem to create a puffed appearance.

Pullover: woollen, long-sleeved top inspired by the knitted garments worn by seamen. Popular in 1920s Europe, when Coco Chanel included it in several of her haute couture collections.

Raglan sleeve: a sleeve extending from the neckline to the wrist.

Rayon: a name for viscose used between the early 1950s and the 1970s.

Redingote: tailored long jacket or coat, usually flared toward the hem and often with a shawl collar. It can be worn with or without a belt.

Revers: lapels; sometimes refers to the turned-over edge of sleeves or skirts.

Romantic look: 1960s and 1970s style of dress, incorporating folk elements and featuring loose cotton dresses, frills and corset tops.

Sabrina neckline: inspired by Audrey Hepburn's clothes in the movie of the same name, this is a square, décolleté collar.

Safari jacket: jacket in a strong, lightweight fabric that is modelled on tropical garments. It is characterized by the colours brown, beige and khaki, and by patch pockets and shoulder flaps. Usually fitted with a belt.

Sailor collar: neckline and collar inspired by naval uniforms.

Sailor neck: zip-fastened turtleneck.

Shantung: irregular, less shiny silk; hand-woven.

Sheath dress: usually knee-length classic dress, collarless and close-fitting, straight and cut from a single fabric piece, with a round or oval neckline; also an evening dress with shoulder straps and décolleté; popular in the 1920s, in the 1960s it became known as the 'Jackie O dress' (after Jacqueline Kennedy Onassis).

Shelf bra: a bra that is built into the garment.

Shift dress: loosely falling, unstructured classic style of dress especially fashionable during the 1920s and mid-1960s.

Shirtwaister: the upper part of this loose dress is modelled on a man's shirt, with a collar, cuffs and buttons to the waist. Popularized by Coco Chanel.

Slinky look: originally fashionable in the 1930s and later revived in the early 1970s; a phrase used to describe sinuous clothes of fluid fabrics.

Slit look: a miniskirt or hot pants worn beneath a midi- or maxiskirt left open at the front; fashionable in the early 1970s.

Smock: narrow, straight dress with front, back and sleeves secured to a yoke collar.

Smocking: fabric tightly gathered with decorative stitching (often created with elastic thread) to form geometric patterns; frequently featured in peasant-style garments.

Spencer: waist-length, short jacket.

Sportswear: generic term to describe comfortable leisurewear.

Swing coat: style of A-line coat, with narrow sleeves and shoulders; shorter than knee-length.

Taffeta: stiffened fine fabric of synthetic fibres or silk often made of changeant (an iridescent material).

Tea gown: loose gown designed in 1864 by Charles Frederick Worth with an intricately decorated front and long sleeves.

Topper: straight, short jacket with sloping shoulders, the front edge forms a right angle with the hem.

Torso dress: simple dress that is gathered or pleated below the hipline with a figure-hugging bodice.

Trapeze line: silhouette of coat or dress with narrow shoulders and a high waist (or no waist at all) flaring out towards the hem. Yves Saint Laurent presented his trapeze line in 1958 and it remained popular through the 1960s.

Tube: garment with a straight, elongated outline that is cut in a casual and comfortable way.

Tulle: lace-like or netting fabric.

Tunic: simple pinafore or dress in a loose, often sleeveless style; the armholes usually form part of the side seams.

Tweed: rough-textured, woollen fabric in a variety of coloured patterns; used especially for suits and coats.

Twist line: narrow-hipped outline with a slightly flared pleated skirt that flares as the wearer moves about.

Umbrella skirt: like an umbrella, this skirt consists of 12 or more sections.

U-neckline: neckline in a U-shape with wide shoulder straps.

V-neck: neckline with an open yoke coming to a V shape midway down the bodice.

Velvet: soft-textured, short-piled fabric; usually cotton.

Vichy check: checked pattern that is like gingham but with larger checks.

Viennese seam: a seam running from one armhole angled across the bust to either the hem or the waist seam, obviating the need for darts.

Viscose: synthetic fibre made of cellulose.

Voile: lightweight, sheer fabric.

Westover: worn with suits in the 1920s and more recently over skirts and blouses, this is a sleeveless, knitted waistcoat.

Wing collar: collar with upper corners covering shoulder seams.

Y-line: garment line designed in 1955–56 by Christian Dior featuring narrow dresses or skirts, wide lapels or other V-shaped necklines to form the letter 'Y'.

Index

Further Reading

Aloha Attire: Hawaiian Dress in the 20th Century, Linda B Arthur Atglen, Schiffer, 2000.

The Art of Zandra Rhodes, Zandra Rhodes/Anne Knight, Jonathan Cape, 1984.

California Casual, Maureen Reilly, PA Schiffer Ltd, 2001.

The Conscription of Fashion: Utility Cloth, Clothing and Footwear, 1941-1952, Christopher Sladen, Scolar Press, 1995.

The Couture Accessory, Caroline Rennolds Milbank, HN Abrams, 2002.

Everyday Fashions of the Thirties As Pictured in Sears Catalogs, Sears Roebuck & Company, Courier Dover Publications, 1986.

The Fashion Year, edited by Brenda Polan, Zomba Books, 1983.

The Fashion Year Volume II, edited by Emily White, Zomba Books, 1984.

Fashions of a Decade: 1940s, Patricia Baker, Batsford, 1992.

A History of Fashion, Elizabeth Ewing, Batsford, 2005.

Hollywood Costume: Glamour, Glitter & Romance, Dale McConathy with Diana Vreeland, HN Abrams, 1976.

Hollywood Knits, Bill Gibb, Pavilion Books, 1987.

In Biba, Delisia Howard, Chris Price and Barbara Hulanicki, Hazard Books, 2004.

In Fashion, Prudence Glynn/Madeline Ginsburg, George Allen & Unwin Ltd, 1978.

In Vogue: Sixty Years of Celebrities and Fashion from British Vogue, Georgina Howell, Penguin Books, 1978.

New York Fashion, Caroline Rennolds Milbank, Abrams, 1989.

The 1940s, John Peacock, Thames & Hudson, 1998.

NOVA 1965-1975, compiled by David Hillman and Harriet Peccinotti, edited by David Gibbs, Pavilion Books, 1993.

The Ossie Clark Diaries, Lady Henrietta Rous, Bloomsbury, 1998.

Ossie Clark 1965-74, Judith Watt, V&A Publications, 2003.

Print in Fashion, Marnie Fogg, Batsford Books, 2006.

Schiaparelli Fashion Review, Tom Tierney, Dover Publications Inc, 1988.

Screen Style: Fashion and Femininity in 1930s Hollywood, Sarah Berry, University of Minnesota Press, 2002.

Twentieth-Century Fashion, Linda Watson, Carlton Books, 1999.

Vanitas: Designs By Gianni Versace, Hamish Bowles, Abbeville Press, 1994.

Picture Credits

The publishers would like to thank the following sources for their kind permission to reproduce the photographs in this book.
Key: t=Top, b=Bottom, c=Centre, l=Left and r=Right

Image Courtesy of The Advertising Archive: 115, 181c, 222, 224, 225 **The Bridgeman Art Library:** /Under the Eyes of New York Skyscrapers, fashion plate from *Femina* magazine, December 1928 (colour litho), Benigni, Leon (fl.1926-29) / Private Collection, Archives Charmet: 29; /Rayon dresses designed by Lucien Lelong, fashion plate from *Femina* magazine, June 1935 (colour litho), Heckroth, Pap (fl.1935) /Private Collection, Archives Charmet: 45 **Camera Press:** 157;/David Steen: 112; 211, 215l, 215r, 216, 217, 220, 228, 233, 234t, 234b, 235 **Christian Dior:** 86-7 **Corbis:** /Michel Arnaud: 184, 193, 204; /Bettmann: 14, 34tl, 34cr, 82cl, 82tr, 110tr, 142cl, 143cr, 143bl, 147, 180cr, 196, 198; /© Condé Nast Archive: 10, 16, 20, 33, 36, 39, 40, 40 (inset), 46, 50, 53, 58cl, 60, 62, 63, 69, 70, 73, 75, 76-77, 78, 79, 82bl, 82cr, 83tr, 84, 86, 89, 92, 94, 100, 102, 103, 104-5, 105, 107, 130, 134, 136, 138-9, 150, 151, 173, 175, 179, 181cl, 218r, 238tl; /Julio Donoso/Corbis Sygma: 25b, 44t, 44c, 182, 186; /Lynn Goldsmith: 206r; /Historical Picture Archive: 28; /Hulton-Deutsch Collection: 35tr, 49, 59cl, 59bl, 66, 111tr, 172; /Douglas Kirkland: 142tr; / David Lees: 110l; /Genevieve Naylor: 74, 83bl; /Philadelphia Museum of Art: 51; / Underwood & Underwood: 47; /Pierre Vauthey/Corbis Sygma: 190; /Condé Nast/ Fair Photo Service: 223, /Fairchild Photo Service/Condé Nast: 236, /© Thierry Orban/Sygma: 213 **Design Council Slide Collection:** /Manchester Metropolitan University © Design Council, endpaper **Getty Images:** /H.Armstrong Roberts/ Retrofile: 181bl; /Loomis Dean/Time Life Pictures: 99; /Pierre Guillaud/AFP: 185,

192; /Hulton Archive: 207tr; /Bill Ray/*Life* Magazine/Time & Life Pictures: p118-9; /Sasha: 58tr; /Topical Press Agency: 35c; /United Artists: 180bl; /William Vanderson/Fox Photos: 58cr; 231l, 231r, /AFP: 218l, 239br, /Gamma-Rapho: 219, /Redferns: 226 © **Jim Lee:** "Ossie Clark/Aeroplane 1969": 133; / "Ossie Clark/ Vietnam/1969": 160 **Kerry Taylor Auctions:** / www.kerrytaylorauctions.com: 212, 232l, 232r **London College of Fashion:** /The Woolmark Company: 127 © **Niall McInerney:** 188b © **Norman Parkinson Archive:** 144 **Réunion Musées Nationaux:** /Page de contre-garde et troisiéme page de couverture (Titre attribué: Troisiéme composition) Delaunay Sonia (dit), Stern-Terk Sarah Sophie (1885-1979) © Photo CNAC/MNAM Dist. RMN - © Droits réservés: 18 **Rex Features:** /David Graves: 116; /Europa Press: 142cr; /Everett Collection: 111bl, 123, 142bl; /Sipa Press: 188t, 197; 230, /Mark Large/Associated Newspapers: 239bl, / Mark Large/Daily Mail: 227, /c.Paramount/Everett: 239cl, /Ken Towner/Associated Newspapers: 221, 229, 238bl, 238r, /Ken Towner/Evening Standard: 236-237, 239cr, 239cr, /Steve Wood: 208 **Roger Harris Photography:** 240c, 241r, 242l, 243l **Scala, Florence:** /Image copyright The Metropolitan Museum of Art/Art Resource: 210tl, 210bl, 210r, 214 **TopFoto.co.uk:** 35cl, 110cr, 124, 143tl, 181cr, 206l, 207bl; /AP: 111tl **Victoria & Albert Museum:** /V&A Images: endpaper, 19, 48, 91, 104, 165, 166br, 167bl, 173 **Zandra Rhodes Enterprises:** /Patrick Anderson: 6tl; /Clive Arrowsmith: 6b; /Robyn Beeche: 6tr, 7, 153

Every effort has been made to acknowledge correctly and contact the source and/or copyright holder of each picture and Carlton Books Limited apologizes for any unintentional errors or omissions, which will be, corrected in future editions of this book.

Authors' Acknowledgements

Emma Baxter-Wright: Special thanks to Lisa Dyer for commissioning me. Dedicated to Dex, O and Dusty Rose. **Karen Clarkson:** Dedicated with love and thanks to Hector, Maggie, Polly, Siggi and Chop. **Sarah Kennedy:** Thanks to Lisa Helmanis, Emma Hodges, Carol McKeown and Jane W. Kellock for fashion memories and positive inspiration. Dedicated to Duncan, Freddie and Findlay, with love. **Kate Mulvey:** Dedicated to Georgia, Myles, George and Oscar, with love.

Publisher's Acknowledgements

The publishers would especially like to thank Cleo and Mark Butterfield for their hospitality, warmth and enthusiasm during the photography process, and particularly for their vast knowledge and expertise in helping to select from their amazing fashion archives. Thanks also go to Zandra Rhodes, for her rare artistry and fervent dedication to fashion heritage. Thanks to Bang Bang Clothing Exchange, 21 Goodge Street, London W1T 2PJ for the images of their shop on pages 240l, 240r, 241l, 243c and 243r, taken by Emma Wright.

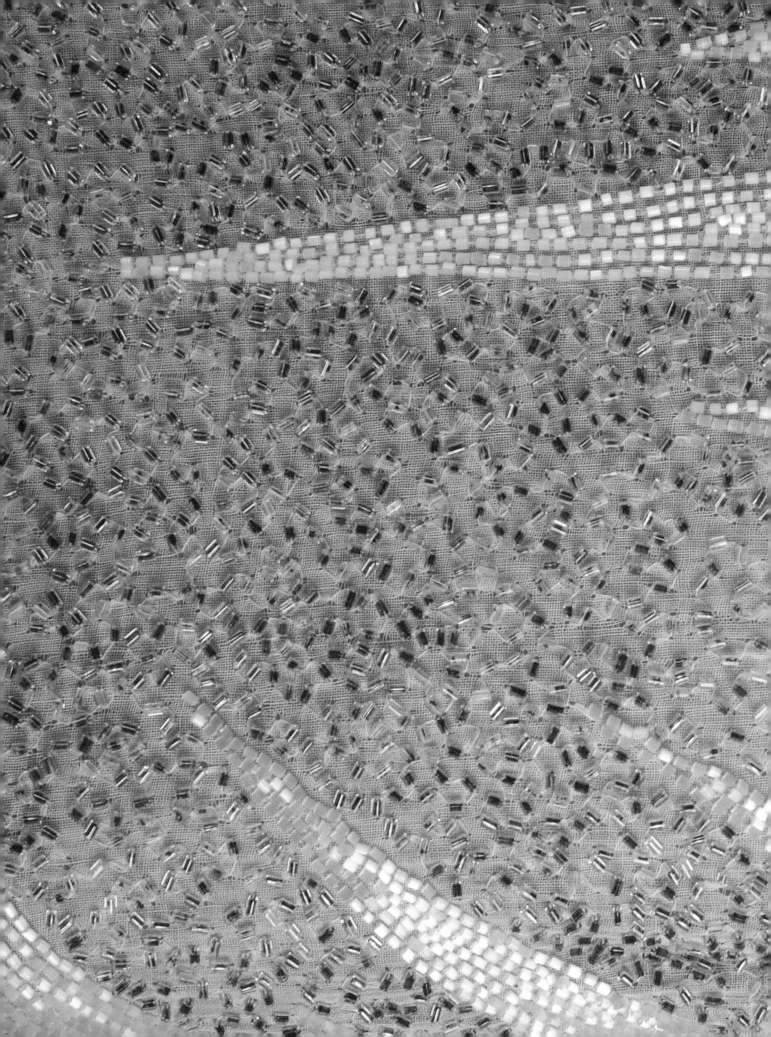